Advanced
Alternative
Medicine
for
Arthritis, Chronic Pain,
and
Injuries

Advanced Alternative Medicine for Arthritis, Chronic Pain, and Injuries

Daniel Nuchovich, MD

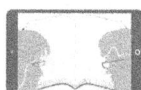

Tablet Publications

TABLET PUBLICATIONS • MELBOURNE, FLORIDA

Advanced Alternative Medicine for
Arthritis, Chronic Pain, and Injuries

Published in the USA by:
Tablet Publications
6300 N Wickham Rd.
#130-416
Melbourne, FL 32940
Phone 321-610-3634
email orders@seaworthy.com
www.tabletpublications.com

Tablet Publications is an imprint of Seaworthy Publications, Inc.

Library of Congress Cataloging-in-Publication Data

Names: Nuchovich, Daniel I., author.
Title: Advanced alternative medicine for arthritis, chronic pain, and
  injuries / Daniel Nuchovich, MD.
Description: Melbourne, FL : Tablet Publications, [2020] | Includes
  bibliographical references. | Summary: "There is more to pain management
  than just pain control." True relief from pain is an outcome, not a pill
  or an injection. It is the result of doing several things right,
  starting from the moment a person decides to act upon the afflicting
  problem. However, this is not always easy, and several barriers, such as
  joint disorders and painful neuromuscular conditions, can stand in the
  way of long-term relief and the return to a good quality of life. To
  make matters worse, some of these barriers are the limited action, or
  inaction, by affected individuals...frequently associated with lack of
  information. Most people don't realize that there is something more they
  could do to relieve their affliction. Most people don't know
  about the variety of therapies they could use to relieve their
  body from joint problems, neuropathies, injuries, and pain. I see this in
  my patients, my friends, and relatives and even in many other doctors I
  talk to. Most resort to some pills, injections, a short course of
  physical therapy, and if no success, surgery, with very little in
  between. They are unaware of the variety of therapy options they could
  use to heal themselves and find the relief they are looking for. Worse
  even, they live in a society that wishes to ignore, and many times deny,
  the variety and profound benefits of the many alternative therapies
  presented in this book"– Provided by publisher.
Identifiers: LCCN 2019051709 (print) | LCCN 2019051710 (ebook) | ISBN
  9781948494298 (paperback) | ISBN 9781948494304 (ebook)
Subjects: LCSH: Chronic pain–Alternative treatment. | Integrative
  medicine.
Classification: LCC RB127 .N82 2020 (print) | LCC RB127 (ebook) | DDC
  616/.0472–dc23
LC record available at https://lccn.loc.gov/2019051709
LC ebook record available at https://lccn.loc.gov/2019051710

Disclaimer

The nutritional and health information provided in this book is intended for educational purposes only and should not substitute for conventional medical care. Nothing listed or mentioned in this book should be considered as medical therapy, advice, or replace medical management. Consult your doctor for guidance on specific health issues and before following this or any program. People suffering from serious medical conditions, severe pain, or worsening health problems should seek professional care or go to the emergency room. The author and publisher specifically disclaim any liability, loss or risk, personal or otherwise, which is incurred as a consequence, directly or indirectly, of postponing immediate medical care or as a result of the use and application of the contents of this book.

The author does not advocate the use of any particular form of health care but believes the information presented in this book and his associated website should be available to the public. However, the medical information is not intended as a substitute for consulting a physician. You should consult a physician if you think you may have a disease or a medical problem, and you should not attempt to self-diagnose or embark on self-treatment of any kind without qualified medical supervision. Nothing in this publication or the website is a promise or a guarantee that pain, arthritis, an injury, or any other condition will disappear or improve. Nothing guarantees the safety or efficacy of any specific treatment.

Daniel Nuchovich, MD

Table of Contents

Disclaimer V

Acknowledgments XI

Introduction XIII

Integrating Therapies 1

Introduction to Inflammation, Pain, and Their Causes 5

    This Happens in the Ideal Situation 6

    Understanding and Treating Arthritic Conditions 8

    Arthritis: A Historic Disease 11

        Risk Factors 11

        Joints and Cartilage in Trouble 16

A Few Basic Concepts 20

    Fats 20

    The Mechanics of a Joint 21

Injuries 25

    A Battle Plan for Neck and Back Pain 25

    Understanding and Managing Common Disorders 40

        Rotator Cuff Injury 41

        Sprained Ligaments 43

        Sprained Joints 43

        Torn and Pulled Muscles 44

        Bursitis 45

        Tendinitis 46

        Elbow Pain 46

        Hip Pain 47

Conventional Treatments 63

    Conventional Treatment and its Limitations 63

    Conventional Approaches to Pain Treatment 65

    Conventional Medical Treatment 67

        Some Conventional Medicine Management Therapies 70

    Our Institute's Approach 73

Alternative Treatments 76

    Why Alternative Therapies are Effective 76

    Alternative Therapies Help Arthritis and Other Painful Conditions 77

Medications 79

Supplements 86

    The Role of Supplements in Healing 89

    Vitamins 91

        Reliable Vitamins? 93

Cartilage Building Supplements..95
Food Sensitivity and Gut Dysbiosis.....................................105
Your Gut and Dysbiosis 109
Food Sensitivity..112
Symptoms of Food Sensitivity 114
Gut Restoration Program 116
Therapies...119
Acupuncture...119
History 119
How it Works...120
Technique 121
Acupuncture for Pain, Arthritis, and Injuries 122
Conditions Effectively Treated with Acupuncture...........123
How to Find an Acupuncturist 124
Chiropractic Care..124
Conditions for which Chiropractic Treatment is Recommended 126
Nutritional Supplements 127
Nutrition Therapy..127
Acupressure 127
Shiatsu 128
Reflexology 129
Craniosacral Therapy...130
Myofascial Release..132
Massage...134
Deep Tissue Massage...136
Swedish Massage 136
Lymphatic Drainage 137
Oriental Massage 137
Neuromuscular Massage...138
European Massage 138
Thai Massage 139
Gyrotonics 139
Reiki...140
Special Exercises 141
Yoga 142
Some of the Beneficial Clinical Effects of Yoga:.............144
Paths 146
Styles...146
Starting Yoga 147
Tai chi 149
History 150

Tai chi in Motion 150
Qigong 151
Feldenkrais 152
Exercise 153
General Guidelines About Exercise 154
Arthritis 155
Helping the Muscles..156
Types of Exercise 159
Flexibility Exercises...160
Strengthening Exercises 160
Aerobic Exercises..160
Sports Activities..161
Tailoring Your Exercise Program 161
Precautions...162
Warming-up...164
Additional Therapies...164
Relaxation Techniques 164
Deep Breathing 165
Guided Imagery 165
Self-talk 165
Mindfulness Meditation...166
Detoxification 166
Homeopathy..166
Nutrition...168
Eicosanoids & the Omegas..168
Fats, Oils and the Production of Eicosanoids........................170
Nutrition and Joint Damage...171
Our Dietary Program Consists of Two Parts 173
The Avoidance Plan...174
Dr. Nuchovich's Alkaline Diet..176
The Jupiter Institute Omega Diet...180
The Mediterranean Diet 181
The Important Aspects of the Mediterranean Diet: 182
The Cardiovascular Advantage...184
Effects on Inflammation and Pain 185
Key Elements of the Mediterranean Diet 185
The Jupiter Institute Omega Diet in Brief.............................189
Foods That Are Best to Eat 189
The Importance of What You Don't Eat 195
Processed Foods...196
Fats: the Bad and the Good 198

The Three Bad Fats...199

The Good Fat...200

Avoid Omega-6...200

Cholesterol and CRP...201

To Lower Levels of CRP...202

The Anti-nutrient Lifestyle..203

Pro-inflammatory Foods..204

An Anti-inflammatory Diet...204

"Mediterraneanizing" Your Diet..205

Hormones, Thyroid, and Adrenals..211

The Hormone Factor...211

Hormone Replacement..216

Hormone Support...217

Hypothyroidism has Several Causes.......................................220

Low Functioning Thyroid Can Cause:......................................221

Thyroid Medications...222

Thyroid Helpers...224

Adrenal Gland Disorder...226

Symptoms of Hypoadrenia...228

Additional Symptoms and Medical Problems............................228

Managing Adrenal Dysfunction...229

Adaptogens...231

Toxins...236

Toxins and Health...237

Hallelujah, the Laws of Salvation...242

How Toxins Hurt You...243

Detoxification..249

Starting Detoxification..250

Gut Restoration Program...250

About Detoxification Programs...251

Detox Products..252

Sleep..255

Finale..267

Appendices..271

Resources for Your Health...271

More Information About Acupuncture.......................................273

Schools of Naturopathy...273

References...274

About the Author..284

Acknowledgments

In my first book, "The Palm Beach Pain Relief System," I acknowledged the teaching, guidance, and support I received from several academic centers, like the Division of Complementary and Alternative Medicine at Harvard Medical School, The Center for Integrative Medicine at the University of Maryland School of Medicine, Georgetown School of Medicine, Southern Illinois University, etc. For this book, however, I acknowledge the positive input I received from many patients who got better following my guidelines and from those far away who read the book, followed its guidelines, and found relief. Their stories of improvement from pain and joint disorders and achieving higher levels of functionality by using my recommendations, and the variations and combinations of the techniques they used, plus the suggestions they made, gave me the idea and encouragement to write this second book. For these reasons, this book is more complete and presents a different approach based on the experiences of many of these people. Let's just say that this book is more mature, more practical, and more effective than the first one.

I thank my editor, Amiel, for his patience and professional work.

I would also like to thank my staff, Linda Grove and Kristi Mahoney, who deal with my patients daily and have been a big help by assisting me in the management of patients with pain, arthritis, and injuries, collecting data as well as in gathering information and comments from our patients.

Once again, I would like to thank my wife Ana. Without her, and her loving and enduring commitment to our family and our office, this new book would not be. I am humbled by her tireless dedication to this project and the success of the Jupiter Institute of the Healing Arts. Despite my cantankerous moods during the construction of this book, she remained an objective, pragmatic and focused contributor.

Introduction

"There is more to pain management than just pain control"

True relief from pain is an outcome, not a pill or an injection. It is the result of doing several things right, starting from the moment a person decides to act upon the afflicting problem. However, this is not always easy, and several barriers, such as joint disorders and painful neuromuscular conditions, can stand in the way of long-term relief and the return to a good quality of life. To make matters worse, some of these barriers are the limited action, or inaction, by affected individuals...frequently associated with lack of information.

Most people don't realize that there is something more they could do to relieve their affliction. This is a very important point and one of the objectives of this book, so I am rephrasing it: Most people don't know about the variety of therapies they could use to relieve their body from joint problems, neuropathies, injuries, and pain. I see this in my patients, my friends and relatives, and even in most of the doctors I talk to. Most resort to some pills, injections, short courses of physical therapy, and if no success, surgery, with very little in between. They are unaware of the variety of therapy options they could use to heal themselves and find the relief they are looking for. Worse even, they live in a society that wishes to ignore, and many times deny, the variety and profound benefits of the many alternative therapies available.

This book is then a mission. It seeks to remedy these stubborn barriers and bring light to the lack of information and confidence towards those therapies while providing you and my patients with the knowledge and the guidance to achieve more than just relief but true healing. It is not based on theories. The management programs I address here are currently helping many of my patients and friends, and I am sure it will help you as well.

I am not giving you a pill. I am giving you something better: an arsenal of information.

Sometime after I started writing this book, I asked myself whether an update was necessary. After all, I had already written one book about the management of pain, arthritis, and injuries, which helped countless patients, and it seemed to be enough. However, my life continued to be in motion and the new experiences and challenges I encountered encouraged me to do more research and try different techniques. As I furthered my studies, it became clear that a second edition with more comprehensive therapies was needed. The addendum grew and grew until I was confronted with this manuscript. I asked myself again: is this new book really necessary?

As I searched for the answer, I encountered a troubled health care environment.

I found that, in conventional medicine, people are not getting what they deserve. They only receive what the doctor knows (or remembers that day), and the recommendation varies according to whether the doctor is in a hurry or not. If patients don't know anything else and have no other source of information, they may not get what they need...or worse, they may end up getting something they don't need.

Moreover, the rate of poor management of pain-arthritis-injury situations is rather alarming. One in every four Americans, or 75 million, has suffered or is currently suffering from pain that lasts longer than 24 hours. Chronic pain is the most common cause of long-term disability, and people are consuming (often abusing) over-the-counter medications of all kinds to help them manage painful disorders, unaware of the side effects. These medications are often over-consumed because of another issue: the health care system in this country has suffered a major setback, causing access to doctors, and time spent with those doctors, to dwindle. The current dissatisfaction with the medical system is widening the gap between people and medicine. Painkiller, opioid, and narcotic abuse, which has become an epidemic, often starts as mismanagement of painful and inflammatory disorders. Add to this the abundance of websites supposedly informing people about alternative therapies but are instead marketing tools to manipulate the viewer towards unscrupulous clinics and doubtful products, supplements, and procedures. Being burned by this "quackery" can create understandable disdain towards many alternative medicine therapies.

Let's face it. For many, the addiction to painkillers, opioids, benzos, and even illegal drugs started with an inattentive, uninformed medical care system.

So, I have found the answer to the question to be yes. This book is necessary. Like it or not, the U.S. is in trouble, painful trouble, and at this time there is no clear solution in sight. However, I am throwing on the table the concept that if people are more informed about their disorders and treatment options, they can prevent themselves from becoming victims of mismanagement.

At this date in time, it is my advice that if you do not have any information about the roots and anatomical structures involved in your ailment, and you have no broad idea of therapy options, a doctor's visit for your chronic or acute painful problem could be ineffective (or even dangerous).

The diagnosis, medications, referrals, and procedures will all lead to a better outcome if you have prior knowledge of your disorder before stepping foot in the clinic. It is becoming more and more clear that an easy-to-read source of medical information might help you, and most individuals, to achieve better outcomes.

I hope you find that this book will easily explain the root causes of common painful ailments, while also introducing you to conventional and alternative methods of treatment that will bring relief.

I wrote this book to be a path, where you will realize that the therapies I present here are designed to provide more than just reduction of pain and dysfunction, but also overall healing and improvement of the problem areas and the body as a whole. This is important since the ultimate goal of therapy is not just relief but healing. Healing the root of the problem is the real goal.

Among the many important topics I address, I emphasize a very important factor: stress. Many studies indicate that the stress created by prolonged severe pain, significant arthritis, and neuromuscular disorders can affect many systems and pathways in the body, causing reduced physical activity, emotional distress, a decline in quality of life, decreased work productivity, depression, and harm to your general well-being. The connection between pain, stress, and the brain can adversely impact recovery and trap the individual in a vicious cycle of declining health. Whether a person gets better or worse might depend on how much that person understands the important correlation between these three factors.

It's quite obvious that the best way to understand pain is to experience pain. After all, how do you describe living with a bad joint to someone who has no idea what it feels like? I came to understand pain, inflammation, arthritis, back problems, disc diseases, tendinitis, by suffering each one of them myself as a result of multiple soccer and basketball injuries. I had all kinds of injuries throughout my body, in my neck, back, knees, elbows, hips, ankles, right foot, hands, and even my chest and thighs. Pushed by my painful frustration with conventional medicine, I started searching in the unconventional field. I read, studied, and tried non-traditional techniques new and old, and discovered a world of alternative medicine therapies. I visited several chiropractors and acupuncturists so I could learn the different techniques each used. I tried massage therapy, yoga, myofascial release, nutrition therapy, herbal products, craniosacral therapy, reflexology, and sauna. I also tried antioxidants, neurotransmitter improvement programs, adrenal relief, detoxification, tai chi, acupressure, and more. It has been a very interesting path of an ever-challenging combination of injuries, therapies, and learning. It seems like with every injury, and every healing, I learned even more and I became more able to help my patients.

I am sure you've heard that knowledge is power, and it's true. Knowledge about your disorder may give you the power to open your mind, choose the correct therapies to help you, and provide you with a flexible attitude to change the outcome of your chronic condition. That is what this book is all about: to allow you to learn. If you are willing to learn, a whole new world of options will unfold before you, and it will empower you to take command of your healing process.

It is important to know that there is no single pharmaceutical product that will heal the affected areas. I know that this is disappointing, but you deserve to know that painkillers will only relieve pain, and anti-inflammatories (including steroids and other injections) will only relieve inflammation, and none of them will heal anything.

At this time, you need to know that there are two common kinds of individual attitudes. First, you have the passive ones, those who don't search for the root of healing and just accept whatever the orthopedist, neurologist, or rheumatologist recommend. Others combine an inquisitive attitude, positive thinking, and flexible actions towards the problem. These latter types do better, heal from inside out, and end up having a better quality of life. I know very well that when we have pain, from whatever cause, it becomes difficult to think. We just want the pain to go away, and we would do whatever to make that happen. But remember that real healing and improvement does not come from painkillers or an impatient attitude, but rather from the knowledge and practice of real therapies. Avoid the passive attitude of just "waiting for things to happen" and ask around, search your environment, learn of new therapies, and try something new. When I look back and see my personal story and the stories of many of my patients, I can tell you that adopting the right attitude can change dysfunction into normal function, and failure into success.

Long ago, a professor of pain management told me that finding relief from painful conditions depends 20% on what happens and 80% on how people react to it, and that healing depends more on how and what the person is going to do about the problem. If you could remember just one thing from this book, it should be this sentence: *"How you are going to be tomorrow begins with what you are doing today?"*

As you advance in the course of this book, a question needs to be answered: is your painful joint or muscle an isolated event, or is it the consequence of a complex metabolic disorder you didn't know about that is affecting your body? And if it's yes, which disorder? Studies show that wrong dietary habits, toxins, and hormone decline do have an adverse impact on the inflammation and degeneration of joints, nerves, and muscles. Even sensitivity to certain foods and low thyroid function can be pretty bad. Anybody over 30 years of age can be affected by any of these or their combinations. Could they be affecting you? Do you know that these factors, that I describe in this book, cause many disabilities, unnecessary surgeries, a decline in quality of life, loss of jobs, etc., to way too many people?

See? There is much more to pain relief than just pain relief, and you will be understanding these questions and finding the answers as you advance through the challenging pages of this book.

About The Program

This program presents a flexible combination of what I have found to be the most effective therapies for the management of pain and painful disorders, such as joint disease, neck and back pain, arthritis, injuries, and inflammation. That is my focus. The success of these therapies did not come to me solely from reading publications, but also from the observations of their practice. Hence, they are based on experience, not just pure theory.

In this book, you will find some unique topics that are essential to your recovery, such as how to deal with the adverse inflammatory effects of toxins and chemicals, that are necessary for the healing of inflamed joints and tissues.

Unlike conventional medicine, my program emphasizes three factors that are essential for healing and recovery:

1) Information about the multiple beneficial therapies.
2) A flexible attitude when trying those therapies, and trying different modalities until you find.
3) Searching into your metabolic puzzle to adjust and correct the possible abnormalities that might block the healing process.

Very important: I present here the program I follow. This book will show you the pathway to design and follow your own program. Use my book as a source of information and as a guide.

Whether you like it or not, the times have changed significantly. The "good old days," when doctors knew it all and took their time with every patient, and health insurance was good for all parties, are over. If you are suffering from arthritis, bursitis, tendinitis, inflammation, or painful injuries of any sort, you can't rely solely on the little time and minimal information your doctor might share with you. On many occasions, you may not even see a doctor but someone with much less training and limited knowledge, such as a physician's assistant or nurse practitioner. Your fate might then be sealed, left only with minimal information, a handful of pills, and an appointment with a specialist in four weeks...who might also be unable or unwilling to give you the time you need. Most of the time, you leave the office without knowing the deep cause of the problem that is affecting you, or what options for further evaluation and treatment are available to you.

Unless you know better, your diagnostic and therapy choices might be very limited, and your chance of future recovery might be slim. You need to gather information yourself and increase your awareness about diagnostic and therapy choices within conventional and alternative medicine. You need to broaden your therapeutic horizon before you engage in procedures that might carry long-term consequences. Even more, you need to have some information in your pocket before your doctor's visit. This book was written with this purpose in mind: to give you what you need to know, loud and clear, so you can use it before and after your clinical appointment. Where else can you find how a pinched nerve, certain chemicals, and food sensitivities can all interact with cartilage degeneration to give you a joint disease? How will you know when physical therapy will not work because your metabolic disorder will block its effect?

And again, when joints, muscles, spine, and nerves can be adversely affected by chemicals, toxins, thyroid and hormonal decline, pollution, and food sensitivities, will you be in a perfect metabolic state to allow your painful area to heal? Will your metabolic puzzle be ready for the badly needed therapies? Where will you learn all this?

1) There is a large gap in the management and treatment of these disorders, but you can help shrink this gap by gathering information. Information is power: the power to recover, the power to heal.

2) This is why I added those special metabolic chapters to this book, each one dedicated to explain the complexities of the metabolism simply and help you in the process of true healing.

Although my main message is that **you don't have to live with pain**, I do have to emphasize that recovery is not guaranteed, but a process that requires your action...and this action should not be in the form of taking pills. If you have seen three or four doctors for your condition, then you might have been prescribed a half-dozen or more medications. Without curing your issues, these pills are causing a range of side effects (such as insomnia, indigestion, or constipation) that can be as debilitating as the pain condition itself. What if it's possible to break that deadly cycle? By treating the cause – rather than the symptoms – of the pain in your joints, muscles, or tendons and ligaments, you can reverse the damage and experience an overall improvement in health, both now and in the long run. There is a catch, however, and you probably know what it is. You must want to do it! Instead of passively taking the pills your doctor gives you, you need to take a proactive attitude and assume responsibility for staking out your path to wellness. I want the healing experiences of others to inspire you to step beyond your belief system, much as I did in abandoning the rigid mindset of conventional Western medicine. You have the inherent potential to heal yourself of the ailments that cause you pain. This book, and the pain relief program outlined within, will provide you with the tools to improve the quality of your life. Now is the time to begin that journey!

Perhaps the secret to finding the true healing and the best relief from the conditions I mentioned above relies on you, and on how much you are willing to learn and open your mind to complementary therapies. When over forty academic centers in the U.S. are now offering alternative therapies, you know the time has come to abandon strict conventional medicine and explore new fields of therapy.

"Alternative medicine" is a term that refers to medical practices or remedies outside of what is considered to be mainstream conventional medicine. The terms "complementary medicine" and "integrative medicine," on the other hand, are used to describe treatment programs that combine conventional medicine with alternative medicine. The aim is to provide the best of each world, using whatever treatment is most appropriate for the individual. This is the medicine of the new century, and it is practiced by open-minded physicians who admit the limitations of their practice and accept the knowledge of alternative medicine practitioners. This is the medicine we practice at our Jupiter Institute of the Healing Arts (www.jupiterinstitute.com). We combine conventional Western medicine with alternative therapies that have proven successful in the treatment of arthritis, chronic pain, and injuries. We also encourage exercise as part of the treatment program. We follow the guidelines of Harvard Medical School, the National Institutes of Health, and the major textbooks of medicine.

Integrating Therapies

*"Many people succeed in healing and relief because they do what
unsuccessful people are not willing to do."*

I t's time for the first step of your journey to a pain-free life. I
recommend that every problem related to pain, injury, arthritis,
or muscular disorder should start with a medical evaluation by a
licensed physician. This doctor should spend unhurried time with
the patient, maintaining a dialogue, listening to the symptoms, and
then examining the patient to find out the details of the afflicting
condition.

I made emphasis on the time because we live in an environment
with a different health care system when compared to the recent past.
Nowadays, many offices and healthcare centers offer a sort of fast-
track medicine, looking to see as many patients in a day as possible
to maximize profits. Often patients are not seen by a physician but by
a nurse, a nurse practitioner, or physician's assistant and, while every
doctor will respect the training and experience these occupations have,
their medical knowledge is limited when compared to a medical doctor.
Within your possibilities, you should start your journey to recovery with a
quality and worthwhile appointment with a licensed physician.

After the medical evaluation and physical exam, the tests begin,
X-rays are taken and evaluated. Blood is drawn and sent away for testing.
Old records from prior doctors may be requested and reviewed. An MRI
might be scheduled, or a consultation with a neurologist, orthopedist, or
another specialist. Each step in this process is giving the physician one
piece of your personal health history. Once the story is complete, and
the condition of the patient is properly diagnosed, a plan of treatment is
discussed.

As part of the conventional medicinal approach, medications such as
non-steroidal anti-inflammatory drugs (NSAIDs) and painkillers may be
prescribed as a trial or for a short time ("Let's see if this helps.") NSAIDs
and painkillers are good, effective, and reliable...only when given in small

amounts, and as long as they are just a part of the treatment and not the entirety.

Ideally, even if he or she is in a solo practice, the medical doctor should be the "team leader," interacting with consultants, chiropractors, therapists, and other caregivers involved in the management of their patients' medical conditions. This is the ideal setting.

For example, in my practice, I often send patients for physical therapy. A physical therapist is trained to assist in the healing of tender joints, sprained muscles, torn tendons, arthritis, neck and back pain, and a lot more. The effects of physical therapy in improving function, decreasing pain and swelling, and stimulating healing are simply tremendous and are almost always beneficial regardless of the type or severity of the injury. I have several local physical therapists that I trust because they have helped me personally, so I often help the patient schedule an appointment with one of them.

Regular exercise is a fundamental part of both the healing process and a healthy life. It would be ideal to exercise in a way that suits your lifestyle and preference, but those who suffer from arthritis and injuries aren't so lucky. Improper exercise can increase damage to the problem area. Exercise instruction is therefore part of my recommendations, and it always comes from one of the alternative caregivers. Why? I am a physician after all, and I've studied all the bones, muscles, tendons, and ligaments, with an understanding of how they work with each other. However, when it comes to exercise, I'll be the first to admit that my knowledge is limited. I choose to defer advice on exercise to a physiatrist, physical therapist, or sports medicine doctor; whoever is the most qualified and within the range of the patient's condition and goals.

In regards to chiropractic care, I find it to be very effective for a great number of painful injuries related to the neck and back. Chiropractic care eliminates pain and restores normal function by correcting imbalances of the spine, joints, and muscles. In addition to being extremely skillful, I've found many chiropractors to also be great team players, coordinating care with the primary care physician and other members of the "team," reviewing X-rays and MRIs, discussing nutritional issues, exercise, and more.

Whenever possible and applicable, I will also recommend my patients to an acupuncturist. Acupuncture is a wonderful healing system that modulates the flow of energy in the body, enhancing its ability to heal itself. Acupuncture is not just a random placement of needles, but rather a complex and very effective treatment backed by over 3,000 years of experience and research.

Often, a change in nutrition is needed for maximum efficiency of treatment. While I will sometimes refer patients to a nutritionist if there are certain dietary restrictions or goals in mind, I have formulated an easy-to-follow diet designed to fight inflammation and increase overall health. This sounds familiar to those who have read my first book, but have no fear; this book features the evolved version of the Jupiter Institute Omega Diet, with all the additional knowledge I've gained in the intervening years. There are many factors, interactions, and substances that can create or relieve inflammation, from omega-3 and omega-6 fatty acids to free radicals and antioxidants, and all play a role in keeping your tendons, muscles, and joints healthy.

Supplements, like vitamins, antioxidants, and minerals are recommended to boost the healing of the tissues. These and other supplements, such as glucosamine, work on the damaged areas of joints, ligaments, tendons, and muscles to promote the circulation of important "building blocks" of healthy tissue and can give a huge boost to recovery. The proprietor of your local health food store is a great resource for learning about and acquiring high-quality supplements.

While this is an example of the team I call upon to treat my patients who suffer from chronic or acute pain, keep in mind that there is no preset therapy program where every patient gets the same treatment. The needs of the individual patient are unique, and so is their path to recovery. A nutritional adjustment might take priority for certain conditions, but it's equally possible that medication and physical therapy are the first steps. Some patients are candidates for chiropractic treatment...and some are not. Both caretakers and patients must take into account that not every therapy suits every person, and that can boil down to the members of the team. Not every acupuncturist is helpful, not all chiropractors have suitable technique, and some physical therapists and even primary care physicians are not going to be 100% effective in your care and recovery.

Conversely, the professionals might be amazing practitioners, true masters in their field but terrible team players. It reminds me of the USA basketball team in the 2004 Olympics. The Americans went into the tournament with an all-star group, including several NBA MVPs and a young LeBron James. They played valiantly and were individually excellent, but their lack of team cohesiveness led to them placing behind Argentina and Italy...teams who were almost entirely "nobodies" by comparison, but their excellent teamwork led the way to victory. Your recovery, the possibility of living a healthy life free from pain, is more important than an Olympic gold medal. That's why finding a primary care doctor who understands the benefits of alternative medicine, and works well with practitioners of alternative medicine, is important.

By the way, this is known as "integrative medicine:" the classic techniques of so-called conventional medicine integrated with the best of alternative medicine. This cohesive approach, now encouraged by the best medical schools and the National Institutes of Health, focuses on tackling the root cause of a patient's problem rather than simply masking the symptoms.

Nevertheless, this ideal setting of qualified professionals working as a team may encounter difficulties in healing many individuals. This happens because of the unique nature of each person; the process of inflammation-degeneration of joints and muscles in each individual is a stubborn process with many variations. Understanding this complex process will help you heal from the inside-out and may have a profound effect on your overall health. I emphasize this approach with my patients and I am emphasizing it now in this book. Let's get started by analyzing the inflammatory process.

INTERCHAPTER REMARK: Now you are starting to understand that there is more to pain management than just pain relief. Just relieving pain does not heal the problem in joint disorders, inflammation, or neuromuscular ailments. Healing will not come from pharmaceuticals or injections but from an integrative approach: combining conventional and alternative medicine. Being seduced by steroids and painkillers could complicate your future.

As you advance in this book you will comprehend that as a joint, muscle, or back are part of your body, healing your whole body will facilitate repair of the ailing part.

Introduction to Inflammation, Pain, and Their Causes

"Lack of knowledge hinders repair."

N ow we're ready to start understanding the intimate process *that affects joints, muscles, and attached structures.*

It makes sense to know your enemies before you go into battle. Therefore, it makes sense to try to understand the root of the problem if you want to treat it successfully. A very common root for the occurrence of pain, whether from arthritis or injury, is the cause of inflammation. From head to toes, ankles to shoulders, neck to knees, any pain you get from a joint, muscle, or ligament is the result of inflammation, and the inflammatory process is the intimate mechanism of what is going wrong in your body.

As painful and disabling as it may result, inflammation is the body's normal response to injury and infection. It is an inherited mechanism of defense and a natural, automatic process that is essential to survival. Every animal, including humans, needs a properly functioning inflammatory response to survive the many assaults from the environment.

When an injury (physical, infectious, or otherwise) occurs, your cells become damaged and release enzymes; these enzymes are chemicals your cells use to say "I'm hurt! Help!" Your immune cells detect these enzymes, recognize the danger, and dispatch different types of cells along with certain other enzymes to the injured area. One family of chemicals, known as eicosanoids, are used by the body to coordinate the defense and repair. Some eicosanoids cause the blood vessels in the surrounding tissue to expand, "opening the gates" and allowing more help to arrive faster. Others will sensitize the nerve receptors in the area, making it tender to the touch. Externally, this causes the area to become painful, swollen, red, and warm, but under the surface, this represents a battle in progress.

There are many varieties of eicosanoids, each designed to carry a specific "message." In this case, we'll divide them in half and say that the message is either "create inflammation," "heal the area," or "attack and repair!"

After the injury, the action begins: a complex defense is mounted by the cells against the lesion. The aggressor, whether it's an infectious bacterium in your throat or a splinter in your skin, is attacked by a swarm of cells and the battle starts. White blood cells (triggered by the "attack!" eicosanoids) surround invading organisms & particles and destroy them, while other cells (summoned by the "repair!" eicosanoids) begin to fix the damage caused in the melee. The process builds on itself; these cells send out signals as they work, causing the body to continue to use eicosanoids to maintain the inflammation and send more help to the area. Once the threat is eliminated and the destruction repaired, the number of eicosanoids sent to the area decreases, and all the typical symptoms of inflammation fade away. The initial inflammation phase led the way to the repair phase. In general, this inflammation process is good; it fights foreign bodies and heals any damage.

This Happens in the Ideal Situation

Nevertheless, things can get complicated. On occasion, this response may be exaggerated and sustained for no apparent or beneficial reason. On those occasions, local events trigger way too many "attack and inflammation eicosanoids" and the messages to repair eicosanoids fall on deaf ears. Many factors can cause the inflammation process to persist and the affected tissues do not heal well. If the immune system is altered, if the piece of glass in your foot is not removed, if your diet is horrible, if the insult to the joint or tendon continues, etc., the inflammatory eicosanoids will dominate bringing on degenerative changes.

I know this is a bit difficult to comprehend, but imagine a beetle suddenly entering an anthill, wandering around, eating the larvae, causing destruction and collapsing tunnels. Its invasion triggers a sudden burst of activity in the ant colony. Soldier ants attack the invader, others focus on cleaning, worker ants repair the damage to the tunnels, all of them communicating for more help as needed, as they work toward a common goal – to kill the beetle and repair the anthill. If things go well, the intruder is killed, eliminated, and the damage repaired. But what if there's too much or too little communication? What if the beetle takes too long to die? Chaos. More soldier ants show up, many more than needed, and start to break up the tunnels even after the invader is dealt with. Or very few worker ants arrive to remove debris and fix the damage. The anthill is left in worse shape than before the beetle walked in, and the result of bad communication is local destruction.

Chronic Inflammation

Inflammation is a complex process, and we will now dive deeper into the nuts and bolts of chronic inflammation, which can cause the type of long-lasting pain that affects your life. The very simple ant-beetle example is a good first step towards understanding how a persistent inflammatory condition can be destructive to local tissues. Grasping this concept is one of the goals of this book and is necessary to comprehend the beneficial effects of the right therapies. Reviewing the process of inflammation-repair will help you understand how medications, nutrition, and therapies can affect its mechanisms and their effects on your life.

Chronic inflammation starts with an initial injury of some kind. The injury can be a single instance of intense mechanical force, like the tearing of a ligament in the knee of a healthy 25-year-old football player after a rough tackle. It can be a relatively minimal injury repeated in an unhealthy joint, such as when a sedentary and obese person climbs a flight of stairs. Whatever the initiating event, the injured cells start to pour enzymes into the surrounding tissues. These enzymes will irritate the healthy cells of the injured spot and cause them to break down, which sets in motion a sequence of events that lead to inflammation. Therein lies the rub: once the inflammatory process starts in the joint, certain proteins might block the formation of new fresh cartilage. Scientists and doctors do not currently understand why this occurs, but we do know that once the inflammatory process has started in the cartilage, it will progress unless something radical is done to shift the trend. This sequence of damage and inflammation, with repair being brought to a standstill, can take place anywhere in the body. If it occurs in a joint, it is osteoarthritis, which affects more than 50 million Americans.

Spreading Inflammation

Until now, we have been discussing inflammation as a local process. An inflamed joint, for example, is arthritis. But now I would like to introduce the concept of inflammation as a systemic issue, affecting your entire body, but originating from a single source. Systemic means "spread and affecting the whole body." (Examples: fever and septicemia are systemic problems; appendicitis and kidney stone are not.).

The concept of "spreading inflammation" (which we can call systemic inflammation) is newer and a bit more complex. We now know that inflammation anywhere in the body can spread to other organs and tissues and cause adverse changes, symptoms, and health changes. Often, we find that the most common source of spreading inflammation is the intestines: your gut. Inflammatory conditions in the intestines can trigger inflammation and diseases elsewhere and can affect joints, muscles, nerves, and even areas that are already hurting. I will explain this later on, but in the meantime, keep this concept in mind as we advance into the field of joint disorders.

Understanding and Treating Arthritic Conditions

With advanced age, most of us will experience some degree of arthritic pain somewhere in our body. While manageable for most people most of the time, those joint conditions tend to get worse and can start to affect daily activities. Many people are told to take over-the-counter pain relief and arthritis medications because "nothing can be done to stop it, anyway." However, this is a matter of choice. Most arthritis can be reversed, and even avoided, with proper measures. I know all too well that when arthritis becomes a degenerative condition, treating only the symptoms rather than the underlying cause is a losing battle.

What is arthritis?

The term "arthritis" is used generally to mean a painful swelling in a joint, without indicating any particular cause. Indeed, the term covers a large group of conditions of different types, and each one requires a different approach and management.

For example, osteoarthritis ("osteo," meaning "bone") is a degenerative joint disease marked by the wasting and breakdown of the cartilage in the joints, leading to swelling, stiffness, and pain. The surrounding tissues of the joint end up affected by the inflammation as well, such as muscle, tendons, and ligaments. As the disease progresses, the cartilage thins and ulcerates (forms small tears or holes), the bone grows painful spurs, and the function of the joint declines. As joint movement becomes increasingly restricted, stiffness settles in. Then the damage gets worse until finally the joint becomes crippled and disabled.

Another is rheumatoid arthritis (RA). RA is an autoimmune disease and involves the body thinking that certain cells are invaders and it tries to defend itself against them through auto-antibodies. The most commonly affected areas include the hands and feet, where the immune system attacks the cells that surround and protect the joints.

In addition to the above two, there are over 100 different types of arthritis, which includes numerous conditions that are easily mistaken as arthritis (but they are not arthritis). A chronically painful knee can be described as arthritic, and it may be due to osteoarthritis...but it could be instead a ligament or tendon injury, gout, bursitis, a tear, or even an infection causing the knee joint to swell and hurt similarly. This issue needs to be clear. Many cases of arthritis are not indeed arthritis, as you will soon find out, but they are called that for practical reasons. Doctors use the term "arthritis" as a general way of saying that a joint is sick, but my goal is to provide you with the information you need so you can understand the differences since they may require different therapeutic approaches. The "arthritic" elbow of a basketball player, a computer operator, a construction worker, or a martial arts expert may look similar, be named similarly, but might be structurally very different and require different treatments.

With that in mind, I've created a simple classification, lumping the arthritic conditions into two groups.

Classification

Group A will contain the arthritic conditions caused by local injury, while Group B is for cases caused by a general (whole-body) disease.

- In Group A, the arthritis is a result of a problem directly related to the joint itself. Sprains, overuse, and bad posture can create injury, which in turn causes inflammation of the ligament, tendons, and muscles near the joints.

- Group B includes the joint conditions caused by a systemic problem, such as an immune disorder like RA, lupus, or psoriasis. In Group B disorders, joint pain is just one of the manifestations of a whole-body disease.

When confronting an achy joint, the first step in management is to figure out whether the condition is in Group A or Group B; essentially, whether the cause is local or general. This diagnosis can only be properly made by a licensed physician through examination and tests such as X-rays and blood work. Most general diseases will cause abnormal laboratory results and X-ray findings that help in the identification. If the medical evaluation shows that a joint problem is related to a general disease (Group B), the patient needs to be seen by a specialist without delay. General diseases such as lupus are serious, and the pain is often just one symptom of systemic disease. Greater and more dangerous health problems will result if the disease is left without intensive treatment. However, those conventional treatments work well with the lifestyle modifications designed to treat Group A arthritis (complementary medicine). So, if you suffer from a condition in Group B, please don't feel as if this book is no longer for you.

Group A: Local causes of arthritis

- Bursitis
- Cartilage or meniscus injury, or inflammation
- Degenerative joint disease (osteoarthritis)
- Infectious arthritis (bacteria, fungus, virus)
- Tendinitis
- Tenosynovitis
- Trauma *Tear *Sprains

Group B: Systemic diseases that cause arthritis

- Cancer
- Connective tissue diseases
- Endocrine disease (diabetes, hyperparathyroidism, thyroid disease)
- Juvenile arthritis
- Lupus erythematosus
- Lyme disease
- Metabolic disease (gout, pseudo-gout, etc.)
- Neuropathies
- Polymyositis
- Psoriasis
- Rheumatoid arthritis
- Vasculitis

In this chapter, we will be focusing on Group A arthritis conditions – those due to local causes – which are by far the most frequent. This initial classification in Group A or B is critical, and a painful joint should always be evaluated by a qualified physician. Once this step is taken, and Group B arthritis has been ruled out, then adequate treatment can be initiated to deal with the sick joint.

Arthritis: A Historic Disease

Arthritis has been causing pain for longer than humans have walked the earth; signs of osteoarthritis have even been found in dinosaur bones. The physicians of Ancient Greece studied arthritis and named it "arthro" meaning "joint" which has come to mean "inflammation." After close examination of skeletal remains, historians have estimated that more than 70 percent of the citizens of ancient Rome over the age of 30 were afflicted with some form of arthritis, and it's believed the famous Roman bathhouses provided relief to their aching joints. Books on the subject started to be written as early as the 16th century. One of the most famous sufferers was the French impressionist painter Pierre-Auguste Renoir, famous for the beautiful Luncheon of the Boating Party and Dance at Bougival, among others. Renoir lived long and died at 78 in 1919, but it's generally regarded that his best paintings date from the 19th century. For the last 20 years of his life, his hands and shoulder were severely crippled with arthritis, robbing this once-prolific artist of his livelihood.

The last fifty years have brought major advancements in the classification, management, and treatment of arthritis. Today, it can be better understood and treated, bringing relief and improvement in the quality of life for millions of people. Research continues in many different fields, including immunology, genetics, and microbiology, to better understand the mechanisms of joint inflammation and deterioration. As these researchers gain knowledge it will lead to new and better forms of treatments, Just like how a better understanding for you will lead to improvements in your health.

Risk Factors

Without a doubt, there are a variety of factors that enhance the chances of developing joint problems, some we can change, some we can't.

Risk factors and likely causes of arthritis

Once you understand the causes of arthritis, you will be able to realize that many of these risk factors can be modified. By changing your lifestyle and eliminating certain behaviors, you can remove some of the causes of your joint problem and put yourself on the track to healing.

As I wrote above, the exact cause of arthritis varies wildly from case to case. Physical injury, such as a joint sprain, can set the stage for arthritis by accelerating the wear-and-tear on the joints. Any physical activity, intense or not, sport- or job-related, can become a risk factor for joint lesions through the effect of repetitive trauma. Walking five miles every day, intense weightlifting, prolonged hours of computer work, repetitively lifting a baby, or playing recreational soccer every weekend are just some of many activities considered as possible risk factors for joint, tendons, and neuromuscular disorders. The very intimate reason for this higher risk is that those activities, and many more, squeeze, tear, hurt local cells causing cellular damage and allowing irritating enzymes to escape from those cells and flood the intercellular space.

Research has shown that degenerative joint disease starts with the breakdown of cells, which triggers active biochemical processes that adversely alter the structure and repair mechanisms of the cartilage and joint tissues. The arthritic process begins when enzymes damage the collagen fibers that maintain the structure of the cartilage, tendons, or ligaments. This damage, and the irritation caused by the enzymes, trigger the inflammatory-repair process that often goes sour.

Let's review those risk factors.

Risk factors that are impossible to change

Scientists have pinpointed several predisposing factors that increase the risk of developing arthritis. These factors might be set in stone, but don't think that your bad luck has sealed your fate. A therapeutic lifestyle can negate the negativity buried deep in your genes.

1) **Genetic Predisposition.** Some people carry a genetic predisposition to developing arthritis. This means they have a gene, or a genetic marker, that makes them susceptible to the condition. If one or both of your parents have osteoarthritis, there is an increased chance that you will develop it at some point in your life. In some families, every generation will have at least one member affected or even crippled by arthritis.

   Researchers have found a large number of different genes that contribute to the development of osteoarthritis. A defect in just one of these genes may lead to the development of abnormal proteins in the cartilage, the growth of misshapen collagen fibers, or problems in a basic structure of the joint. Most commonly, the rogue gene will affect either the strength or the repair capacity of the cartilage, turning daily wear and tear into long-lasting damage.

   However, there are a growing number of scientists and other professionals, with the research to back them, who believe that gene expression can be altered through healthy lifestyle choices.

2) **Ethnicity.** Beyond individual genes, as listed above, it is possible that whether a person develops arthritis may depend on their ethnic background. Different ethnic groups have different rates of developing joint problems, some showing a higher incidence of osteoarthritis, and some lower. There is evidence that Asians, especially Chinese, have lower rates of osteoarthritis in the hip, but higher rates in the knee. African-Americans tend to have a higher overall rate of osteoarthritis than other races. If your family background means an increased risk of developing arthritic conditions, it is more important for you to follow the protocols and counteract it. If you are African-American, let's say you have a 10% increased chance of developing arthritis, but by taking steps to lower your risk by 20%, you've essentially "defeated" your genetic obstacle.

3) **Age.** It shouldn't be surprising to you that the risk of developing arthritis increases with age. The older the person, the more "mileage" the joints have undergone, and increased wear and tear is hard to avoid. Every year after your 45th birthday you elevate your risk higher and higher. As mentioned before, you can greatly decrease your chances of developing arthritis by adopting healthy habits. It's never too late (or too early) to take steps towards better health and to ensure a long and pain-free life.

Risk factors and likely causes that you can do something about

While there is little that we can do about the risk factors above, there are several risks that can be actively counteracted. Some changes are easier than others, but even the difficult ones are worth taking steps towards because it's all for the sake of your health.

1) **Joint Abuse.** Erosion is a simple concept: a simple action, performed many times a day over many years, will gradually wear away at the materials involved. This is also true for your bones and joints. Whether sports or work-related, repetitive activities will start to damage the joint structure, causing cartilage breakdown and faulty repair functions. Joint degeneration and osteoarthritis, as you know, follows. In these cases, the affected joints will be the ones involved in the repetitive activities, such as a typist's wrist and fingers or a construction worker's hips and back. Professional marathon runners (knees) and tennis players (elbows) are also good examples.

Osteoarthritis resulting from sports injuries is on the rise, and it seems to no longer be restricted to athletes as more people are using their leisure time to play sports and engage in vigorous exercise. Sports activities that begin in the teenage years and continue through adulthood carry a greater risk of causing osteoarthritis.

2) **Weight.** Obesity can also cause complications due to mechanical action but in a slightly different way. If a person is carrying excess weight, their bones and joints must work harder to support those extra pounds. This is especially true for the joints of the lower body: the hips, knees, and ankles. Even if you're not engaging in work or exercise involving repetitive stress and strain, the extra weight puts extra stress during normal activities such as walking and climbing stairs. As the damage advances, minor daily movements like shopping or walking the dog may trigger acute joint inflammation and pain. Even attempts at fixing the obesity can backfire: an overweight and sedentary person suddenly deciding to start walking a mile a day is a great breakthrough in their health, but the damage to their joints can cause painful inflammation that will force them back into their old unhealthy lifestyle.

3) **Nutritional Causes.** Cartilage is not just a lifeless layer of rubber but rather a living tissue that is continuously being renewed. To keep it fresh and functional, the cartilage is in a constant process of breakdown and repair. Special cells are continuously digesting old cartilage and creating new cartilage. To make new cartilage, these cells need special nutrients that come from the foods we eat and digest. Hence, the process of breakdown and repair seems to be influenced by nutrition, and recent publications report that nutritional deficits can adversely affect the biochemical and biophysical strength of your cartilage.

Among the nutritional causes of osteoarthritis, we find several culprits:

a) **Free Radicals.** A free radical is a "damaged" oxygen molecule that destroys healthy connective tissue. Free radicals are harmful to all bodily tissues, including the cartilage, and they are generated in response to any type of stress (chemical, physical, emotional, and mental) but they are also introduced to the body by exposure to environmental toxins in the air, water, and food. The adverse effects of free radicals are twofold: direct damage to cells and the impediment of healing mechanisms.

b) **Nutrient Deficiency.** To build new cartilage, the body needs raw materials in the form of nutrients. Unhealthy dietary habits can deprive the body of these essential nutrients and cause weakness in the cartilage structure. Certain eating habits, such as those associated with what I call the Standard American Diet, are known to cause adverse effects in the joints. A diet rich in bad fat and processed carbohydrates, but poor in omega-3 fatty acids, is a clear contributor to osteoarthritis. Those who eat lots of fast food and no fresh salads or fruits deprive their bodies of healthy essential fatty acids and antioxidants.

c) **Food Sensitivities.** There are indications that reactions to certain foods play a significant role in the onset and progression of osteoarthritis. Foods that most commonly appear on food sensitivity tests, and therefore the most likely to create arthritic conditions, include dairy products, beef, yeast, wheat, eggs, oranges, peanuts, green beans, vegetables of the nightshade family (peppers, potatoes, tomatoes, eggplant), chocolate, sugar, and corn. This doesn't mean you have to toss everything out of your refrigerator! Not every arthritis patient has food sensitivities, and vice-versa. We suggest that you consider the possibility of a food sensitivity problem. Your local health food stores and naturopathic and anti-aging physicians will usually have information on the subject, including possible testing outlets. An Internet search can be very enlightening in helping you find local options.

d) **Metals and Minerals.** In many patients with osteoarthritis, high levels of copper, mercury, and aluminum are found in their blood. It is believed that their negative effects result from their interference with the absorption and use of vitamins and antioxidants. Imbalance in minerals such as selenium, boron, manganese, zinc, and calcium can also cause disorders in the cartilage structure. What can you do about it? Eat a variety of raw vegetables and fruits, and gather information (again, from health food stores and natural medicine doctors) on a daily supplement plan that suits specifically what your body needs

4) **The Indirect Effect**. It's also possible that arthritis in your hand may have its root in a distant part of your body: the spine. If a person has a degenerative or inflammatory process occurring in the spine, the nerves coming out of the spine will be squeezed and become irritated. If an irritated nerve goes to a muscle, the irritation will be transmitted to the muscle, and the muscle will not work well – it will either be too relaxed or too tense. This abnormality in the muscle will translate into an abnormal motion of the joint, which will eventually end up harming its cartilage and ligaments. It all starts in the spine. That is how arthritis in the neck can cause osteoarthritis of the

shoulder, or spinal arthritis in the lower back can cause arthritis of the hip and knee. That is the indirect effect.

5) **Combinations of Factors.** Putting aside the factors (genetic, ethnicity, and age) that are mostly unavoidable, a combination of any of the above risk factors will compound their effects. Imagine an obese man working in building construction: constantly going up and down stairs wears on his knees and his excess weight is accelerating that abuse, while his diet of fast food generates bad eicosanoids and free radicals, promotes inflammation, and does nothing to heal the damage (no antioxidants or omega-3). Therefore, he stands a much higher, compounded chance of developing arthritis. Taking care of just one risk factor will do much more than eliminate its negative contribution. Or imagine a tennis player who has multiple diseased discs in his cervical spine and has a diet based on a typical Standard American Diet. His cervical neuropathy will cause an indirect effect on his shoulders and elbows, the excess activity will make those joints suffer and his bad diet will interfere with the repair process. Do you think that some pills and perhaps a couple of cortisone shots will fix the problem?

Joints and Cartilage in Trouble

In a healthy joint, the cartilage, ligaments, and tendons work together to shield the joint against friction and impact; daily wear-and-tear is minimal, and local tissue repair is successful. However, if part of the joint is not healthy (due to injury, bad posture, toxins, nutritional deficiency, etc.) daily repair will not be successful. The small micro-damages will not be fixed before the next day of use, and inflammation sets in and persists. Further damage occurs: the cartilage thins and erodes, muscles go into spasm, ligaments swell. Friction creates more heat, which creates more injury, and the inflammatory process is accelerated. A vicious circle begins, creating more and more pain and spasm in local muscles, which in turn creates tightness and restriction in movement and further tissue damage. The cartilage becomes trapped in a cycle of inflammation-causing damage and damage causing inflammation. Whether the process begins as a slow degeneration of cartilage and extends to tendons, muscles, and ligaments, or it starts as tendinitis or ligament injury and moves to the cartilage, the result is similar: pain, swelling and cartilage disease. Continuous inflammation leads to degenerative joint disease (osteoarthritis). The inflammation triggered by this process is a complex cellular and biochemical reaction. If the cause that precipitated the inflammation is eliminated and the cartilage is healthy proteins, eicosanoids and cells will work together to fix the damage. However, if the agent that caused the injury is still present, if the injury recurs, or if the cartilage is not healthy (perhaps because the person is not healthy), the inflammatory process will continue. Dysfunctional repair and degeneration ensue, which institutes the development and progression of osteoarthritis.

Repair

If the injuries are small and far apart and the healing process is adequate, there will be no progression into osteoarthritis. Successful repair will prevent it. However, if the injuries are too severe or frequent – such as with a tennis player, hard labor worker, or a basketball player – the repair process may not be quick enough to prepare the joint for the next activity and repair will not be successful. On other occasions, the injury may be small but the repair process is defective, pushing the joint into osteoarthritis. Regardless of whether the injury is small or large, the repair process is the main factor in the healing of the joint and the prevention of arthritis. Let me rephrase this extremely important concept: whether the joint will heal or will develop arthritis depends on the repair process. Explaining the causes of a defective repair process is one of the primary aims of this book.

Whether a joint will heal or will be pushed into arthritis depends on the efficiency of the body's natural repair process.

Sorry, but there was no way to make the last few pages any simpler. We've been dealing with a very complex mechanism that you need to grasp if you want to understand why integrative medicine works.

Arthritis is not just a passive erosion of the joint, but an active process of inflammation, degeneration, and unsuccessful repair.

At this time, it is important to repeat the sentence for the management of arthritis: Arthritis is not just a passive erosion of the joint, but an active process of inflammation, degeneration, and unsuccessful repair. We need to comprehend that the inflammatory-degenerative process of arthritis is not like a tragedy people watch on television, to which they may say "Oh, it's awful...but there's nothing I can do." With arthritis, there is something that sufferers can do, but they must assume the responsibility of doing it. Of course, they can shield themselves behind the excuse that it is too difficult to understand, or too complicated. Well... yes, it's a bit complicated, I agree. But what's the alternative? To keep taking pills until the day the orthopedic surgeon is standing over you with a scalpel? Once the complex process of arthritis is understood, it will be clear that taking anti-inflammatory pills will not fix it. A comprehensive management regimen such as the one offered by the Jupiter Institute Arthritis and Pain Program, can treat the intimate mechanism of arthritis and provide a beneficial effect in addressing the root causes of the arthritic condition. I invite both patients and doctors to engage in similar approaches to combat this disabling disease.

But if you don't understand it, how can you fix it? Hence, the importance of this book.

Using the points of our program, a significant improvement, and even a reversal of the arthritic process can be achieved. Studies show that adopting an anti-inflammatory diet like our Jupiter Institute Omega Diet can have a favorable effect on healing the degenerative and inflammatory processes of arthritis and injuries. This favorable effect can be enhanced with certain supplements and vitamins, like a special combination of Boswellia compounds mixed with antioxidants and an extra-refined omega-3 oil that we use in my office with great success. I describe this with more detail in the supplement chapter. Research also shows that both chiropractic and acupuncture treatments have a positive effect in healing painful joints and injuries, and many books have been published showing how certain exercises, physical therapy, and the alternative therapies I describe in the next chapters aid in the repair process of the ailing tissues. But when all these therapies are combined and integrated, the sum of the whole is a lot more powerful than any of the individual components by themselves. The beneficial effects are tremendous, and the impact of decreasing symptoms and improving the quality of life is enormous.

INTERCHAPTER REMARK: Now you know something new, that any painful joint, nerve or muscular problem, and any painful situation, revolve around an inflammatory process; and all repair efforts must be geared in that direction. Inflammation needs to be somehow understood and taken care of. As you visualize the different forms of arthritis, you can appreciate that eicosanoids, (molecules difficult to understand), and free radicals, need to be appeased. There are all kinds of repair efforts, but all must be focused on the inflammatory problem.

While you try to recover from whatever is hurting you, keep in mind THE INDIRECT EFFECT and the INFLAMMATION process. They need to be taken care of, but don't expect your physician to help you with that: YOU may need to manage them and get the right professional to help you.

You also acquired very important concepts: that a painful joint or muscle might have its roots in the cartilage, the ligaments, a tendon, a distant nerve, or might even be related to a systemic or metabolic disorder that needs to be explored. Most importantly, the concepts of joint abuse, food-related disorders, lack of nutrients, and the indirect effect must be kept in mind at all times.

A Few Basic Concepts

This chapter is devoted to a few basic concepts, some that we covered in the first two chapters, and others that will be explained in more detail later on.

Fats

Omega Fatty Acids

It's hard to go anywhere without hearing about omega-3 nowadays; there are even television commercials advertising oil capsules boasting incredible amounts of the stuff. But what is it exactly?

To keep things simple, they are a type of fatty acid, which is an acid molecule with a fat molecule attached to it; the term "omega-3" defines which molecules are where. Fatty acids are present throughout the body and are necessary for every part of cell metabolism. Omega-3 fatty acid specifically, is found in high concentrations in the human brain but is also found in every tissue where it is involved in creating anti-inflammatory molecules. You can see where I'm going with this: omega-3 reduces inflammation. Almost every nutritional choice in this book is aimed at increasing the levels of omega-3 in your bloodstream, which will in turn reduce inflammation wherever it is.

Like all the "essential" fatty acids, omega-3 is not created by the body and must be obtained through diet. The only cells that synthesize omega-3 are found in green plants, such as flax and seaweed. Consuming these plants, or high-quality cold-pressed oils extracted from them, is a great way to supplement your diet. Fish that eat a diet composed primarily of algae and seaweed (specifically oily fish like salmon, tuna, mackerel, and sardines) have high levels of omega-3 in their flesh, which makes them the perfect dinner when you're fighting damaging inflammation.

But aren't there other omegas? After all, how can we have omega-3 without omega-1 and omega-2? They do exist, but they're not as important. The one other omega you must be aware of is omega-6 fatty acid. While omega-6 is also essential, it promotes inflammation and (unlike omega-3) is found in very high amounts within the average American diet. Think of omega-6 as the "anti-omega-3. While omega-3 breaks down to create anti-inflammatory molecules, omega-6 works to create pro-inflammatory molecules.

It is important to keep a good ratio of omega-6 to omega-3, and that means a small ratio. A typical American diet has a ratio as high as 20:1; only five percent of the omega fatty acids consumed are omega-3. While it's practically impossible for the ratio to be equal, it's a good thing to keep in mind: increasing more omega-3 is always good and can help limit the damage caused by inflammatory foods. For example, you can soften the blow of a cheeseburger by starting your meal with a fresh salad drizzled with flaxseed oil (it's delicious!). Omega-6 is likely very prevalent in your diet already, so the easiest way to balance the ratio is by adding foods that are rich in omega-3!

Free radicals and antioxidants

Free radicals are molecules generated by the metabolic processes of the body. They possess an unpaired electron, and that makes them a powerful component in the organic chemical reactions that take place many times every second in living tissue. In normal situations, every cell in our body uses oxygen, glucose, and fat to produce its vital energy. This energy is used by the cell to function and fulfill its role in our metabolism. As a by-product of the energy production, some free sparks of electrons escape and bounce around like ping-pong balls. These sparks are called free radicals and they can damage the inner structures of the cell. To control this damage, they need to be neutralized by antioxidants, and your body does this automatically as soon as free radicals appear. In excess, free radicals damage cells by causing too many reactions with other molecules. The damage is known as oxidation, similar to metal rusting when exposed to water and air.

Think of free radicals like you would chlorine bleach: you need a little bit to get stains out of your clothes, but too much will ruin your entire wardrobe. Injuries and inflammation disrupt local metabolic pathways and cause an increase of free radicals, damaging the surroundings like a leaking bottle of bleach. An excess of free radicals causes the inflammatory process to last longer and be more damaging. If your body is full of free radicals, even the good effects of omega-3 in your diet will be neutralized. Free radicals are definitely "bad guys" in the context of inflammation.

The Mechanics of a Joint

A joint is more than just a place where two bones come together: it's a marvel of organic engineering. The most important element in a joint is cartilage, which covers the connecting ends of the larger bones and surrounds the smaller bones often found within the joint itself. This smooth, tough, rubbery material works as a shock absorber, preventing the bones from rubbing against each other. Surrounding the joint is a strong cylindrical sheet that attaches to the end of each bone: the joint capsule. You can visualize it by putting your two fists together inside the sleeve of a shirt. The capsule keeps the joint in a closed and sterile environment and is filled with synovial fluid. Clear and similar in consistency to an egg white, this slippery fluid acts like oil in an engine, protecting all the moving parts by decreasing friction.

Anchoring to the bone from either side of the joint, ligaments hold the joint together and keep it well-aligned. Tendons are fibrous cords that attach muscle to bone and pass through the outer part of the joint, also helping to hold it together. Bursae (singular: bursa) are small sacs filled with synovial fluid that provide an extra cushion in certain areas between the joints and tendons, facilitating their sliding and relieving friction between these structures.

Cartilage

Cartilage within a joint (articular cartilage) is a dense, rubbery material that covers the two heads of the bones. It is whitish and extremely tough. Its major constituents are water, collagen (a fiber-like protein), and chondrocytes (cells that create collagen and other proteins), all mixed creating tissue with strong structure. The firmness and health of the cartilage are crucial for the proper function of the spine and joints. With the painful disorders this book discusses, you will be hard-pressed to find a paragraph that doesn't involve managing the metabolic harmony of this cartilage.

The major function of the articular cartilage is to coat the bones and absorb shock. The proteins in the cartilage act like sponges, holding water during rest and pushing it out under pressure. This system absorbs the mechanical force, allowing the cartilage to give and flatten against pressure instead of cracking and breaking.

An important feature of the inside of the joint is lubrication. The cartilage surface, wet with synovial fluid, is slippery, allowing the joint surfaces to slide back and forth with very little friction.

The Spine

The spine, also called the vertebral column, is composed of thirty-three vertebrae stacked on top of one another. Each vertebra has a hole through the middle, each hole forming part of a long tube that holds the spinal cord in place. On either side, there are small holes that allow nerves to branch off from the spinal cord and extend to the muscles and essentially everything else below the neck. The spine plays an extremely important role in our bodies as it supports the upper body's weight, provides posture while allowing for movement and flexibility, and protects the spinal cord. The spinal cord is obviously important; together with the brain, it forms the central nervous system (CNS) and is mainly responsible for sending instructions from your brain to your muscles ("put your hand in cold water") and messages from your sensory nerves to your brain ("the water is cold").

Pain

It's no doubt that you've heard the phrase, "know thy enemy." Our enemy is "pain." Familiarity with how pain occurs – and all the ways it rears its ugly head – is important in understanding your condition and will help you defeat this nefarious foe.

There are many causes of pain, but for simplicity, we must divide them into two groups:

1) Pain is one symptom of a more complicated issue, especially those relating to a problem outside the muscles, bones, or joints. This includes conditions such as kidney stones or angina, tumors, infections, toothache, etc.

2) Pain that is itself the main symptom and arises from either chronic or acute inflammation in the musculoskeletal system.

While the pain arising from the first category can be just as crippling, this book is unfortunately not written with those conditions in mind. While the guidelines and information in this book (especially in the chapters on nutrition and supplements) can be enjoyed and utilized by anyone in their quest for better health and wellness, they are not intended for those conditions and will not have any direct effect on that type of pain.

Within the second category, we divide again: acute pain and chronic pain. Acute pain is essentially "new" or has an onset within 30 days. After 30 days, if the pain is still present and the sufferer has adjusted their daily life around it, then it becomes chronic pain. Acute pain is usually debilitating and caused by trauma, and chronic pain is associated with inflammatory conditions. In the spine, for example, a fall off a stepladder can result in a slipped disc, which is immediately painful (acute pain), and can be treated with physical therapy or surgery. However, an arthritic condition can degenerate the vertebra, causing inflammation which pinches the nerve and creates pain that while not as sharp and debilitating as a slipped disc, can last for decades. This is chronic pain.

Depending on its severity, chronic pain can be a persistent nightmare, dominating the sufferer and causing physical, mental and emotional weakness and even depression. Chronic pain, like arthritis, needs to be understood, which means that we must look for, find, and address its root causes to achieve healing. Chronic pain is a multifactorial disorder requiring the coordinated efforts of a treatment team since the resources of a single practitioner are generally insufficient to properly identify and treat all of the involved factors. This is a critical point that needs repeating. Doctors and patients must understand and accept the fact that a solo practitioner is generally unable to address the variety of causes of chronic pain and the resulting problems and symptoms. Just one or two treatments of a single therapeutic approach are typically unsuccessful at treating a chronic pain condition. Rather, chronic pain conditions require the combined efforts of a team over time. Here are examples of single therapy approaches that are typically unsuccessful: A woman with neck pain taking only painkillers and anti-inflammatory medications; a man who has had shoulder pain for eight months receives one cortisone shot and takes Ibuprofen. These are just two examples of how treatment can be confined to symptom management, while the underlying condition worsens. In both of these cases, there is no particular broad therapeutic approach that addresses the cause of the pain or that promotes the healing and repair of the condition. Pain means injury and injury demands repair. Repair demands a plan of treatment and not just pills. The success of any treatment plan depends on a thorough understanding of the causes of the pain – by both the patient and the doctor. Furthermore, doctors must understand that the causes of chronic pain should never be addressed with a pill, and patients should understand as well not to push doctors to give them a miracle pill but rather to present to them a variety of therapy options. Once this understanding is firmly intact, a comprehensive approach needs to be applied and followed. Without it, healing will be unlikely. The comprehensive approach must include complementary medicine for long-term relief, and both patients and doctors must open their minds to embrace and use it.

INTERCHAPTER REMARK: Understanding the dynamics of a joint and its attached structures will help you understand how to heal it.

A little message: the mechanics of many joints depend on the integrity of the spine.

Injuries

Broken-eggs and metabolism?

A Battle Plan for Neck and Back Pain

Expanding on what we just learned; the spine consists of thirty-three separate vertebrae divided into five regions. Vertebrae are separated by cushions, known as intervertebral discs, which are made of cartilage and allow a degree of motion between one vertebra and the next. Remember the spinal cord and its role in communicating with the rest of the body? To send those messages, it relies on nerves extended through small holes in each vertebra. Each hole is formed by a tiny gap between two vertebrae in an area exposed to (and in contact with) the intervertebral disc. There lies the flaw in this design: if you've suffered from back pain, you've understood how delicate this feature is. Any inflammation, whether from an arthritis condition or injury, can irritate, pinch, or squeeze the nerve at the point where it exits the vertebra. Whether irritated or pinched, the nerve conduction is stimulated, and pain is felt. This is neuralgia; ancient Greek for "nerve pain."

Neck pain caused by trauma.

Fractures and dislocations of the spine must be considered first in any person with a recent history of neck pain or injury. Therefore, an X-ray of the spine is needed in every case of significant neck pain, and after an injury or accident. Many terms are used interchangeably to refer to the typical soft tissue injury of the neck, including "whiplash injury," "cervical sprain," and "neck sprain." In the case of neck sprain, the ligaments that hold the vertebrae together are sprained or overstretched, often by the head snapping backward. If the injury is severe, one vertebra may slide forward out of place and compress the spinal cord. This creates an urgent situation that requires a visit to the emergency room. However, if the sprain is mild, the person will just feel pain and stiffness in the neck area. Whiplash injury is a severe strain of the neck caused by sudden violent movement, damaging muscles, tendons, and ligaments. The spine is such a thick web of ligaments, tendons, nerves, and muscle fibers that it is easy for an injury to damage all four of these structures at the same time. Imagine a bunch of uncooked spaghetti that suffers a blow: not just one strand cracks but several, and on different levels. Similarly, whiplash may create many simultaneous micro-centers of injury. Although job and sports-related injuries may occasionally cause these problems, most instances of whiplash result from rear-end automobile collisions. The typical injury occurs as the head is first flexed and then forcibly overextended beyond its normal range of motion. Significant injuries will affect not only muscles, ligaments, and tendons but also the joints and cartilage of the spine, as well as the nerve roots. There are multiple types of injuries including sudden elongation of nerves and ligaments, muscle tears, ligament sprains, and cartilage, and tendon injuries. Although one particular muscle or ligament may take the brunt of the damage, typically many very small areas of injury result.

Broken-eggs – use this example for every muscle, tendon, and ligament injury.

Since cells are torn and damaged, each of these micro-injuries triggers the inflammatory process. Just like when an egg is cracked and the egg white leaks through the crack, torn and damaged cells leak their inside protoplasm and enzymes, which scatter among the surrounding cells and irritates them. This process ends up damaging neighboring cells. In a slow and continuous chain of events, cells that were first damaged die, and those that were unhurt begin to sustain damage. Those cells eventually die, freeing their protoplasm and enzymes, and hurting more cells in addition to previously unharmed cells. The destruction spreads and increasing numbers of cells become injured and die. This process generates tissue irritation (inflammation). As the inflammatory process progresses, it extends over a larger area, worsening the swelling and progressively increasing the heat and pain. Local irritation and tissue damage can also cause muscle spasms. When this happens, blood flow is reduced, causing even more suffering among the cells. The intense inflammatory process continues, triggering the production of eicosanoids in large quantities, which attracts more white blood cells. These white blood cells arrive at the inflamed area and draw in even more enzymes and eicosanoids. After several days, each one of the micro-injury areas will have transformed itself into a complex center of inflammation. This explains why sudden neck injuries caused by auto accidents, jobs, or sports activity hurt even more after a few days. These events are the result of the 'broken-eggs effect."

The majority of conventional medical treatments involve – almost exclusively – the prescription of muscle relaxants and pain relievers. While these pharmaceuticals may result in the temporary remediation of symptoms, they do not address the underlying causes of ongoing inflammation and, therefore, cannot heal the injury. Most injuries trigger a complex biological and physiological response that requires a multi-disciplinary approach. Anti-inflammatory nutrition, chiropractic care, physical therapy, and other forms of alternative treatments work synergistically to eliminate underlying inflammation in the body – and in the micro center of the injury – which allows for permanent healing.

Reviewing the relationship between anatomy and the pain process will help you understand the value of the treatment plan described at the end of this chapter.

Neck pain not due to trauma

The cervical spine – the spine in the neck area – is unique. It has a motion capacity unlike any other part of the spine. It can flex and extend, rotate, and bend to the sides. Thanks to this mobility it also has a unique exposure to all types of injuries caused by falls, sports, work-related accidents, and poor posture. Many of these injuries result in micro-injuries in the ligaments, joints, and cartilage of the spine that accumulate over time. After many years of silent progression, these lesions slowly cause the discs to flatten and bulge. The ligaments give way, tear, and calcify, and the cartilage of the joints deteriorates. This is a process called degenerative disc disease, and it may remain silent without symptoms for many years. However, as the condition progresses, a trigger event finally occurs bringing attention to the weakness. The trigger events can be a fall, an accident, a job-related injury, poor posture, sleeping on the couch, whiplash, or other physical strains.

The inflammation caused by this event ends the silent period of this process by activating the symptoms of pain, stiffness, and decreased mobility. Because the cervical spine contains a tight bundle of nerves, the pain caused by the degenerative disc disease may be felt in the neck, but may also radiate to the shoulders, arm and even to the hands. On many occasions, the alarming symptom is not the pain but rather the tingling, numbness, and even weakness of the arm. Whatever the symptoms are and whatever the cause that triggered them, the initial steps in management are an evaluation by the doctor and a review of the

X-rays of the cervical spine. Then – and only then – a treatment program can be decided. Treatment options may include medications, physical therapy, traction, injections, integrative medicine, massage, exercise, or a consultation with a specialist. Part of the evaluation may include an MRI exam and the measuring of nerve conduction velocities. As the treatment modality is decided, patients and physicians must be aware of two things. First, there is an old degenerative process, which means that a complete return to normal is not possible. Second, there is an ongoing inflammatory process in the spine, which means there are areas of swelling, cell injury, eicosanoid activity, and heat. Since the degree of inflammation and cell injury varies from case to case, treatments vary as well. One thing is for sure: an anti-inflammatory program, with anti-inflammatory medication and an anti-inflammatory diet, is essential if one wants to focus on tissue repair and not just masking the symptoms.

Neck pain can be the result of four main causes:

a) A traumatic injury, such as in a whiplash or fall, in an otherwise healthy neck.

b) A traumatic injury in the neck, already affected by a degenerative arthritic process. (This explains why sometimes a small injury can cause such a storm of pain and disability.)

c) A non-traumatic injury that has been evolving for a long time and finally starts to produce symptoms (and pain or tingling starts for no apparent cause). It may be scoliosis of the spine or an extremely slow, progressive bulging disc.

d) A non-arthritic and non-traumatic condition, such as a cyst, tumor or neuropathy, etc., affecting the neck or its structures.

The first step in evaluating the cause of neck pain, therefore, is to see a doctor for an X-ray of the cervical spine to rule out a traumatic injury, and to make sure that it is an injury and not an arthritis-related problem.

An X-ray will also help to determine whether the problem is indeed (a), (b), (c), or (d). The X-ray findings will determine the treatment. Additional evaluation includes an MRI, complete blood tests, and possibly even a second opinion from a consultant. So far so good. However, if the distress is caused by (b) or (c), there is likely an old and/or new injury process occurring in the cervical spine, which also means that there is an active inflammatory process in one or more locations in the spine. There could be more or less pain, and there could be more or less degeneration or bulging of the discs. But, for sure, there is an inflammatory process somewhere in the spine. From our previous discussion, we know that at the center of these inflammatory pockets the cells are being injured and are pouring their enzymes onto surrounding cells. Eicosanoids are interacting with proteins and cells; there are swelling and heat, there are numerous white blood cells and waste products, and cartilage is being eroded because its fibers are disintegrating. If you could look at the process under a microscope, it is like the disrupted anthill that I mentioned earlier, teeming with ants frantically moving everywhere.

The purpose of the inflammation is twofold: as a defense against further injury, and as a reconstructive force for the injured area. Inflammatory cells, proteins, enzymes, and eicosanoids all interact in the process. The eicosanoids, which are produced by cells from omega fatty acids, can be of the good type or the bad type. As described in the previous chapter, the good eicosanoids will try to decrease inflammation and promote repair while the bad type will do the opposite. The ratio of good to bad eicosanoids will depend on the magnitude of the injury, the state of health of the tissues, and the nutritional value of the foods consumed by the person. Whatever treatment is chosen, it must take into account both the cause of the injury as well as this inflammatory process. This is a critical point. There may be more or less injury, there may be more or less degeneration, but for sure there is a degree of inflammation. And now, combining this fact with what I mentioned in the first two chapters, the inflammation in the spine will be affected by the overall inflammation status of the whole body.

Remember I told you inflammation travels through the body and can become systemic? Hence, advanced gut inflammation or dysbiosis (refer to page 109), combined with an omega-6 lifestyle (which I will be explaining over and over) will enhance the fire in the spine, discs, nerves, etc., while a healthy gut combined with a healthy, omega-3 anti-oxidant rich lifestyle, will have an anti-inflammatory and repair effect.

If the pain and disability are just treated with pills, or with pills and massage, then the root cause of the problem is not being treated. When the real cause of the problem is neglected, and the symptoms are masked with pills, the problem continues to grow and worsens with time. Those who suffer from injuries or arthritic conditions in the neck should not rely on pills for treatment. It is acceptable to take medications for a short time; however, this should not be the main and only therapy utilized for healing, but rather part of the global treatment plan.

Again, the main treatment should target the cause of the problem and the inflammatory process. The cause of the problem can be treated with:

- Cervical collar
- Chiropractic manipulations
- Exercise
- Injections (which can be extremely helpful in the right hands)
- Manual manipulation
- Massage
- Physical therapy
- Special pillow (sold at chiropractor's offices)
- Traction

The inflammatory process should be treated with an anti-inflammatory program that includes:

a) A short course of anti-inflammatory medication

b) An anti-inflammatory diet (as you will see later on)

c) An omega-3 lifestyle

d) Avoiding the omega-6 lifestyle, and

e) Supplements, including omega-3s and antioxidants, known to be powerful anti-inflammatory agents. Here I need to make a brief stop and address the supplement issue. There are many supplements in health food stores and many more on the Internet. I tried many of them with disappointing results and got all kinds of side effects. Don't buy them. Based on reliability and my past experience, I only recommend the ones I get from laboratories recognized by the Anti-Aging Academy, which I describe later on. I found a great deal of success with "Joint-Aid," a special combination of purified Glucosamine with Boswellia and certain brands of certified-organic and purified fish oil (most fish oils are unreliable so we are careful with the ones we recommend).

Let me elaborate and repeat. The idea that we can fight inflammation by just taking anti-inflammatories and/or cortisone (Prednisone, Medrol, etc.) is an outdated concept. Just as penicillin was used when it was initially discovered for every bacterial infection, nowadays we know better and have different options. So, now that we understand the entire inflammatory and injury process much better, we must modernize and update our treatment programs so that the painful conditions that afflict people can be eradicated.

But wait, it gets better.

An inflamed area, affected by chronic degeneration, tends to accumulate toxins and free radicals, therefore a detoxification program is frequently helpful. This kind of program, explained in more detail in another chapter, will not eliminate or cure the problem, but for sure will help in the anti-inflammation and repair process.

The same area blocks the flow of our bio-energy, creating a high-pressure area that causes pain and interferes with healing. Hence, acupuncture, craniosacral therapy and the alternative therapies I explain later on can be very effective.

If the hormones and thyroid of that person have declined too much, nerves will be more sensitive, and muscular recovery will not be that good. Natural hormone replacement (as I explain in a separate chapter) and thyroid support do offer a significant benefit in the recovery process.

And there is more. If the adrenal gland is dysfunctional, the repair will be hampered. This is already too complicated and needs a separate chapter.

And last, but not least, if you have a significant food sensitivity problem this may affect the inflammation and repair of a problem joint, inflamed tenosynovitis, a torn muscle, and even a surgical site. For instance, if you are very sensitive to dairy, wheat, and eggs, and you continuously eat those foods, the gut toxicity these foods create will leak from the gut and shower your metabolism and your problem area with undesired particles.

As you can see, repair is a complex process, and neither a pill nor an injection will do it. It is not just one of the above options that will get you better: it is their integration. That's the key. That's where you need to open your mind.

As you can see, several factors need to interact to decrease inflammation and favor repair, and as you take this necessary path and you start to get better, after a while you will realize how you separate yourself from the "common wisdom" of conventional medicine. Then one day you'll wake up and you'll feel you are better and you'll understand even more the concept of integration.

Low back pain

Low back pain is a frequent complaint and may be localized above the buttock area or on the buttocks. It is generally intense, affecting one side more than the other. The pain may radiate down the thigh or leg (what is known as sciatica), indicating that one or more nerve roots are being pinched. The cause, most likely, would be the same as that triggering the back pain. Like any arthritic condition, low back pain may be activated by general disease or by a local cause. Numerous general diseases and metabolic disorders can affect the lower back, along with localized spinal disorders, ranging from cysts and tumors to fractures and genetic disorders. Most of the local causes are related to acute ligament sprain and muscular strain, or acute worsening of an old disc problem.

The first step in the management of low back pain is an evaluation by a medical doctor.

The second step is to decide whether blood tests are needed, which should occur when there is suspicion of a generalized metabolic or rheumatologic condition such as anemia, lupus, rheumatoid arthritis, or infection, for example.

The third step is an X-ray of the lumbar spine and, on occasion, an X-ray of the pelvic bone as well. In dynamic medical offices, with physicians attentive to the patient's concerns, blood test and X-ray results may be obtained within 48 to 72 hours – or less – and a determination can be made about the cause and treatment of the problem. Major diseases need to be ruled out first. These include tumors, cancers, metabolic diseases, congenital disorders, severe osteoporosis, Paget's disease, rheumatoid arthritis, old fractures, pelvic disorders, kidney diseases, vascular disorders, and other conditions.

If all of these diseases have been ruled out, the focus will be on the spine and related areas. If the findings in the X-ray suggest spine and vertebral disease, treatment can be initiated according to the symptoms of the patient and the X-ray findings. A CAT scan or an MRI is not routinely necessary. Whether they are advised depends on the doctor's evaluation. The most frequent cause of low back pain is what is known as a bulging disc, or degenerative disc disease. In most cases, the problem has been brewing for years, with slow protrusion or herniation of the disc into the spinal canal, with a slow displacement of the vertebrae forward, backward, or with the slow progression of scoliosis. Other slow-motion events that have taken years to deform the problem area include calcification of ligaments, mechanical nerve root compression, flattening of the discs, traumatic tissue breakdown, loss of mobility between the vertebrae, and degenerative arthritis of the different parts of the vertebral joint.

All of these conditions are the result of multiple areas of microtrauma injuries and lesions due to heavy lifting, falls, accidents, poor posture, sports-, or work-related stress. The effect of these injuries and lesions accumulate through the years; gravity and body weight also aggravate the situation. Eventually, one of two things happen. Either a trivial event (such as standing up, sitting down, bending over or taking a short walk) triggers severe back pain, or a fall, accident, sports injury or job-related injury triggers a cascade of events: pains, spasm, inflammation, heat, and gait disorder. In either one of these scenarios, a new disc herniation (bulging) with new inflammation has been added to an old chronic process. While the disc herniation causes mechanical compression of the nerves and tissues, the new inflammation brings swelling, cellular disruption, enzymes, and eicosanoids. Good and bad eicosanoids will be present but in a ratio that depends, among other things, on the magnitude of the injury, the state of health of the person and his/her nutrition. This picture varies from case to case. In some people, there is more inflammation and less herniation. Others show a large herniation of the disc but only a small amount of inflammation. In either case, treatment has to focus on the two main processes: herniation and inflammation. Hence, some part of the treatment should be concentrated on relieving the bulging while other parts of the treatment should focus on relieving the inflammation. Simply taking anti-inflammatories and pain medications will provide no healing and may mask a serious problem.

Remember, while pills relieve the symptoms of the problem, the real cause of the problem is not being addressed, so the actual condition is likely to worsen with time. Neck and back disorders may have different symptoms, but they have one thing in common: the presence of injury and inflammation. The inflammatory process, described already in detail, is usually characterized by a cascade of broken cells, scattered enzymes, good and bad eicosanoids, and repair cells, and is accompanied by swelling and heat. The inflammation present in each one of these lesions shares responsibility for the pain and swelling of the problem area. Free radicals, as we've seen before, are harmful molecules that damage the cells and prolong the healing of the injury. Antioxidants, on the other hand, are "good" molecules that neutralize free radicals. Antioxidants are, therefore, called anti-inflammatory molecules while free radicals are pro-inflammatory. Among the cells and proteins of the inflammatory cascade, eicosanoids, free radicals and antioxidants do their share in helping or disrupting the healing process. The winner of this inflammatory battle determines whether the healing process is shortened or prolonged. Any treatment of low back pain or neck pain must take the inflammatory process into account. This will greatly influence the healing process and determine whether or not the inflammation subsides or remains.

By the way, combining refined, concentrated fish oil with special antioxidants, as we do in our office, has a beneficial effect on eicosanoids.

Sciatica and arm pain

Pain in the upper or lower limbs can be very misleading. It can be caused by an injury or disease in any part of the limb, including muscular disease, arthritis, and tendonitis, or bone disease. Pain can also be caused by an irritation of the nerve that feeds the limb. In this case, even though the pain is felt in the limb, it is a radiated pain. The problem is indeed at the spine. Such is the case with shooting pains down the arm, or with an achy or numb arm. This is akin to sciatica, whereby pain in the leg is caused by a compression or irritation of the roots of the sciatic nerve in the area adjacent to the spine. The pain can be constant or intermittent, sudden or progressive, sharp, or dull. It is characterized by pain radiating down the arm or leg, which at times can be felt as a stabbing or an electrical sensation. The arm pain in these cases is known as a pinched nerve, neuritis or neuropathy, and its equivalent in the leg is called sciatica. Both represent a similar condition – an irritated nerve.

These two conditions have an inflammatory process in common: at the root of the nerve. There may also be a traumatic, mechanical, or metabolic condition at that level, but either way, local inflammation is present. This means that treatment should focus on relieving both the causes of the nerve irritation and the local inflammation. These conditions are triggered by bulging (herniated) discs, spinal stenosis, ligament sprain, spinal arthritis, muscular irritation, etc. Each requires a different treatment approach. The local inflammation indicates that tissue damage is in progress at the center of the problem. This process is active, with inflammatory cells, swelling, good and bad eicosanoids, heat, enzymes, and attempts at repair.

As with all the painful conditions described in the previous pages, any treatment program that attempts to bring relief must consider this inflammatory process and try to heal it. You simply cannot heal a significant inflammatory process and a bulging disc area with pills or a little bit of physical therapy. If nothing is done for both the relief of the inflammatory process and the reduction of the bulging, there will be no real improvement.

The plan for neck and back pain, sciatica and arm pain
(Effective for shoulder and hip pain as well)

Indeed, the plan is plan B, since plan A should be your first step: to see a medical doctor. Don't hesitate. A physician needs to establish whether a serious disorder could be present, like a fracture, severe scoliosis, invasion of bone by malignant disease, bone disease, significant spinal stenosis, bone tumors, infectious disease, severe misalignments, and possibly conditions that might require surgery. You need to rule all these out first.

The doctor should also establish whether an X-ray, CAT Scan or MRI might be needed and whether a short course of anti-inflammatories, mild painkillers, and rest could take care of the problem.

However, make sure the doctor listens to you and addresses the problem properly. If the visit ends too quickly with a prescription of painkillers or just a referral to an orthopedic doctor, maybe you should see someone else.

If everything is okay and nothing major is going on, you can get started with our plan.

The plan to heal all these conditions is part of our Jupiter Institute Arthritis and Pain Program. It embraces a prescription of anti-inflammatory medications for a short course, which we will review in the medications chapter, as well as anti-bulging weapons (techniques aimed to correct the disc bulging) and an anti-inflammatory diet, which we call the Jupiter Institute Omega Diet, discussed in detail in the diet chapter.

I describe all this NOT for you to come to us, but for you to read, review, analyze, and establish a plan to manage your disorder. I talk about my personal experience and the experiences with patients to send you the message that, doing it well, this path may be successful.

At this time, I am sure, you are a bit more familiar with the concepts of inflammation and integration so the following information should be easier to comprehend.

Highlights of the battle plan are:

Anti-inflammatory weapons

A) Anti-inflammatory medications

    A.1 Anti-inflammatory diet. The diet is aimed at increasing the intake of anti-inflammatory omega-3 fatty acids and antioxidants while decreasing the intake of pro-inflammatory omega-6 and free radicals. This means staying away from an omega-6 lifestyle and embracing an omega-3 lifestyle instead. As you will see later, that means, adopting an omega-3 lifestyle, with an alkalized Mediterraneanized way of eating.

    A.2 Dietary supplements. Supplements including omega-3, omega-9, antioxidants, and vitamins, all known to have a powerful anti-inflammatory effect. I found that Boswellia AKBA mixed with turmeric and antioxidants (see the Chapter on Supplements) to provide a very powerful anti-inflammatory effect and many of my patients take them with great results. The effect is even better when we combine it with our detoxification program. Combining all these products with certain types (but not all) of omega-3 fish oil provides even a stronger anti-inflammatory effect. Most products from supermarkets, pharmacies, and health food stores are not reliable.

B) Anti-bulging weapons

B.1 Chiropractic manipulation. No other profession will provide such a beneficial effect in reducing the mechanical effect of a herniated disc.

B.2 Physical therapy. Not just any physical therapy, but rather a treatment protocol administered by a therapist who follows the instructions of a chiropractor, who also knows what they are doing. It is best to have a skilled chiropractor and physical therapist working together as a team.

B.3 Traction. There are several kinds of traction devices. Some can be very effective, some are useless.

B.4 Massage therapy. This can be effective in relaxing the muscles and allowing the spine to decompress. It can be a great complement to both chiropractic and physical therapy. I review this form of therapy in another chapter.

B.5 Exercises. They can be very helpful, but they need to be instructed by a chiropractor or a physical therapist. The wrong kind of exercise can aggravate disc problems. Go carefully.

B.6 Back brace. Get one and use it 1-2 hours at a time, once or twice a day. Wear it if you are going shopping or for a walk.

B.7 All these treatments should be integrated, that is, you should try to do all of them. They should also be complemented by acupuncture, a natural modality that heals the injured area physiologically and energetically.

This is the path to real healing. It is the course we follow and the one that we encourage both patients and doctors to adopt. I urge you to design a similar program for yourself if there is no team currently available in the area where you live.

C) And more, like applying the nutritional and alternative therapies I mention in this book, and a variety of therapies and healing techniques like Tai chi, Gyrotonics, Qigong and Craniosacral therapy, all directed to complement the above therapies, but each one capable on its own to bring on relief to the above ailments. They improve the flow of your bio-energy, known as "chi" or "Qi," relieving areas of abnormal pressure and energy block, allowing them to improve inflammation and aiding in repair.

D) And even more. Dealing with your Metabolic Puzzle. This might be a bit difficult to understand and accept, but I will explain it all in subsequent chapters. Suffice it to state that your metabolism as a whole controls your healing.

There are several factors to take into account when we are struggling with a painful, degenerative, or inflammatory condition (although most people are not affected the same way):

- ✓ Bad diet, with lack of nutrients and excess of omega-6
- ✓ Low levels of B vitamins and folic acid
- ✓ Excess stress hurting the adrenal gland function (Adrenal Stress)
- ✓ Drug, alcohol and/or painkillers abuse
- ✓ Chemicals in food, water, and environment
- ✓ Presence of inflammation or infection
- ✓ Low functioning thyroid
- ✓ The adverse effect of food sensitivities
- ✓ Dysbiosis and gut disorders
- ✓ Poor sleep
- ✓ Hormone decline (in both men and women)
- ✓ Exposure to toxins and the need for detoxification
- ✓ Abnormal lab work (showing kidney or liver disorder, low potassium, anemia, etc.).

These factors may or may not be present. They all reflect your metabolic panorama, and, if they are present, they can affect the revitalization and recuperation of cells and tissues. They don't affect everybody the same way, but for sure they can increase inflammation, interfere with healing, disrupt recovery, and even prolong pain and dysfunction. They are part of the metabolic puzzle you need to find out about.

These factors are very important and I address them separately in the next chapters.

I will just give a few quick words about detoxification and hormones before I continue with the management of some common disorders.

As mentioned above when addressing neck problems, some other therapies might be helpful.

Detoxification may help by removing toxins accumulating in the problem area. As I wrote earlier, this will not eliminate or cure the problem, but it will help in the anti-inflammation and repair processes. More and more testimonies are showing the beneficial effect of a methodical detoxification program, and our patients find our program to be simple yet very effective. Combining detoxification with our Glucosamine-Boswellia has provided many of our patients with amazing results and we were even able to spare some patients from surgery.

If you are unable to do anything else (for lack of resources or time) you can try two days of taking detoxification products combined with anti-inflammatory medicine, twice a day, a combination that might bring you some relief allowing you to buy time until you see your doctor.

Improving hormone decline with natural hormones, correcting low thyroid function with the right medication, and addressing adrenal gland disorders with the right supplement may improve the inflammatory process. This will allow the muscles and tendons to be more functional, will decrease the over-sensitivity of nerves, and for sure would aid in the anti-inflammation and repair process.

Food sensitivities can have an adverse effect on repair, as I addressed above.

For example, the case of a person with a pinched nerve in the neck, with resulting numbness and tingling on the right arm and pain in the wrist and hand, with the problem persisting despite physical therapy, chiropractor, the usual medications and a neck brace. Or a second case of a man with back pain, radiating ache all down the leg with pain in the foot. We'll assume that the X-rays and MRI are not showing anything bad, and conventional NSAIDs are not relieving the symptoms. Or a third case of a woman with chronic knee pain and or another woman with persisting left hip pain, both having been evaluated by doctors and are not responding to simple conventional care. They should all consider evaluating the metabolic puzzle I mention above. There might be dietary, nutritional, hormonal, toxic, thyroid, etc., factors at play of which they are unaware and might need to be evaluated and treated. I will be describing the importance of those factors as we advance.

Alternative options

Very frequently, as you probably realize, the spine is involved directly or indirectly, as a causative agent. You should be aware that when treating many limb injuries and joint and neuromuscular disorders, treating the spine would help in the healing process. Alternative medicine practitioners know that for centuries, different therapies have been created in different countries to work on and relieve the spinal situation of affected individuals. Herbal Medicine, Reiki, Yoga, Kinesiology, Ayurveda, Alexander Technique, Nutritional Therapy, Chelation, Feldenkrais, Reflexology, and Qigong are just some of the many alternative therapies that could be integrated to whatever conventional care you receive.

Again, the key is not to use just one of those therapies but to try to use them all, to integrate them. Repair is a complex process and requires complex management.

The success of those therapies varies from person to person according to their needs and conditions.

Again, not every treatment is for everybody.

For neck or back pain, with radiating pain down the arms or with sciatica, Martin will need a chiropractor and an acupuncturist, but Bob will not, and will do well with just traction and physical therapy. Susan will do better with physical therapy and massage, but Martha will do better with Gyrotonics and acupressure. For all of them, a metabolic evaluation, including all the key factors I mentioned above under "metabolic puzzle," might be needed before, during, or after the 3rd or 4th therapy session.

I once combined chiropractic treatment and Tai chi and it was effective. See? We are all different. In other people, just rest, anti-inflammatories, my omega diet, and a neck and back brace might be all that's needed.

Moreover, you have to be careful where you go. If you go to a bad chiropractor (many of them are) and also to a bad physical therapist (as I have met a few) and you get non-Chinese acupuncture by someone who just took four weekends training, you may not get better and claim that those therapies are bad and useless. Therefore, you need to select, ask around, meet people, research the market, make phone calls, and find out who is good and who is not.

Understanding and Managing Common Disorders

The process of injury and its consequent inflammation is complex. After a significant lesion caused by sports or from a motor vehicle accident, the human body sometimes responds with a series of musculoskeletal events causing a sudden and rapidly advancing inflammatory and degenerative process. Once the chain reaction starts, it is difficult to stop the process using conventional medical therapies based on pharmaceutical drugs. Use your imagination: it is like someone took a step on a floor full of eggs. Some of them are broken, some are badly cracked, some are just slightly cracked. Their content, full of enzymes, is oozing to the outside hurting other eggs. This is what happens when you get whiplash in the neck or a torn muscle or ligament, where some cells are broken, others cracked, and oozing material is all around. This material expands damaging more cells (the "broken-eggs" effect), creating an epicenter of inflammation, that brings on pain. Pain brings on muscle spasms, that causes decreased blood flow, which then causes some of the cells to suffer even more and die. This ends up causing more oozing material, more damage, and more spasm, so the process continues, slowly expanding.

You don't fix this with pharmaceuticals or anti-inflammatories (NSAIDs). You need to learn what to do for each one of the different lesions.

This chapter focuses on the various acute lesions including rotator cuff injuries, sprained joints and ligaments, torn and pulled muscles, tendinitis, and bursitis. These conditions have in common a similar inflammation and tissue disruption process, including "the broken-eggs" effect, (broken cells), inflammation, a biochemical mess, and pain. Each of them requires prompt evaluation by a doctor – an orthopedist, an internist, a general practitioner, or a chiropractor. All require some form of treatment, such as physical therapy, rest, massage, medications, manipulation, or a combination. Also, all these injuries require an anti-inflammatory program. Each one of these lesions (injuries) is not just an area of broken tissues but rather a small center where an inflammatory storm has begun. Although inflammation can be decreased and controlled with anti-inflammatory medications, such as Naproxen, Motrin, Aleve, Ibuprofen, Celebrex, etc., these medications will not promote the beneficial effect of the eicosanoids in the healing process.

Our purpose here is to show how a person can influence the eicosanoid system so it will assist in the healing of the injury. Once the process of inflammation is understood, people in any of these injury groups can positively influence the healing process: they can reduce inflammation thereby promoting a faster recovery. Yes, a person has control over the repair of their injuries.

The message continues to be the same: help your eicosanoids and decrease the inflammation with alternative medicine.

Rotator Cuff Injury

The shoulder is one of the largest joints of the body and is formed where the humerus (upper arm bone) fits into the scapula (shoulder blade), like a ball and socket. The whole shoulder includes the clavicle (collarbone), as well as cartilage, numerous ligaments, tendons, and many muscles that cross it like bridges and hold it together. Some of those muscles are particularly important in keeping the joint in place and are grouped with the name "rotator cuff."

Any weakness in the rotator cuff muscles makes it easy for the joint to lose alignment and hurt the inner structures of the joint. Injuries to the rotator cuff muscles are usually secondary to sports activities, work, falls, or gardening. A rotator cuff injury can also occur when falling on the arm, lifting heavy objects, and abusing the shoulder through improper or excessive weightlifting, sports activities, and repetitive manual work. When this occurs, the rotator cuff muscles become stretched, and the joint loses its alignment and squeezes the tendons, causing pain and inflammation. Typical symptoms include pain, stiffness, shoulder-arm weakness, and loss of motion. A rotator cuff tear is a more advanced injury, more painful, and more disabling. It requires extra intense and prolonged therapy, and, on occasion, even surgery. When the rotator cuff is injured as in any injury to muscles, an inflammation process starts in the area of the lesion. Hence, management should include visiting a doctor, getting an X-ray to rule out a fracture, and getting physical therapy, but also paying particular attention to the inflammatory process. Severe cases of rotator cuff injury require appointments with a doctor, and an orthopedic surgeon as well as getting an MRI. Some severe cases require surgery, no joke. Don't postpone or try to diagnose yourself: go to a doctor soon.

The proper treatment of rotator cuff injuries that don't require surgery is a good example of integrative medicine.

If the X-rays are negative, and the MRI does not look that bad, the first step is to stop all aggravating activities to that shoulder and rest the joint. Then continue with:

- Physical therapy treatment
- Exercise instructions given by the therapist
- Prescription of anti-inflammatories
- Anti-inflammatory diet (i.e. our Jupiter Institute Omega Diet)
- Chiropractic evaluation for possible manipulation to decrease muscular tension in the neck and back
- Supplements like omega-3 gel caps and antioxidants (natural healers)
- Consider acupuncture
- Myofascial release and Tai chi may help a lot
- You may also try the many therapies I mention in the next chapters.

Strongly consider acupuncture, with or without electrical stimulation, since it can expedite the healing as well.

Practicing yoga could make it worse, but Tai chi, Qigong, and craniosacral therapy will help.

People who follow this integrative approach stand a much better chance of faster and better healing.

I had a painful frozen left shoulder with a rotator cuff tear, a product of basketball injuries. Regular physical therapy did not help. I was told by four orthopedic doctors and a rheumatologist that surgery was my only option. Sure. Well, I fixed it with a special kind of physical therapy, acupuncture, a product called "Joint Aid," another product called "Collagen-Plus," chiropractor's treatment, and special exercises. I regained full function, full range of motion, and the pain went away. Let me ask you: next time I get shoulder pain, who do you think I should see? And, what do you think I recommend my patients with shoulder pain do?

One of the problems that often occurs is that people wait too long to seek help, and by the time they see a doctor the whole joint is messed up. Then, in addition to the tear, there are additional abnormalities like cartilage erosion and ulceration, joint effusion, cartilage and ligament degeneration, bursitis, spurs, local muscle inflammation, and degeneration (myositis), lots of swelling and even a frozen joint. The whole clinical picture looks bad and orthopedic procedures and surgery seem the only viable option. The combination of the management therapies I continue to emphasize may save the day: rest, physical therapy, chiropractor, acupuncture, and anti-inflammation integrated with other alternative modalities (massage, detox, etc.) can lead to recovery without pharma or surgical procedures. I had a frozen shoulder with surgical complications that I mentioned above and that is how I recovered.

Sprained Ligaments

A ligament is a bundle of fibers that acts as a bridge between the two bones of a joint, attaching and holding them together. A sprain is defined as the stretching or tearing of a ligament caused by a forced movement. When it is simple, there is a minimal disruption of the fibers of the ligament, causing swelling, pain, and joint stiffness. A severe sprain may cause total rupture of the ligament with marked swelling and joint instability. Although sprains are more commonly found on the ankle, they also occur in the knee, lower back, and neck.

To get the idea of a sprain, imagine a bundle of spaghetti suffering a sudden blow. Although the bundle itself may not break completely, much of the spaghetti will tear, breaking many fibers. Each one of these fibers is like a cell and the tearing will create a micro-spot of injury as I explained earlier, which will generate a micro-spot of inflammation, swelling, heat, and pain. This brings eicosanoids and white blood cells into the area. The white blood cells bring even more eicosanoids with them and the process of inflammation and repair continues.

Again, the first step is a diagnosis by a physician, chiropractor, or physical therapist. If it is not severe, you can use physical therapy and the alternative medicine therapies I mention here. Don't mask symptoms with medications.

Acupuncture with electrical stimulation is a big help. If no major medical treatment is needed, the combination of physical therapy and acupuncture can be very effective. No yoga.

AT ALL TIMES, give the part involved time to heal. Rest. Relax. Eat a proper diet.

Sprained Joints

A joint sprain is an injury to the ligaments of the joint. It happens most commonly after a sports injury or a fall. A mild or Grade 1 sprain simply stretches the ligament and causes pain and swelling. A moderate, or Grade 2 sprain, partially tears the ligaments and is much more painful and disabling. A severe, or Grade 3 sprain, is a complete rupture of the ligament and requires surgical repair. When a jogger steps off of a curb and twists the ankle, simply stretching the ligament without tearing it, that is a mild – Grade 1 – sprain. When a soccer player is hit by a blow to the outside of the knee pushing the knee inside, the blow causes severe stretching and even rupture of the medial ligament, which is a grade 2 or grade 3 sprain.

For grade 2 and 3 sprains, see a doctor, (rheumatologist or orthopedic) first. Don't waste time. X-rays, MRI, and orthopedic appointments may have priority.

After you are done with doctors, consider a combination of physical therapy and acupuncture, which can be very effective. Gentle massage and anti-inflammation will help as well. Chiropractor treatment to work relaxing the muscles can help in recovery. No yoga at this time. Supplements with glucosamine, bio-cell collagen, and turmeric may be of great help (I review them in their respective chapter).

Again, the longer people wait to seek help, the more the injury will expand to adjacent tissues, causing inflammation and degeneration. See a doctor early.

Torn and Pulled Muscles

Muscle pulls and tears commonly occur in the major muscles of the arms and legs, and they represent different degrees of the same type of lesion. The injury occurs from a sudden over-stretching of the muscle beyond its limit. The degree of over-stretching determines whether the muscle is just pulled or torn. In a pulled muscle, many areas suffer cell damage and cell rupture with small areas of inflammation in multiple sections of the muscle. In a torn muscle, some areas are separated. The degree of separation depends on the magnitude of the injury. Inflammation will be present in each one of these areas.

Severely torn muscles and ligaments might need surgical repair.

Don't accept injections.

If not so severe, then don't massage, don't pull the affected muscle. Rest, then see an acupuncturist or physiatrist. Very gentle physical therapy combined by acupuncture with electrical stimulation can work wonders. No sports for two-three weeks.

I learned a lesson when I got a horrible hamstring tear. The muscle tore and bled inside and the next day my whole thigh was all black and blue. I knew that my chances to ever run or walk without a limp where slim. I did not want to see an orthopedist or a rheumatologist but I knew what I had to do. I needed someone to perform a miracle, allowing the fibers of the muscle to reunite and stick together strongly. I made a lot of phone calls, asked many questions, and finally one of my patients gave me the name of the magician, a very humble but excellent Chinese acupuncturist. He gave three extended sessions of acupuncture augmented with electrical stimulation and some strange smelling Chinese herbs that I took without asking what they were. In two weeks, my thigh was like new and I was able to walk all over Lisbon without pain. Keep in mind my example.

Hurry up! Tears, sprains, and injuries need to be evaluated and treated while they are fresh. Don't wait. See a doctor, orthopedic, podiatrist, rheumatologist, etc., to have it diagnosed and possibly X-rayed. If it is not a major injury, you will have plenty of time to choose your favorite alternative therapy.

Bursitis

Bursae are sac-like cavities filled with oily fluid located near the joints at sites where friction occurs. They may lie between two tendons, between a tendon and a ligament, or between the tendon and the bone. Bursae facilitate normal movement and minimize friction between the moving parts. Inflammation of these bursae, called bursitis, may happen suddenly, or over some time. And it is very painful.

Bursitis happens frequently in the shoulder but may also occur in the elbow, knee, heel, and other joints. The cause of this type of bursitis is usually overuse, injury, exercise, gout, infection, or local inflammation. If there is arthritis in neighboring areas, inflammation from there can spread into the bursa and cause bursitis. Symptoms of bursitis are pain, localized tenderness, stiffness, and limitation of movement. Swelling and increased local temperature also occur. On occasion, bursitis may spread to tendons, and cause tendinitis. Excessive friction plays a major role in the development and progression of bursitis, which is why it typically presents in joints and areas such as the shoulder, elbow, hip, knee, and heel, which experience more force from daily activities. Because bursitis is an inflammatory process, treatment must focus on mitigating and eliminating this inflammation. Excessive usage of the affected joints will increase friction and worsen the inflammation. Therefore, in addition to anti-inflammatory treatment, rest is essential.

Physical therapy, acupuncture, acupressure, chiropractor's treatment, and cold packs are a good therapeutic combination. Tai chi and Qigong may be helpful and so is craniosacral therapy.

Tendinitis

When a tendon is inflamed the condition is called tendinitis. When this inflammation involves the tendon sheath (synovia) it is called tenosynovitis. If this occurs at the level where the tendon is passing near or over a joint, the pain and swelling may give an erroneous impression of an arthritic condition. Indeed, this disorder is called para-arthritis (para = next to) and requires a different kind of treatment. The typical causes of tendinitis and tenosynovitis are overuse, daily wear and tear, exercise, injuries and repetitive microtraumas related to work or sports activities. Some general diseases may also cause these conditions, and require further investigation. Rest and cold packs might be all you need. If no success, physical therapy, acupuncture, and chiropractor's treatment are good therapeutic combinations. Tai chi and Qigong may be helpful and so is craniosacral therapy.

Elbow Pain

Unless a trauma was involved, usually an X-ray is not necessary. If you just wait and don't take care of it, with time it will get worse. Therefore, start with identifying the cause of your elbow pain.

Overuse of the forearm and wrist muscles, or repetitive or prolonged lifting, gripping, or even the way you hold the steering wheel can be the cause. Or the cause can be overusing the muscles at the gym, carrying heavy boxes, lifting too much weight, playing golf or tennis, and even gardening. Fishing and racquetball could be the cause, or perhaps the way you work with the computer or laptop. Think about all these, since you need to prevent it from happening again.

The problem occurs when there is a strain or partial tear in the muscle and tendon tissues that are attached to the elbow joint, causing intense pain in the outer elbow area.

A good doctor, chiropractor, or physical therapist can help you diagnose what the cause of your elbow pain may be. Lateral epicondylitis and medial epicondylitis are the most common sources of elbow pain, and very frequently a cortisone shot in the hands of an efficient specialist can be very effective and terminate the problem.

However, on occasion, additional testing is needed.

The problem could be an arthritic elbow caused by gout, or it could be pseudogout, in which the cartilage of the elbow suffers a breakdown, which appears similar to other forms of arthritis, with joint inflammation and pain. The crystal deposits and characteristics of arthritis in pseudogout are very similar to those in gout. Hence a proper diagnosis is important to begin appropriate therapy. In case of significant inflammation, a rheumatologist or orthopedist might need to do some needle aspiration.

You may need to see a doctor and have blood work done to rule out gout or a swollen bursa, which is like a big cyst at the tip of the elbow. If you have a large elbow bursa, a special treatment by an orthopedist or rheumatologist is the only way to take care of it.

Once metabolic problems are ruled out, if a cortisone shot does not help, the next phase is to see a physical therapist. Don't waste your time with braces and pills. The longer you wait the worse the problem will become.

Myofascial release combined with physical therapy works best. Acupuncture and acupressure may help but not always. Yoga and massage won't help. Chiropractor treatment, Qigong, and supplements will not help.

Hip Pain

Hip pain is a different situation. People tend to simplify the problem by saying "oh, I have arthritis in my hip."

Well, pain in the hip may not be arthritis at all. It could be tendinitis, myositis, bursitis, neuropathy, or another cause.

The nerves that go to the muscles surrounding the hip come from the lower back. Therefore, pain in the hip can be secondary to pinched nerves in the spine, a radiated pain. This could be caused by disc disease, scoliosis, severe osteoporosis with a vertebral fracture, or even a spinal tumor.

Go and read again what I wrote in the Injuries Chapter "The plan for neck and back pain, sciatica, and arm pain." The same plan is effective for shoulder and hip pain, it will help you understand that the problem might be in your spine.

Perhaps the pinched nerves are tensing and irritating the muscles of the hip, and the hip pain may not be arthritis but muscle pain. Perhaps it is a torn muscle around the hip caused by the overstressed muscles.

Perhaps it is none of those, but some tensed muscles around the hip are causing bursitis and tendinitis because there is too much friction. Bursitis is the painful swelling of bursae, which are like sacs attached to the joint, like fluid-filled little bags that cushion your tendons, ligaments, and muscles. When they work normally, bursae help the tendons, ligaments, and muscles glide smoothly over the bone. But when the bursae are swollen, the area around them becomes very tender and painful. Trochanteric bursitis is swelling affecting the bursae of the hip.

Perhaps the cartilage of the joint is all eroded and ulcerated. Perhaps it is not. How can you tell? You need to consider all those possible diagnoses, and the first step is to find a professional that will help you get a good diagnosis.

Start by seeing your doctor and getting X-rays of your hip and spine. You may need an MRI and perhaps some blood work to rule out metabolic disorders.

Don't waste your time doing exercises that may end up doing more harm than good. Anti-inflammatory medications will give you relief of course but will cure nothing.

Get a good evaluation by a physician, orthopedist, or rheumatologist. Again, keep in mind that it may not be the joint but rather muscle pain, bursitis, tendinitis, etc. Sometimes a physical therapist or a chiropractor will give a better diagnosis.

Depending on where the pain is located, we can get an indication as to what may be causing it. If your pain is on the inside or the front of your hip or groin, then the cause may be in the muscles, the nerves, or even in the hip itself. As I remarked above, remember that the hip, like any other joint, represents two bones meeting together and a lot of muscles, tendons, ligaments, fascia, bursae, and connective tissue surrounding the joint. "Pain in the hip" can be caused by any of those structures that are outside the joint and could be due to bursitis, tendinitis, ligament tear, muscle sprain, nerve irritation, fasciitis, or any combination of those disorders, BUT NOT REAL JOINT DISEASE. Therefore, be selective in who you see and who is diagnosing and treating you. I have seen a lot of misdiagnosis and mismanagement regarding hip pains. Pain on the buttocks and upper thigh may be due to the muscles, and other soft tissues that surround your hip joint. Again, I repeat, your pain may be coming from the hip itself or it may be coming from your lower back and pelvis.

Spine and hip X-rays may shine a lot of light into the root of the problem.

Once you are done with doctors, consider the same approach I wrote about earlier under "The battle plan for neck and back pain, sciatica, and arm pain." Combining chiropractic treatment to relieve nerve and muscle tension with acupuncture to improve nerve, muscle, and tissues might be all you need. Using a back brace for 1-2 hours once or twice a day may be a good idea if the problem comes from the spine. Taking a very mild anti-inflammatory for a short time and supplements with glucosamine, collagen, turmeric, and fish oil help a lot.

Consider adding Tai chi, and also getting a memory foam mattress. Targeted massage and myofascial release may be of benefit as a combination of the therapies mentioned in this book. Qigong and reflexology could help. In addition to Tai chi, there are other alternative therapies out there and I describe them in a separate chapter.

A good physical therapist could show you all the things you are doing wrong and teach you some very important exercises. Consult one, or tell your doctor to refer you to one.

No yoga, no biking, no running, and no long walks.

Don't be seduced by an orthopedist if you have not tried these therapies first.

What all of these conditions – bursitis, tendinitis, tenosynovitis, and sprains – have in common is the inflammatory process. In each of them, there is an injury, swelling, white blood cell activity, increased temperature, cellular disruptions, pain, and a repair process that has been activated. Furthermore, there is an activated eicosanoid system in all of them. Inflammation does not occur to cause pain. Inflammation is triggered by the disruption of local tissue and is the body's attempt to heal the injury.

As you are probably thinking, very frequently the spine is involved one way or another, sometimes directly, sometimes indirectly, sometimes as a causative agent, sometimes as a consequence. This should clue you into realizing that with many injuries as well as joint, muscular, and tendinous problems, treating the spine would help in the healing process. Alternative medicine practitioners know that for centuries, different modalities of therapies have been created in different countries to work on and relieve the spinal situation of affected individuals. Yoga, Kinesiology, Reiki, Ayurveda, Reflexology, and Qigong are just some of the many alternative therapies that could help you in your search for relief and better quality of life.

I explain many of these therapies in another chapter.

Indirect Causes

Now read this slowly and twice, since it describes how a disc problem in the back can give you arthritis in your shoulder, hip or knee even if you don't know that you have a spinal disc problem.

As I wrote previously, arthritis, tendinitis, and bursitis may also have their origin in a different area of the body. Now that you have a better understanding of anatomy and you read some of the general concepts about a pinched nerve, you can better visualize that if a disc disease (inflammation, bulging, etc.) squeezes (pinches) a nerve coming from the spine, the nerve will be irritated. This irritates the area of the body that is served by that nerve. If the irritated nerve is connected to a muscle, the irritation is transmitted directly to that muscle, causing it to become tense. This can create problems in neighboring joints. Moreover, nerves not only stimulate the muscles inducing contraction, but they also nourish them, maintaining their health. This is important because all muscles have a nerve that stimulates their contraction but also keeps them metabolically well. Hence, if a nerve is pinched at the level of the spine, the irritated nerve will not only affect the contraction of that particular muscle, but it will also make that muscle metabolically ill, causing some of the fibers to degenerate and be substituted by scar-type fibers that don't contract. When this happens, five bad things can occur:

1) As I wrote previously on the "indirect effect" (see page 15), the muscle can become too tense or too relaxed. If the nerve tenses the muscle, the muscle will pull the joint together approximating the bones too much, which will cause excess rubbing and friction. Friction will induce heat and inflammation and degeneration of the joint and later on pain and swelling. If the muscle ends up too relaxed, it will cause joint instability, hurting the joint. As you can see, neither too tense nor too relaxed are good, and both can give you joint problems.

2) When a muscle or its tendon crosses over a joint – like a bridge - to connect to another bone, there is usually a little bursa to facilitate sliding and avoid friction. When a muscle is tense, it is partially contracted. This contraction causes stress pressure on the bursa, squeezing it, irritating it and causing it to inflame, triggering bursitis, which can be very painful.

3) The irritated nerve may alter the metabolism of the muscle it goes to, creating inflammation, degeneration, and pain in the muscle. This is called myalgia.

So now you have arthritis, bursitis, and muscular pain, all because of a pinched nerve that you don't know about. This can occur even if you have NO neck or low back symptoms.

4) The hurting, inflamed and metabolically altered muscle may be tense and with loss of elasticity, becoming more susceptible to tear in case of any abrupt demand. In these cases, any unusual effort may cause the muscle to rupture. This muscle tear can be partial or total.

5) The process of nerve-muscle irritation may occur slowly, causing some of the muscle fibers to degenerate and become fibrous, carrying much less elasticity. The muscle then becomes much less flexible, tense, and unable to distend, which tends to hold the joint in one place. This causes a decrease in the range of motion or even a frozen joint.

These five events are very important to understand and explain how spinal nerve irritation can end up causing arthritis, muscular pain, bursitis, loss of flexibility, tendinitis, muscular tear, frozen joint or any combination of the above five disorders, or even cause all of the above problems at the same time. We see this rather frequently in people with chronic shoulder problems. We also see this with hip and knee problems.

Understand this well, because unless you relieve the nerve irritation, you will not get better. Understanding all of this is essential to comprehend why conventional medicine alone will fail in the short or long run and why alternative or integrative medicine will help you.

This sequence of events may occur in other joints as well.

I have been addressing this and I will continue to explain it from different angles, so allow me to repeat it in another way just to make sure. Even though you may not know that you have disc problems in your spine, those bulging, inflamed and degenerated discs might be irritating the local nerves, and then those irritated nerves may cause excessive tension in the corresponding muscles, creating tension around a joint, indirectly triggering bursitis, tendinitis, inflammation, a frozen joint, or even arthritis.

This is how a disc disease in the spine that you may not even be aware of, may give you bursitis, tendinitis, or arthritis in your shoulder or hip.

Again, this is an extremely important concept, and I have to insist: please read it again.

This is how a neck problem can result in a hurting shoulder, hands, or even in pain down the arms. This is why some people wake up at night with numbness or pain in the arms or stiff achy fingers.

A low back spinal problem may end up hurting the hip or the knee or cause tense or torn hamstrings, bursitis, stiffness, pain, and heat in the hip causing gait disorders. Ignoring this will impair recovery. And again, this is why conventional medicine alone, with painkillers, muscle relaxers, prednisone, injections, opioids, and anti-inflammatories will fail, and why you need to use the integrated modalities of therapy I review in this book.

The spinal process at the root of all of the above is usually very slow. Many years of neck trouble may result in shoulder pain, and the neck may be symptomatic (with pain and stiffness), or relatively symptom-free – perhaps exhibiting only a slight decrease in the range of motion. Other times, a person is asymptomatic (without symptoms). Then one day they develop bursitis, tendinitis, or arthritis in the shoulder, which may or may not be related to a neck problem. (For example, the problem may be related to a partial tear in the rotator-cuff that, after years of suffering, finally gave way and tore.) In any case, my point is this: the symptoms may present themselves as bursitis or arthritis of the hip or shoulder, or as tendinitis in the knee, but the root of the problem may be in the spine – at the origin of the nerves that extend to the hip, shoulder or knee. An abnormality in the spine and vertebrae is then the indirect cause of the problem.

That's why anyone who has pain in the shoulder or arm, or the buttocks, hips, or thighs, must have a spinal evaluation, which will require X-rays. If the spine is affected, a correlation can easily be made by tracking nerves to their corresponding body areas using an anatomy book. This may help to quickly identify the real cause of the problem, and the treatment of this cause may accelerate and improve the cure. If an issue with the spine exists but is undiscovered, treatment is likely to proceed in the area displaying symptoms without addressing the root cause of the problem. This is likely to prolong and complicate the inflammatory and degenerative process. Scar formation, calcification, stiffness, chronic pain, and disability may require excessive use of medications, physical therapy, injections, medical appointments, and – in some cases – result in surgery. The idea of an indirect cause may seem surprising at first. But in medicine, the cause of the pain is not always located where the pain is felt.

Here are some examples. Pain in the back can be caused by a gall-bladder stone (which is in the front). A kidney stone can be felt as pain in the groin. Heart trouble can be felt as a pain in the left arm. A tumor in the spine can be felt as a weakness in the leg. These symptoms are called "radiated symptoms." To emphasize that they may also be part of the cause of the inflammatory and injury processes, we call them the indirect cause of the problem.

For pain in the knee, hip, leg, thigh, arm, or shoulder, ask your doctor to also order X-rays of the corresponding spine.

Let's go back to shoulder pain.

At this time, after what you read in this chapter and the previous chapter, you should be ready to understand and manage this common problem.

Just like it happens with the hip, the pain in the shoulder can have many causes. Just saying "I have arthritis in my shoulder" does not illustrate the panorama.

The shoulder might just be achy, have a decreased range of motion, or be partially frozen. It might have an effusion, severe degeneration, and may be associated with ulceration of the cartilage, tendinitis, and even tenosynovitis, which by now you should be understanding how they occur.

A bit of a warning: Keep in mind that left shoulder pain can be caused by heart problems and even a heart attack.

There can be a muscle tear in the shoulder, total or partial, in one, two or three of the muscles passing by the joint or attached to it, there could be a partial separation or dislocation, myositis (degeneration of some of the muscles), bursitis or capsulitis (inflammation of the joint capsule). There can even be severe arthritis and bone spurs. We reviewed all these events previously.

Two, three, or more of these problems might be present at the same time, making shoulder pain a difficult disorder to treat. An X-ray might show part of the problem but certainly, an MRI will show it all.

Be careful now about your next move. Many patients and doctors I know decided on what I think was unnecessary surgery.

Cortisone shots will not help the problem. Pills will only mask it. Physical therapy will help very little. Orthopedic doctors for sure will want to operate.

What to do then?

It is OK to use a short course of anti-inflammatories while you decide what to do. Will they help? They may.

Get many opinions. Go and see your doctor, and then see a rheumatologist and at least two orthopedic doctors. Get the opinion of a physical therapist as well. Gather opinions and information.

KEEP IN MIND that what I wrote in the Injuries Chapter under "A Battle Plan for Neck and Back Pain," and for sciatica and arm pain, is also effective for shoulder and hip pain.

The Indirect Effect. The pain in the shoulder may be caused by bulging discs in the neck pinching the nerves that go to the shoulder and causing them to tense up. The extra tension causes friction, heat, and inflammation, which bring on effusion, tendon, and cartilage damage. The tension on the muscle causes myositis of the muscle (degeneration) and finally the debilitated muscle tears, as previously explained.

Therefore, your treatment should consist of good physical therapy, and special exercises taught to you by the physical therapist. Make sure you know about the physical therapy center you go to. Don't go to an unqualified one or you will regret it. I know from personal experience. Ask your doctor if they know these therapists? Have you or members of your family been treated there? Do you know that center? What do your patients say about that place? Find that out. If you see that your doctor gets upset because you ask those questions, well maybe you should see another doctor who won't get upset.

You want to go to a place where they take Physical Therapy very personally and do an excellent job. I send most of my patients to a local therapist who has treated me, my wife and my daughters and I tell my patients loud and clear "I am sending you to the therapist that has healed me." Think about it. Isn't that the right way of practicing medicine?

You should strongly consider chiropractic manipulation to improve the neck and shoulder dynamics, decrease nerve irritation, revive nerve conduction, and relax the muscles. Massage, of course, is helpful. Acupuncture can do a fantastic job, improving energy and blood flow to affected shoulder areas, reviving nerves and muscles, and stimulating local healing.

Again, the question: Will a short course of anti-inflammatories help? I am not sure about that. Certainly, they will help you feel more comfortable and relieved, but how will you know you are getting better if you are masking the symptoms? How will you know XYZ treatment is effective if you are suppressing the symptoms? See the point?

So then, here comes a big question: what would you think about the doctor you are seeing for the shoulder pain if he/she just gave you anti-inflammatories, painkillers, a pat on the back, and denies you alternative medicine? Or just muscle relaxants and prednisone? Think about it. Do you think this doctor will help you? What if this doctor just gives you a few pills and sends you to an orthopedist?

And what would you do if this doctor of yours gives you sixty Percocet or some other opioid painkiller in large quantities? Is he not only not helping you but also opening the door to addiction?

See how careful YOU have to be?

See how YOU have to be informed, aware, and alert about the next steps in your management?

Suppose you had a car accident, you are in pain, your shoulder hurts, your neck is stiff and tender, you can't sleep, you feel overwhelmed, and you need something done. Then the doctor gives you a Medrol pack and narcotics. Will you take them? Will you be alert enough to know that is not only not going to cure you but possibly push you into addiction?

Be very careful: many addictions started just that way.

Be careful: many unnecessary surgeries started that way as well.

And don't blame it all on the doctor: IT IS YOUR RESPONSIBILITY, TOO.

The core therapy is physical therapy, chiropractic treatment, acupuncture, and anti-inflammation.

Tai chi and Qigong will bring added benefits and assist in the healing, try them if they are available.

Yoga and gym are not recommended, they could aggravate the problem. Acupressure will not help, but gentle massage will.

Get a chiropractor's pillow.

Practicing a program combining a) detoxification, and b) supplements like the extra-refined concentrated fish-oil, organic turmeric, Boswellia-AKBA compound, and antioxidants, as we teach in our office. They provide significant relief and aid in repair. I describe those specific products in another chapter (see the chapter on Supplements).

If the MRI shows cartilage wasting or erosions, take supplements designed to rebuild the cartilage (which I describe in another chapter).

Certainly, adopting a diet like the alkalinized Mediterranean diet (the Jupiter Institute Omega diet) will help a great deal.

Going back to knee pain, this is a common problem not often diagnosed or treated properly. There are too many structures involved in this complex joint and each one can suffer damage.

Let's start with fractures. These are rather uncommon since this joint is designed to sustain all kinds of injuries without breaking.

Metabolic disorders can trigger a knee problem, like gout (crystals of uric acid in the joint), or osteomalacia (caused by softening of the bones occurring due to inadequate levels of phosphate, calcium, and vitamin D).

Chondrocalcinosis is another metabolic disorder that can affect the knees. It is caused by deposits of calcium pyrophosphate crystals, and is also known as CPPD (Calcium pyrophosphate deposition disease) – this disorder might be associated with Wilson's disease, hemochromatosis, hyperthyroidism, and hyperoxaluria, and can even result from arthritis. If it causes a sudden arthritis attack, it is then called pseudogout.

Rheumatoid arthritis, an autoimmune disorder, may affect the knee, debilitating and inflaming it.

Other metabolic knee disorders are Paget's disease (interferes with your body's process, where new bone tissue gradually replaces old bone tissue), severe osteoporosis (caused by advanced abnormalities in calcium, vitamin D and phosphorous which can lead to tiny fractures), and osteoarthritis (which occurs when the cartilage on the ends the bones wears off, ulcerates and tears away).

They all damage the knee and trigger pain, inflammation, increased local temperature, and stiffness.

As in other joints, tendinitis, bursitis, and muscle tears can affect the knee.

Lupus and Lyme disease can also hurt the knee. Certain bone tumors and even cancer can affect it as well.

Two special structures of the knee, the meniscus and cruciate ligaments, can cause severe problems. The meniscus is like cartilage wedges inside the joint and the cruciate ligaments are two very strong structures that hold the joint together. They both can suffer slow or sudden damage, and when these occur, the whole function of the knee is compromised, creating misalignment, malfunction, pain, swelling, stiffness, and increased local temperature. A torn meniscus can be severe, locking the knee. A tear on the anterior cruciate ligament (ACL) is what is called an ACL tear, and it is particularly common in people who play sports that require sudden changes in direction.

Side, back, and frontal ligaments can tear and that can cause pain, stiffness, and swelling as well.

A loose body may be present inside the joint, like a piece of bone or cartilage, causing pain and hurting the knee function.

Tendinitis of the patella, more frequent in those practicing sports, is another problem causing similar symptoms of pain and stiffness.

Like I described before, the knee problem can be caused by a distant factor as well, like:

a) Hip misalignment
b) Scoliosis of the spine
c) Spinal disc disease irritating the nerves that go to the thigh, agitating them, increasing friction, causing heat and subsequent inflammation, bursitis, tenosynovitis, cartilage degeneration, and a world of complications.

Yes, it is a complicated picture with a variety of possible diagnosis, and none seem to be good. Moreover, any given person can have two, three, or more of these disorders at the same time, and the fact that one of these problems is found does not even rule out the others. That is, Martin comes in and complains of "knee pain" and he is found to have some mild meniscal problem, but at the same time he has bursitis, chondrocalcinosis, tendinitis, and an imbalanced knee secondary to a bad spine. While Bob has the same complaint of "knee pain" and he has cartilage joint degeneration, mild knee effusion, partial cruciate ligament tear, meniscal wasting, partial tear in the lateral ligament and he does not tell you that he did something that he shouldn't. See? By just saying "knee pain" we are not pointing at any diagnosis. A workup by a physician is needed, which includes lab work and X-rays.

Nevertheless, with knee problems, something in particular happens: people want a quick solution.

I see this over and over. Every time they take a step, it hurts. They want the pill, the X-ray, and to get better in five minutes or see the orthopedic doctor soon and perhaps get an injection. They want instant relief, and I understand that.

However, what needs to be done next is a proper evaluation by a professional. However, running to an orthopedic doctor may not solve the problem and may add procedures that could have been avoided. Also, most general doctors, have neither the proper training nor the time and patience to deal with knee problems, especially if the patient is demanding a quick solution and relief. So my advice is "Everybody stay calm and no one will get hurt."

Get lab work to rule out metabolic disease, and get an X-ray of the knee. If it's suspected, also get an X-ray of the pelvis and lower spine. A short course of anti-inflammatories can be given in the meantime. A few days of prednisone or Medrol can be given to buy time and because when someone is in pain she or he can't think.

Once X-rays are reviewed, if they look bad, get an MRI of the knee.

According to the MRI decide the following: a) just rest, take cartilage building supplements, avoid exercise or straining the knee; or b) see a physical therapist to have a proper evaluation and therapy, while you continue with rest and supplements; or c) if there is effusion, see a rheumatologist to have some of the joint fluid drained and analyzed, to help in diagnosis. If a rheumatologist is not available, an orthopedist can do the procedure; or d) see an orthopedist (if you need one, you need one).

Seeing a rheumatologist early in the process is a great idea. Try to do it sooner rather than later.

As part of the workup by physicians, some abnormalities may be found and might need to be taken care of. For example, it may be gout. Or if rheumatoid arthritis was found, that needs to be taken care of with special medications.

Perhaps the knee joint is so bad that an arthrocentesis needs to be done by the orthopedist, for diagnosis and management. There is no way to predict who is going to have a good or bad knee.

Once you are done with doctors: a primary doctor, an internist like me, a rheumatologist and/or orthopedic doctor, and nothing major was found, you can get started with management, it is best to combine:

1) Cartilage building supplements and natural (non-pharma) anti-inflammatories, and special glucosamine-collagen combinations, which I describe in another chapter

2) Physical therapy

3) Acupuncture

4) An anti-inflammatory program (diet and supplements).

Rest the joint and your body as much as you can. Give yourself time to heal.

To this, you can add reflexology, Tai chi, or Qigong. I explain a lot about various alternative medical therapies in the chapter on Therapies.

Acupressure and myofascial therapy will not help. Yoga: abstain. Don't go to the gym, and don't go running or playing sports. You are going to need that knee for the rest of your days. Don't get cortisone injections, they don't heal anything and they just mask the problem.

Do the exercises the physical therapist tells you to do, and no others.

Jupiter Institute Omega Diet: very important, start now, as soon as you finish reading this sentence.

If the spine or pelvis are tilted, you may need to see a chiropractor. In some offices, you can get chiropractic treatment, physical therapy, and acupuncture at the same time.

Chinese herbs could be an excellent choice, so if you have a chance to get them from a Chinese acupuncturist (from no one else!), get them, I did that a few times and they helped me.

Stem cells and special compound injections can be very effective if done by proficient professionals. Ask around in your area before you commit to those treatments.

Do things right and take the time to do them. Knee replacement is just around the corner.

After Surgery

There are all kinds of surgeries and all kinds of instructions and restrictions to be followed according to the surgical procedure the patient received.

The number one priority is to follow the instructions given by the surgeon. Some surgeries, like digestive system surgery, require strict dietary control. Follow them (if the doctor was kind enough to give them to you).

Non-digestive system surgeries may still require dietary control according to the medical condition of the patient and the additional medical problems present. Low salt diet, protein restriction diet, and low potassium diet are some examples of restrictions when the cardiovascular system or the kidney function is compromised. A low carbohydrate diet for diabetics and a low-fat diet are more examples.

Again, dietary restrictions should be according to the instructions of the doctors involved in the management of the patient.

ONLY when the patient is told he/she can have a normal diet, then our concept of healing should be applied. Then, it is time to remember that any surgery, orthopedic or not, means that tissues were cut and cellular lesions have occurred. Hence, an inflammatory-repair process has initiated in the site of surgery, and the best outcome the patient can wish for is the successful healing of the affected tissues or organs. Even if this was an orthopedic surgery the tissues need to be healed promptly and successfully. Then, the best medicine you can take is the foods you eat, and the best healing dietary program you can follow is the alkalinized, Mediterraneanized, Jupiter Institute Omega Diet, described in another chapter.

Take into account that your tissues were cut and body fibers were separated and that the site of surgery needs to repair itself. The best you can do is to rest and eat foods that will encourage healing and allow the affected tissues to reunite and re-attach themselves. You don't want to eat an anti-nutrient diet but rather a healing diet and the best nutrition you can do is our omega diet; that and lots of rest. Give yourself time to heal and don't be stubborn.

Wrist pain and wrist stiffness

Unless you had a significant injury, X-rays are not needed. Some doctors like to divert attention using names like "carpal tunnel" or tendinitis. I have found that wrist pain is generally the result of a neck problem. When there are disc disorders in the cervical spine and the nerves are irritated, they may cause the muscles of the forearms to work under tension. This tenses the tendinous cords at the level of the wrist, creating friction, heat, and pain. If you want to find relief, start with an X-ray of the cervical spine, and then go see your chiropractor.

Physical therapy will not help. Injections will not help either. Acupuncture, if combined with chiropractic treatment, does help.

Finger pains and locking fingers

In general, unless you had a severe injury, fall or trauma, no X-rays are needed. Cortisone shots will hurt a lot and will not help.

The best success I found is with a professional hand therapist, not just a physical therapist but a HAND therapist.

Make sure the wrist, hand, and fingers are not hurting because of disc disease in the neck irritating the nerves that go all the way to the hand, causing stiff muscles and excess rubbing of the joint. This triggers inflammation, heat, cartilage degeneration, and subsequent arthritis. Consider getting a neck X-ray and visiting a chiropractor.

Take natural anti-inflammatories as well, for a short time. Glucosamine and bio-cell collagen might be of help, but, again, it is with hand therapy and a chiropractor where you will find relief.

You may need some blood work to rule out a metabolic disease like rheumatoid arthritis.

Ankle, foot, and toe pain

Go and see a podiatrist. They know best.

Avulsion fractures, ligament tears, fasciitis, and bursitis, are all very common and annoying and the sooner you can get healed the better. Podiatrists know their magic well and no one else will help you as they will.

INTERCHAPTER REMARK: Now you have your basic knowledge of joint and spine structures and a description of common lesions. Injuries will occur to us throughout our lifetime, unavoidably. Successful healing might depend more on our knowledge and action than on conventional medicine and pharmaceuticals.

Moreover, you can appreciate that things are a bit more complicated than expected. Confronted with a painful joint, neck pain, or injury, factors like the indirect effect, the broken egg effect, metabolic disorder, and even hormone imbalances HAVE to be taken into account as they can perpetuate the painful process and hinder any repair effort. You will not fix them with painkillers or with steroids.

Neck pain, back pain, direct and indirect effects, and inflammation, can improve and even reverse when people integrate alternative therapies. Depending on different situations, the adverse effect of toxins, hormonal decline, and spinal disorders need to be kept in mind.

People, in general, should resist the use of painkillers, narcotics, and be wary of their addictive effect. Only the informed mind will be able to make the right choices.

Conventional Treatments

Conventional Treatment and its Limitations

Millions of people suffer from pain, arthritis, bulging discs, or injuries, sometimes from all four. The standard medical treatment has simply been to prescribe medication to reduce the symptoms, such as anti-inflammatories (Advil, Aleve, Ibuprofen, Naproxen, Celebrex, Vioxx, Bextra, Indocin, etc.), muscle relaxants (Soma, Skelaxin, Parafon, Valium, etc.), and pain medications (Tylenol, Darvocet, Lorcet, Codeine, Vicodin, hydrocodone, Percocet, etc.). These pills just supply a "mask of relief," and they don't heal. Worse, as the sources of the problem – cell damage and tissue degeneration – are not being treated, the damage worsens.

See how tricky the situation gets? As medications give relief, the person gets the false feeling that the problem is healing and a wrong sensation of safety. However, since nothing will be done to provide real healing the person will continue to do adverse joint motions, and the result will be a worsening at the very roots of the problem. As the joint or part of the body deteriorates, more medications are needed and new prescriptions are given. People then increase the white pill from twice a day to four times a day, the red tablets from two to three times a day, and so on. Very often, the doctor dismisses the patient with a pat on the back and one or two prescriptions, saying "I'll see you in a month." Soon the patient is taking three or four different medications. As he or she continues to complain, more professionals become involved in his/her care, including perhaps a rheumatologist, an orthopedic surgeon, a neurologist, a pain clinic specialist, and sometimes even a psychiatrist. Injections and steroids will follow sooner or later. Sleep or the digestive system may be affected, so an appointment with a sleep clinic or gastroenterologist may be the next step. Lab tests and X-rays will be done as well. As the condition fails to improve and as pain persists, patients become overwhelmed with medical appointments and pills. They lose their independence, become slaves to their condition, and find themselves trapped in the maze of the medical system. Pain relief is important, of course, but some even become addicted to pain pills. Over time, the failure to treat the real roots of conditions will lead to further progression of pain and joint problems. In the end, surgery appears to be the only possible solution. I know that well since it happened to me.

Over twenty years ago a neurologist told me, "Daniel, your neck is getting worse, your arm is getting weak and you are not responding well to painkillers. You are going to need surgery...for your own good."

"Surgery? I'm afraid. Is there any other way?" – I asked.

"No, Daniel. I see no other way. It's going to be for your own good. I am sending you to the neurosurgeon."

Well, I never went to see that neurosurgeon.

For my own good.

I did what you are reading about. I got better. I still run and exercise. I never had the surgery. My neck and my arm improved, and I enjoy life.

But even if the patient gets surgery, and even if the surgery is successful, the deterioration of the tissues may have progressed so far that pain and disability persist and the freedom the patient seeks remains beyond reach. If you could look back and see the evolution of your suffering joint, or of the joint of your spouse, parents, or relatives, you would observe something like a slow-motion picture of progressive degeneration. This very slow deterioration will have been years in the making, with the joint tissues slowly but surely affected by the process I describe in this chapter. As you read this, ask yourself: "Why has the doctor just kept giving pills and painkillers and done so little to improve the joint all those years?" And, "Why was an orthopedic doctor consulted so many times while he just kept switching pills and giving those cortisone shots, to no avail?" Or, "Why have none of these highly trained specialists ever told me to try something unconventional or pursue an alternative course to prevent the joints from wasting away like this?"

Here are two even more interesting questions: "What could have been done three or four years ago to stop the degenerative wasting before that joint deteriorated so badly?" I want you to remember this question, and another: "What can be done today so that in one or two years the problem joint will cease being a problem?" I'll tell you what can be done: understand the process of arthritis, injury, and pain, look for the answer in this book, then accept that conventional medicine alone is not enough to take care of these problems. Be receptive to alternative medicine options. Then develop an active attitude and assume responsibility for being the caretaker of your joints. As a starting point, we are going to explain the process of arthritis.

Conventional Approaches to Pain Treatment

Conventional medical treatment is very effective and should not be put aside in our eagerness to adopt alternative therapies. The combination of physical therapy and medications that I explain in this chapter provides our patients with prompt relief. Moreover, many times this relief is long-lasting and improves the quality of life.

There is no single standard conventional medical treatment for arthritis, pain, and injuries. Instead, there are many treatment options and modalities depending on the person and the type of problem. Different conditions, both acute and chronic, may involve slight or severe inflammation, very mild or advanced osteoarthritis, a clear history of a recent injury or no injury at all. The pain felt by sufferers may be mild and in a small area, or intense and covering the whole arm or leg. This brings us to the following conclusions:

1) Treatment must be adapted to the patient and not the patient to the treatment. Rather than two or three structured treatment options for all cases, a wide variety of treatment options should be offered, coordinated, adapted, and tried in each case. Both doctors and patients must understand this and keep an open mind when facing these challenges.

2) Treatment should be provided not by one person but by a team. This team should include a primary care doctor (who could be an internist, family or general practitioner, or chiropractor), and a group of other professionals. These could include a physical therapist, nutritionist, orthopedic doctor, chiropractor, rheumatologist, neurologist, and massage therapist, who may or may not be consulted according to the patient's needs. Other possible members of the team, depending on the patient's condition, could be an acupuncturist, reflexologist, podiatrist, and the manager of the health food store. Both patients and physicians should have an open mind about calling on other professionals within both conventional and alternative medicine.

3) The primary care doctor should not be the sole provider of medical care to the patient. Rather, he or she serves as the team coordinator. He or she will evaluate the patient and decide which of the above-listed consultants will be called in. He or she will explain the diagnosis and provide counseling to the patient, choose medications, arrange

for appointments and follow-ups, and coordinate the care with the other professionals. He or she will be the captain of the ship, exercising command and control but understanding that treatment will not succeed without the efforts and goodwill of crew members.

4) The use of medications, vitamins, and supplements should never be liberal. Excessive use of anti-inflammatories should be avoided, and the use of painkillers, although sometimes needed, should be controlled strictly. Vitamins and supplements should be limited to certain reliable brands. Careless use may provide no improvement and might even be harmful due to adverse reactions.

5) Patients and doctors alike need to increase their awareness of the alternative medicine providers in their area. Integrative centers that combine conventional and alternative medicine already exist in many cities of the United States. If integrative centers are not available, it is necessary to become acquainted with alternative medicine practitioners in the area. These practitioners need to be acknowledged, recognized, met with (in person), and even invited to be a part of an extramural team so that better choices are offered to the suffering patients. These practitioners are not competitors to the doctors since they cannot treat the hundreds of conditions that only physicians can treat. They are, instead, doctors' helpers, assisting the physicians to achieve the main goal – to heal the patient.

The Arthritis and Pain Program of the Jupiter Institute of the Healing Arts (www.jupiterinstitute.com) was created with the idea of providing relief and healing to conditions like pain, arthritis, and injuries. It is an idea that works, although not every time. We invite physicians to follow our model, or the many other models like ours across the country, and to broaden the scope of their treatment options by counseling their patients about alternative medicine.

Patients need to read, learn, participate, and understand that healing and being pain-free requires personal effort and commitment. Healing will not come from a pill bottle or a surgeon's knife. Patients need to accept the fact that while pills provide relief, they are also hiding the problem. Although patients may feel better while taking the pills, their condition will be worsening if left untreated at its cause. Patients need to remember: Pain is a message you should not ignore!

Conventional Medical Treatment

Conventional medical treatment for arthritis, pain, and injury consists of a combination of the following:

- Cortisone shots
- Exercise
- Medications
- Physical therapy
- Surgery

1) **Physical Therapy** - also known as physical medicine and rehabilitation, is the most widely used treatment for arthritis, injuries, and certain pains. It focuses on the reduction of inflammation and the recovery of function and attempts to suppress symptoms though physiologic healing. This patient-oriented emphasis on function rather than symptom suppression makes physical therapy the best treatment for all kinds of neuromuscular and skeletal disorders. The role of physical therapy in treating pain, arthritis, and injures has expanded significantly over the last several years. Physical therapists work more closely with physicians and chiropractors, and improved communication has enhanced both treatment effectiveness and pain relief. Physical therapists have learned that early and effective application of pain-relieving modalities combined with patient education reduces many problems associated with pain, enabling individuals to resume their normal lifestyle much sooner. Physical therapists are a mandatory addition to any therapy team as their knowledge and effectiveness makes them a vital component in any treatment plan.

Some of the physical therapy modalities include:

- **Heat therapy** - This can be applied using moist heat packs, paraffin baths, hot packs, heat lamps, and hydrotherapy.
- **Ultrasound** - Ultrasound treatment can be given alone or using phonophoresis, which includes the addition of a steroid lotion that is forced into the tissues to increase treatment effectiveness. This technique uses an ultrasound device with a hand applicator.
- **Short wave and microwave diathermy** to provide deep heating of tissues.
- **Cold therapy (cryotherapy)** - In this technique, cold packs are applied superficially to reduce blood flow, lessen muscle tone, and decrease swelling. Treatment is rendered using ice, chemical packs, or refrigerated units.
- **Transcutaneous Electrical Nerve Stimulator (TENS)** - This is a small, cigarette-pack-sized device easily concealed in the pocket

or under the belt and connected with wires and patches to the problem area. It provides pain relief but does not cure or heal.

- **Iontophoresis** - This therapy introduces substances through the skin and into deeper tissues using electrical paths.
- **Vibration** - This therapy is used to relax muscles in painful disorders.
- **Traction** - Traction is indicated for injuries of the cervical and lumbar spine. It can be accomplished through manual traction, mechanical traction, or gravity traction. It is contraindicated in organic lesions of the spine: X-rays should be taken to eliminate these causes before starting treatment.
- **Compression** - The following are types of compression: ace wrapping, garments, and gradient pumps.
- **Massage** - Massage stimulates nerve receptors producing muscular relaxation; it also improves blood flow to the muscle and stretches adhesions. Massage relieves pain, decreases swelling, and reduces muscle spasms.
- **Electrical stimulation** - Electrical stimulation speeds recovery in injured muscles. It also decreases spasm and pain.
- **Education** - The encounter between patient and therapist is unique. The patient has the special opportunity of being counseled on numerous aspects related to healing including exercise, avoidance of improper sports and incorrect posture, prevention of injuries, medications, and possible needs for consultations. Each one of these brief therapy sessions is a golden opportunity for the patient to receive some of the vast knowledge and expertise of the therapist.
- **Therapeutic exercise** - These are exercises taught by the therapist that the patient must perform at the therapy center or at home. They correct impairment and improve musculoskeletal function.
- **Aquatic therapy** - Pool therapy can be extremely beneficial, allowing exercise and improved relaxation.

Physical therapy is perhaps the most important of all patient treatments for neck and back pain, arthritis, and injuries. By utilizing combinations of the above treatment modalities, therapists help to improve function, decrease stiffness, relieve pain, and facilitate healing in the problem area. A course of physical therapy typically lasts only a few weeks, although long-term therapy may sometimes be recommended. Some excellent books are listed on our website (www.jupiterinstitute. com) for those who want to learn more.

A WARNING: physical therapy can be great or it can be frustrating, depending on who does it.

I've had physical therapy many times and I can tell you that it can be excellent when done right by a well-trained professional. However, not all therapists are the same, and some of them might not have the skills to provide relief. In that case, patients treated may feel that "physical therapy does not work for me." Therefore, if your experience with this therapy is not providing results, ask your doctor to send you to another therapy center. Make some phone calls, ask your neighbors and friends, and find another therapy place. Or perhaps you need to combine it with some of the alternative therapies. The point is that well-done physical therapy is very helpful, and if you don't find it helpful, then perhaps that therapist is no good, or you might need a combination of treatment or perhaps you might need to go back to your doctor.

2) **Medications** – Suffice it to say that I am not against medications (which I frequently provide to my patients), but rather I affirm that they should never be the sole treatment and should only be used for a short time.

3) **Exercise** - helps keep the joints healthy while assisting in the healing process of joints, ligaments, and muscles. However, certain exercises may be harmful to a joint or part of the body affected by arthritis, inflammation, injury, or pain. Going for a five-mile walk with a sore knee or going to the gym to lift weights with an aching shoulder are common but unwise mistakes that need to be avoided. Improper exercise may amplify the damage and on occasion make it irreversible. Physical therapists and chiropractors are the ideal professionals to consult about exercise. They can help you learn the exercises that may help in the healing process and those that should be avoided. Note that physicians, like general practitioners, orthopedic doctors, internists, rheumatologists, etc., are generally too busy to teach exercise to their patients, and, in general, they don't know much about PROPER exercises. You can find additional information about exercise in numerous books at the library and bookstores.

BY EXPERIENCE I tell you here: follow the exercise guidelines given by physical therapists and chiropractors. They know best.

4) **Cortisone shots** - are injections of anti-inflammatory steroids that may help relieve pain and inflammation in a specific area of the body. They are most commonly injected into joints, such as your ankle, elbow, hip, knee, shoulder, spine, and wrist. On occasions, a small

amount of local anesthetic is injected at the same time to provide quick pain relief. They can produce miracles by providing sudden relief from agonizing pain. Cortisone's ability to almost fully alleviate extreme pain is extraordinary, but some critics state that there are some negative effects to consider. The side effects that a cortisone shot can trigger may counterbalance or outweigh its ability to reduce pain and inflammation, therefore, balance your decision well. As you think about it, consider how urgently you need the relief, can you wait a little longer? Or are you desperate because you just can't stand the pain anymore? Keep in mind that cortisone shots do not heal, most of the time they just temporarily take the pain away and decrease inflammation. In some cases, however, a well-done shot can disrupt the damage-inflammation-pain cycle spreading into the hurting tissues which can be a very blessed relief.

I had cortisone shots in the past, in my neck, in my elbow, etc., and they helped me a great deal.

If you need them, and you decide to get them, don't make them your sole therapy but rather combine them with other therapies.

5) **Surgery** - On occasion, if all treatments fail, surgery is the only choice. The treating physician will then be in charge of recommending an appointment with an orthopedic doctor. Surgical procedures have come a long way. The greatest surgical advances in the treatment of arthritis are joint replacement and arthroscopic surgery. Numerous joints can now be treated or replaced using new refined surgical procedures. Orthopedic surgery is an excellent profession that provides relief to an enormous number of patients. When appropriate, orthopedic surgery can be highly successful in providing relief.

Some Conventional Medicine Management Therapies

1) **Neural blockade** - This is a procedure in which the signals of a regional nerve are deliberately interrupted for pain relief and local anesthesia. The procedure uses equipment that includes a sterile field, needles, syringes, and sometimes catheters.

   1a. Central nerve block - involves spinal and epidural techniques to stop or reduce pain in the legs and abdomen. It is usually used for procedures or surgery. Pain is numbed when local anesthesia enters the vertebral canal, where the spinal cord and nerves are. It is generally used for abdominal surgery (bowel, liver and gallbladder), gynecological procedures, and in certain orthopedic and thoracic surgeries or procedures.

1b. Peripheral nerve block - is an already common anesthetic practice used in many surgical and dental procedures. It is accomplished by injecting a local anesthetic near the nerve controlling sensation or movement to the area of the body requiring surgery. Peripheral nerve blocks are generally done to control pain arising from a nerve, also known as neuralgia. Nerve injury can be caused by trauma, compression, ischemia, or toxic exposure to a nerve. The block involves the injection of a local anesthetic combined with a steroid in proximity to the injured nerve to decrease the conduction of pain signals along the nerve. This therapy can be a very successful way to abruptly control pain and on occasion, the benefits are dramatic, with an enormous relief of an intense painful disorder.

1c. Facet nerve block - involves injecting a small amount of local anesthetic combined with a steroid medication in the proximity of the facet area of the spine. This procedure can anesthetize the facet joints on the side of the spine and block the pain. In the hand of an expert, a facet joint injection is a relatively simple procedure and is usually performed in an office or outpatient clinic or ambulatory surgical center.

2) **Epidural steroids injection** - is a technique in which a combination of a local anesthetic mixed with corticosteroids is injected into the spine. The injection reaches the epidural space, between the spinal cord and the spinal canal and is done to relieve pain and occasional dysfunction. This is not a healing procedure but mainly done for pain relief. It is a minimally invasive procedure that can help relieve neck, arm, back, and leg pain caused by inflamed spinal nerves. Its effects are improved if combined with other forms of therapy.

Although much has been discussed and argued about this technique, when performed by proficient hands in a patient struggling with severe pain, the results can be wonderful and can even bring tears of joy.

Regarding the above injection therapies, yes, they are effective. They are not curative but they bring on relief. Only those patients who have been affected by intense pain, day and night, day after day, can understand the feeling when the intense fire of pain suddenly disappears.

3) **Physical Medicine and Rehabilitation** - also known as physiatry or rehabilitation medicine are a combination of different therapies designed to relieve pain and improve stiffness, injuries, spinal dysfunctions, neuropathies, and tendon and ligament disorders. It aims at enhancing and restoring functional ability and quality of life.

I already described this modality above, under "Physical Therapy."

Depending on the injury, pain, illness, or disabling condition, some therapists may treat their patients using the following procedures/ services: ultrasound, thermotherapy, massage, acupressure, stretching, joint manipulation, manual procedures, nerve stimulation, electrical stimulation, and target exercises.

4) **Occupational Therapy** - is a combination of techniques designed to assess and evaluate the impairments and physical needs of an affected individual, and accordingly target and manage interventions to develop, recover, and maintain meaningful activities, ambulation, and occupations of that individual. Patients might be suffering from painful disorders, congenital problems, stroke, traumas, fracture, surgery, developmental or emotional disorders. Occupational therapists work with those patients, providing specialized therapy and assistance to help them regain the ability to confront activities of daily living, improve mobility, and lead a productive and independent life.

5) **Trigger point injections** - is a local procedure of injecting a steroid and anesthetic combination in small areas where pain originates (trigger point). It is used to treat pain and spasms. It is an effective treatment modality for inactivating the root of the pain and providing prompt relief of symptoms like neuralgia, myofascial pain, and acute muscle spasms. It is not a healing technique but provides relief while other therapies focus on healing.

6) **Spinal Decompression** - is a type of traction therapy applied to the spine in an attempt to relieve the pressure of disc and vertebrae over a nerve root. The goal is to relieve pain and promote healing of the intervertebral disc. It attempts to create a negative intradiscal pressure to promote retraction or repositioning of the herniated or bulging disc material. Common indications include lower back pain, sciatica (leg pain), or neck pain caused by a herniated disc, bulging disc, or degenerated disc. There are several kinds of devices on the market but the best ones are the ones offered at a physical therapy center.

This technique should NOT be used in cases of pregnancy, broken vertebra, patients who had spinal fusion or disc implant, patients who had back surgery, osteoporosis, infection in the spine, spondylolisthesis, spinal stenosis, spinal tumors, or patients taking blood thinners.

Because of these contraindications, and many others, I recommend patients refrain from buying their own devices and use only the ones offered at physical therapy centers. You may find wonderful devices on TV, with unknown individuals making beautiful promises. Don't buy any of that stuff. Go and see a physical therapist.

This should be called "non-surgical spinal decompression," since there is also a surgical spinal decompression

7) **Surgical decompression (laminectomy)** - is a different thing. It is a surgical intervention in which the surgeon removes the bony roof covering the spinal cord nerves to create more space for them to move freely and therefore relieving the compression. It is used when the narrowing of the spinal canal and the hole through which the nerve passes are causing chronic pain, numbness, and muscle weakness unrelieved by other means. This narrowing (stenosis) is often caused by spinal arthritis, enlarged joints, bulging discs, and thickened ligaments. It is not an ideal solution, but sometimes there is no other choice.

8) **Orthopedic surgery** - includes all the surgical interventions you hear about, including shoulder, knee, hip, and hand surgeries. Comprehensive descriptions require a whole separate book.

9) **Medications** - as we address in the Medications chapter.

Our Institute's Approach

We use medications as part of our treatment program, combining acetaminophen, anti-inflammatories, and painkillers since they provide quick and effective relief. On occasion, we use corticosteroids as well (most of the time Prednisone). They are all part of our medical treatment, but we don't prescribe all or any of them to every person. We do not prescribe them every time, and we do not give them in large doses. We use these corticoids (aka corticosteroids) because they provide unique relief and immediate comfort to the suffering patient, giving us time to coordinate the plan of treatment.

Some patients need additional short-term use of stronger painkillers (like Ultram (Tramadol), Vicodin, or similar), which we prescribe and recommend as long as the patient understands that they are provided to buy time until we complete the workup and start the various forms of therapy.

On many occasions, I have given a combination of treatments to a patient when he/she walks into my office in severe distress because of bad neck pain, painful shoulder, sciatica, frozen hip, etc. Take a look at this combination:

- 15 mg of prednisone
- B-Complex (with methylated folate and methylated B-12)
- 1/2 Vicodin (of the 7.5/325 tablet)
- 500mg Tylenol
- ½ Adren-AM (an adaptogen to improve a struggling adrenal gland)
- 1 Max-Adren (an adrenal gland strengthener)
- 2 of our Detox-Vitamins
- 2 capsules of Joint-Aid (a multi-ingredient capsule that relieves joint pressure)

Then make the patient rest. Usually, in about 45 minutes, pain and distress are easing up, joints feel better, muscles are not tense and there is a significant amount of relief. We can then start making plans for X-rays, further evaluation, and management.

Using medication with physical therapy also provides a prompt reduction of pain, giving the patient more time to think and make plans (you cannot think well when you are in pain). We then proceed to discuss the treatment plan with the patient, which includes the integration of chiropractic care, acupuncture, exercise, physical therapy, nutritional treatments, supplements, and an emphasis on fighting inflammation by immediately adopting an omega-3 lifestyle and avoiding the adverse omega-6 anti-healing lifestyle.

Regarding the need for Rheumatologists, Neurologists, and Orthopedic Physicians. A WARNING

As much as I believe in and encourage alternative medicine, there is no substitution for the professional opinion, and possible therapy guidance or suggestions, from Rheumatologists, Neurologists and Orthopedic Doctors, in conditions like:

- advanced spondylosis
- ALS
- assessment of complex pain disorders
- autoimmune disease
- brain disorders
- cancer and metastasis
- cancer pain

- cluster headaches
- complex cases of chronic pain
- complex migraines
- differential diagnosis of complex neuropathies
- dysautonomia
- extrapyramidal disorders
- hereditary disorders
- hidden or avulsion fractures
- Lupus
- muscular or joint disease
- myelopathy
- myofascial pain syndromes
- myopathies and myositis
- neuropathies
- orofacial pain and temporomandibular disorders
- osteoporotic fracture
- psoriatic arthritis
- reflex sympathetic dystrophy
- rheumatoid arthritis
- rheumatoid spondylitis
- spinal cord compression
- stroke-related joint disease
- traumatic pain disorders
- tumors
- unusual causes of low back pain

All of these in addition to the variety of neuromuscular disorders, stroke and its complications, multiple types of joint and muscular disorders, and all those "conventional medicine problems" that fall under the management of conventional medicine physicians.

INTERCHAPTER REMARK: Conventional medicine provides different methods of therapy, which can be effective in providing relief. Their beneficial effect and their prompt efficacy in providing relief should not be negated. However, they have little effect on the real healing process.

Alternative Treatments

"Are you going to wait until those who don't know anything about alternative medicine give you the OK?"

That is an interesting question; can you answer it?

When you combine several repair approaches, the benefits of the different elements multiply. Hence, if you combine avoiding the omega-6 lifestyle, engaging in a healthy lifestyle, participation in appropriate exercise, and use of a positive combination of chiropractic care, acupuncture treatments, and physical therapy, arthritis will improve, joints will heal better, inflammation will decrease, injuries will heal, and pain will be much better controlled.

You need to understand the very root of the inflammation degeneration process so you can perceive why focusing on it may tilt the repair process in your favor. Your health may depend on how you use this information and the actions you take.

I understand that I am presenting strange concepts in this book: yin, yang, Qi, and body energy flowing in the body through meridians. Strange ideas indeed, difficult to understand and impossible to see. But what are all these energy things? Should you believe in them?

Well, you better start to understand this. Conventional medicine is just a few centuries old, while alternative therapies based on body energy manipulation are much older.

The more you open your mind to these concepts and explore them through the Internet, library, and bookstores, and then you try them, the more relief you will get and the better your quality of life.

Why Alternative Therapies are Effective

Have no doubt: alternative medicine therapies are very effective. We use them in our Jupiter Institute of the Healing Arts for one simple reason: they work. We explain to our patients and readers how integrating them with conventional medicine provides relief and enhances repair in individuals suffering from pain, arthritis, and injuries. Alternative medicine offers patients another avenue to gain control of their disease.

Alternative Therapies Help Arthritis and Other Painful Conditions

Alternative therapies are a group of different treatment modalities, developed in different countries, and supported by extensive experience. Not all alternative therapies are indicated for arthritis, pain, and injuries.

I did not write about all the different alternative medicine techniques, but rather the most common ones and those that I received opinions and background information about from my patients and friends. On the other hand, you should not drive yourself insane trying all kinds of therapies. Your goal is to take care of arthritis, injuries, and inflammation and with what I describe here I am sure you will have more than enough.

Here are some of the most highly recommended forms of alternative medicine that provide benefits in the treatment of arthritis, pain, injuries, neck and back pain, muscle and tendon pain, bursitis, and fatigue:

- Acupressure
- Acupuncture
- Chiropractic care
- Nutritional supplements
- Nutrition therapy
- Reflexology
- Tai chi
- Therapeutic massage

Some other forms of alternative medicine may provide additional benefits to individuals suffering from these conditions as well as other illnesses and may improve their general well-being. These therapies are:

- Ayurvedic medicine
- Craniosacral therapy
- Herbal medicine
- Homeopathy
- Meditation
- Qigong
- Reiki
- Yoga

We urge you to learn about these therapies as you may find significant relief, healing, and reduction of distress in one or more of them.

There are some other non-therapy regimens designed to improve the metabolism, providing a significant benefit in helping control arthritis, inflammation, injuries, and recovery from surgery or traumas:

- Adrenal management
- Detoxification
- Hormonal improvement

I will be addressing these three in the chapter on Hormones, Thyroid, and Adrenals, so don't miss that info since these three approaches are known to bring on unexpected benefits.

Keep all the above management options in mind.

At all times remember to be aware of all these options and be, yourself, the commander of YOUR treatment.

Check local practitioners, ask questions, exchange opinions, demand, request, research, and don't just passively accept what you are told by a practitioner with limited conventional knowledge who just spends sixty seconds with you.

Recommendations

Follow these steps when considering alternative medicine or integrative medicine: Make an informed decision. Get information from local bookstores, libraries, and the Internet. Again, ask around, research your environment, contact professional organizations, use common sense. Unconventional therapies are remedies that may or may not be successful; weigh the risks and benefits. Ask your doctor to assist you as you explore other alternatives to your treatment plan. Do not expect a miracle cure. Have realistic expectations and patience. Get an accurate diagnosis. Make sure you know from your physician what type of conditions you have, so you know what you are treating. Don't hesitate to ask questions. Ask questions like whether and how a particular therapy will help your condition. Check references. Talk to others who have similar conditions and have gone through the same treatment.

Be suspicious if the practitioner cannot show you a professional license, asks you to stop your medications, promises you a cure, or tells you not to tell your doctor. Even if you pursue alternative medicine for your conditions, do not neglect conventional medical therapies if you need them. You might have a condition that requires prompt medical care by a physician, and you must act on it.

Don't assume that because I recommend and emphasize alternative medicine, I neglect the importance of conventional medicine. I do not. I am an internal medicine practitioner after all.

INTERCHAPTER REMARK: Alternative therapies relieve pain, inflammation, and injuries at a slower pace, but their benefits in healing are far superior to conventional medical choices. These therapies focus on healing, rather than masking the problems with false relief. The best therapy is to combine a short course of conventional medicine with a long course of alternative therapies. Integration is the key.

Medications

Just as there are a variety of symptoms among people with arthritis, injury, and pain, there is a broad variety of medications to help control the symptoms. None of these medications heal; they merely decrease or eliminate the symptoms and provide temporary relief. However, anti-inflammatory medications, by slowing the process of inflammation, may occasionally prevent further damage caused by inflammation in the problem area.

In many circumstances, medications enhance the effect of physical therapy and increase the effectiveness of the treatment. The combination of Tylenol and an anti-inflammatory medication decreases the stiffness, swelling, and pain caused by osteoarthritis, allowing millions of individuals to be able to have days of normal activity. Without these medications, these people would be prisoners of their daily stiffness, pain, and disability. As much as these medications have been criticized, the benefits they provide are tremendous. Although there are numerous arthritis and pain medications with exotic-sounding names, those most commonly used fall into one of these categories:

- Acetaminophen
- Corticosteroids
- Muscle relaxants
- Narcotic painkillers
- Non-steroidal anti-inflammatory drugs (NSAIDs)
- Topical pain relievers

Acetaminophen

You are probably familiar with acetaminophen. It is sold over-the-counter with brand names such as Tylenol, Datril, Panadol, etc. Many pharmacies have their own brand of acetaminophen. Acetaminophen is a painkiller but is not anti-inflammatory, so it decreases pain but does not decrease inflammation. However, it is very effective for osteoarthritis pain, and among the safest drugs a patient with arthritis pain can take. Considering the millions of doses consumed every year, it causes remarkably few side effects. Acetaminophen does not act on the inflammation process of the joint and does not interact with the eicosanoids as the anti-inflammatory medications do. It works in the nervous system, decreasing the sensation of pain. Not messing with the eicosanoid system has both positives and negatives. The positives are that it does not interfere with the stomach eicosanoids, avoiding all the stomach problems that anti-inflammatories cause. The negatives are that it improves neither the eicosanoid imbalance nor the inflammation process at the problem areas. Although not always effective, acetaminophen offers certain advantages:

1) It is less expensive than prescription medication.

2) It is easily obtainable over-the-counter, found in grocery stores, and pharmacies around the world.

3) It is gentle on the gastrointestinal tract and much less likely to cause a stomach to bleed or ulcerate than some other medications.

4) It will not raise blood pressure even after years of use.

5) It is less likely to cause diseases of the liver or kidney after many years.

6) It is less likely to interact with other medications.

Despite its admirable safety record, acetaminophen can cause serious illness, liver damage, and even death in large doses. Regular users need to know that they face an increased risk of liver and kidney damage. The risk of organ damage increases if the person consumes alcohol. Problems with acetaminophen almost always result from doses higher than the recommended 4,000mg a day. It is critical to note that even moderate doses can be dangerous for older people and those with liver disease. Most importantly, this medication (or any of the others) should not be used as a long-term strategy for managing pain. A full treatment program like the one outlined in this book is essential for the eradication of both pain, arthritis, and injury.

Non-Steroidal Anti-Inflammatory Drugs (NSAIDs)

NSAIDs have become the most popular choice for physicians and patients when dealing with arthritis and pain. These first-line medications carry pain-killing properties, but they also slow down the production of the bad eicosanoids described earlier, which decreases the inflammation response. NSAIDs are effective for arthritic and injured patients and for all who suffer from pain. They come in over-the-counter products, prescription medications, and even in injectable form. Intravenous NSAIDs are frequently given in the emergency department for numerous painful conditions. NSAIDs have two names, one being the generic or pharmacological name and the other the brand name given by the pharmaceutical manufacturing company.

The following are the most common NSAIDs being used, which are divided into three groups.

1) Salicylates, Aspirin, Sodium Salicylates (Salsalate, Trilisate).

2) Non-selective COX inhibitors:

Acetic acid derivatives: Sulindac (Clinoril), Diclofenac Sodium (Voltaren), Diclofenac Potassium (Cataflam), Tolmetin (Tolectin), Indomethacin (Indocin), and Propionic acid.

Acid derivatives: Ibuprofen (Motrin, Advil), Ketoprofene (Orudis, Oruvail), Fenoprofen (Nalfon), Oxaprozin (Daypro), Naproxen (Naprosyn, Aleve, Anaprox), Flurbiprofen (Ansaid), Oxicam derivatives Piroxicam (Feldene), and Meloxicam (Mobic).

Others: Etodolac (Lodine), Ketorolac (Toradol,) Nabumetone (Relafen), Meclofenamate (Ponstel), and Diflunisal (Dolobid).

3) Selective COX Inhibitors:

Celecoxib (Celebrex), Rofecoxib (Vioxx), and Valdecoxib (Bextra).

The anti-inflammatory action of the NSAIDs occurs at the level of the eicosanoids, also known as prostaglandins. We describe the whole inflammatory process in the chapter on Inflammation. Inflammation, whether located in cartilage, ligament, tendon, or muscle is a complex process of cell injury. "Good eicosanoids" are trying to decrease inflammation in the joint and heal the tissue while "bad eicosanoids" push for more inflammation and further tissue damage. In this inflammatory process, arachidonic acid, which is a byproduct of omega fatty acids, interacts with the enzyme Cyclo-Oxygenase (COX) to produce eicosanoids.

There are two types of COX enzymes, COX-1 and COX-2. If the arachidonic acid interacts with COX-1, then good eicosanoids, which decrease inflammation and promote harmony in the local healing process, are produced. However, if the arachidonic acid reacts with COX-2, then bad pro-inflammatory eicosanoids are produced, intensifying, and prolonging the inflammatory process. Aspirin and all other NSAIDs non-selectively block both COX-1 and COX-2, reducing the total amount of all eicosanoids and blocking the inflammatory process. This decreases the swelling and pain, lowers the local temperature and lessens stiffness. It is important to note that NSAIDs decrease the entire inflammatory process, including the repair process. NSAIDs also decrease eicosanoid production in other areas. A lack of eicosanoids in the stomach, for example, causes a reduction in the secretions of the stomach's protective lining, making it susceptible to its own acidic juices. This is why NSAIDs can potentially cause stomach irritation, gastritis, ulcers, heartburn, and even stomach bleeding. The use of NSAIDs is also linked to kidney damage. The last group, selective COX inhibitors, work by selectively decreasing the action of the enzyme COX-2, therefore blocking the production of the bad pro-inflammatory eicosanoids and decreasing the swelling. This action results in the reduction of inflammation and pain. COX-1 enzymes produce the protective mucus that coats the stomach and intestines. Regular NSAIDs have an adverse effect on both COX-1 and COX-2 enzymes, thereby decreasing this mucus secretion and thus promoting gastrointestinal irritation. However, COX-2 inhibitors do not affect gastrointestinal COX-1 enzymes, so the protective mucus is not harmed. That is how Celebrex, Vioxx, and Bextra (the new COX-2 inhibitors) provide anti-inflammation without hurting the stomach. So, why was Vioxx removed from the market? Because it was hurting the COX enzymes that provide anti-inflammatory protection in the coronary arteries and the heart, thus breaking the balance between eicosanoids and promoting coronary artery and heart disease. Celebrex and Bextra can cause coronary disease and heart attacks in the same way.

Advantages of COX-2 inhibitors: COX-2 inhibitors are no more effective against pain and inflammation than standard NSAIDs. Their advantage lies in the lessening of gastrointestinal side effects, including irritation. They can also cause kidney damage like the other NSAIDs. However, COX-2 inhibitors are much more expensive than other NSAIDs. Mobic and Relafen offer the advantage of providing mild COX-2 suppression, thus causing less gastrointestinal irritation in those who use them.

Side effects: Most side effects of NSAIDs are due to their inhibition of the "good" eicosanoids throughout the body. (See the description of "good" and "bad" eicosanoids in the Injuries Chapter) NSAIDs may disrupt the eicosanoids of the immune system, causing a severe allergic reaction, in addition to high blood pressure, stomach irritation, and bleeding. They can even trigger nausea, cramps, diarrhea, constipation, drowsiness, nervousness, asthma, dizziness, heart disease, and kidney disorders. The possibility of side effects depends on how long the patient takes NSAIDs and how high the dosage. NSAIDs cause over 100,000 hospitalizations and lead to 16,000 deaths every year in America. If you want to learn more about the medications we recommend, we post the titles of several other books on our website (www.jupiterinstitute.com). Additional information about these medications may also be found in local libraries, bookstores, and the Internet.

Two more disadvantages: There is growing evidence that NSAIDs may inhibit the synthesis of cartilage proteins, a vital part of the joint structure. This means that the same pill a person takes to relieve the symptoms of arthritis may cause further damage to an already arthritic joint. The second disadvantage is the "wasting" effect. By decreasing and eliminating the symptoms of arthritis (pain, swelling, and stiffness), NSAIDs provide a false sense of improvement. Patients may then make two mistakes: they will not take care of a bad joint and will continue performing activities that damage it, aggravating the injury even more. Considering this, NSAID use may worsen osteoarthritis and injured areas in the long run. Advantages of NSAIDs: they provide fast relief of pain, stiffness, swelling, and disability. As a result, they are a good choice when treating numerous musculoskeletal disorders. Whether alone or combined with Tylenol, NSAIDs offer handy and practical relief to headaches, pain and inflammation, improving the quality of life.

There are ways to prevent or minimize the adverse reaction caused by NSAIDs:

- Take them with food.
- Take them with a full 6 oz. glass of water.
- Do not lie down for at least 30 minutes.
- Do not take an excessive dosc.
- At the first sign of stomach disturbance, take over-the-counter Pepcid or Maalox.
- Call your doctor as soon as possible if you feel any abnormal symptoms.
- Do not mix them with alcohol.
- Avoid taking them for a prolonged time.
- If you feel the need to take NSAIDs for longer periods, inform your doctor.

Using Aleve, Motrin IB, Advil or Ibuprofen is a very good idea on many occasions since it brings alleviation of symptoms without having to call a doctor or asking for assistance. But be extremely cautious with the amounts you take and the length of time you take them. Adverse reactions are like a tiger stalking you in the dark; any step can be a fatal one.

Corticosteroids

Corticosteroids, also known as steroids, include Prednisone, Medrol, and the Steroid-Packs. They also come in injectable form and may be injected locally ("cortisone shots") or given intravenously. Steroids have a strong anti-inflammatory effect, which is much needed for many injuries, intense inflammation, and pain conditions. They work very well. The main goal of using steroids is to stop the damaging effects of inflammation and the distress of severe pain. In these two areas, they do an excellent job. However, unless particular conditions require otherwise, steroids are short-course medications, used mainly to avoid an attack, crisis, or sudden injury. They should be administered only by a physician.

Narcotic painkillers

"Painkillers" are by definition all those medications that decrease pain. We have already described the minor painkillers such as acetaminophen, aspirin, steroids, and NSAIDs. We will now describe the major painkillers, also known as narcotics. Narcotics provide fast and effective pain relief, which is at times a very important issue when taking care of arthritis and injuries. They have an important role in the overall management of the suffering individual as they eliminate symptoms, allowing the person to resume a normal life and be able to sleep.

Some of the most common narcotics, alone or in combination are:

- Codeine (Tylenol #3 & #4)
- Fentanyl (Duragesic)
- Hydrocodone (Vicodin, Lorcet, Lortab, Vicoprofen, Annexa)
- Hydromorphone (Dilaudid)
- Levorphanol
- Meperidine (Demerol)
- Methadone (Dolophine)
- Morphine (MSI, MS Contin, Kadian)
- Oxycodone (Roxicodone, OxyContin OxyIR, Percocet, Roxicet, Tylox)
- Oxymorphone (Numorphan)
- Propoxyphene (Darvon, Darvocet)

The disadvantage of narcotic painkillers is that they mask symptoms, fooling a person into thinking that the problem is healing when it may be getting worse. Besides, they have an enormous number of side effects, including addiction, sedation, constipation, and respiratory depression. The list of the adverse reactions and drug interactions is very long and will not be presented here, but it is the responsibility of both the doctor and the patient to be aware of it. Doctors should instruct patients thoroughly about the side effects, but patients should not shield themselves behind the excuse of ignorance by saying "My doctor never told me." Books on the side effects of medications are found in most bookstores and libraries. The Internet has plenty of information, and it is the responsibility of the patient to consult these information sources.

However, as much as their use may be criticized, narcotics are often needed and recommended when treating severe pain. When used properly, they do provide relief and they do assist in the healing process. The type of narcotic, its dosage, and the length of treatment depend on the individual.

In cases like severe, painful, acute arthritis or cases of injuries, combining rest and immobilizing the problem area together with some NSAIDs and low dose painkillers and even some Tylenol, will decrease pain and suffering, lowering the distress and facilitating recovery. So again, a short course of proper painkillers, let's say codeine or hydrocodone, may be indicated and beneficial.

About painkillers: Beware! If a doctor offers you a large number of painkillers as the main option, be extremely careful. That prescription may give you comfort but will mask the real root of the problem while possibly leading you into addiction. The doctor doing that might be irresponsible but IT IS YOUR RESPONSIBILITY TO DECIDE WHETHER TO ACCEPT THAT PRESCRIPTION OR PROMPTLY LEAVE HIS OFFICE AND GO SOMEWHERE ELSE.

Topical pain relievers

These provide only local pain relief. They provide no healing. Some individuals apply them liberally to their problem areas and obtain a reduction in inflammation, pain, and stiffness. This does not mean they provide any healing benefit to the injured tissues.

Muscle relaxants

These medications are often used to treat muscle spasm associated with the injury of muscles, bones, and joints. Other than in cases of severe spasm, they provide no benefit and generally should be avoided. In some recovery situations, like after surgery or car accident, these medications might be of benefit to help the muscles rest. In general, I don't use them or recommend them.

INTERCHAPTER REMARK: Medications are just one of your tools to get better. They might be very good and successful tools for you to get the relief you need, but they SHOULD NEVER BE YOUR ONLY TOOL. They should be part of a plan or program. Narcotics, and opioids, can be addictive and although they provide pain relief, doctors and patients MUST be very wary and responsible for their use.

Supplements

"Supplements? There shouldn't be a problem here.
Most men and women know what to take.
Do they? Well, they don't."

Eicosapentaenoic acid (EPA) and docosahexaenoic acid (DHA) *are the omega-3 fatty acids in fish that provide tremendous health benefits to joints, organs, and the cardiovascular system. However, qualities vary greatly depending on the species of fish, whether the fish was farm-raised or caught in the deep cold ocean, and whether it is eaten raw, cooked, or canned. Consuming fish with a good content of omega-3, twice a day, will work even better if the individual integrates it as part of a Mediterranean dietary plan. The benefits of this diet in the anti-inflammation process is just wonderful.*

Fish and Fish Oil

Here we encounter a bit of a problem. In many other countries, natural food consumption provides omega-3 and the dietary intake of omega-6 is not that bad. Keep in mind that fats containing omega-6, and diets promoting the omega-6 pathway, cause inflammation while omega-3 is anti-inflammatory. Therefore, the omega-3/omega-6 ratio in those countries is rather acceptable or not that bad. However, in the USA, the omega-3 content in food is poor while the dietary intake of omega-6 is high, hence, the omega-3/omega-6 ratio is bad. That's why Americans need to complement their diets with additional omega-3 in the form of FISH-OIL CAPSULES.

As you will understand later on, there is a huge omega-difference between a burger and fries in the U.S. and a steak and a salad in Argentina.

FISH OIL CAPSULES ARE AN ESSENTIAL PART OF MY ANTI-INFLAMMATORY MEDITERRANEAN DIET, that I like to call "The Jupiter Institute Omega Diet" for a precise reason: we are not in Greece or Sicily, and it is not easy for the average worker or homemaker to follow the common dietary guidelines of those regions, or prepare meals like in the southern part of Spain, France, etc. It is not even easy for me to prepare all those dishes since either I don't have the time or the products are not available or some of the dishes go against our habits, etc. So, my dietary program tries to adapt the concepts of a Mediterranean diet to the reality of life in the United States. And as part of this adaptation is the intake of concentrated and purified fish oil capsules. That is part of the "Mediterraneanization" of my dietary guidelines.

But not just any fish oil is good, so be careful with this.

Most fish oils and salmon oils you can find over-the-counter and in health food stores are contaminated with toxins and even chemicals. This is important, because in this day and age, the regular amounts of EPA and DHA (the main ingredients of the fish oil) are too small to satisfy our needs, and we have to take concentrated fish oil. The ideal amount of EPA and DHA in capsules with concentrated fish oil is EPA 300-450mg and DHA 280-360mg. To accomplish this, the fish oil needs to be concentrated, but if this fish oil already contains toxins and chemical impurities, those are going to be concentrated as well! That is bad because you will be getting an extra load of contaminants. Therefore, we all have to be very careful with the brands we take. Concentrated fish oil is not enough, it has to be purified, and it has to be guaranteed by responsible and reliable laboratories. Otherwise, I will not recommend it, I will not take it, and I will not let my wife, my kids, my patients, my friends or even my dogs take it. That is the reason I only use brands from laboratories recognized by the American Academy of Anti-Aging Medicine, the American Association of Naturopathic Physicians, and that are IFOS certified. The International Fish Oil Standard program (IFOS) is the most important international organization that certifies the purity, freshness, and potency of the different brands of fish oil. It protects consumers from bad, cheap and contaminated products. If a fish oil product is not IFOS certified, do not take it.

Yes, they cost more. Good things often do.

I just don't trust any other brands than the ones I describe here, and you should do the same. There are too many beautiful yet unreliable websites, too much lack of consumer protection, too much marketing manipulation, and too much misinformation, so I am careful with what I take.

Here is the list of those laboratories and their products:

Laboratory	Web Site	Products Name
Carlson's	www.carlsonlabs.com	Elite Omega-3
Douglas	www.douglaslabs.com	Quell Fish Oil, Opti-EPA
Metagenics	www.metagenics.com	OmegaGenics EPA-DHA 720
NuMedica	www.numedica.com	Omega 780 EC (Enteric Coated) (anti belching) Omega 950, Omega 600 EC
Nu-Vitals	www.jupiterinstitute.com	Super Omega Ultra Pure
Ortho Molecular	www.orthomolecularProducts.com	Orthomega 820
Prothera	www.protheraincom	Marine Fish Oil
Protocol For Life	www.protocolforlife.com	Ultra Omega-3
Pure Encapsulation	www.pureencapsulations.com	EPA/DHA Essentials
Thorne Research	www.thorne.com	Omega Plus
Xymogen	www.xymogen.com	OmegaPure 820, OmegaPure 600 EC (Enteric Coated to improve stomach tolerance, anti-belching)

Any of the above products is excellent. If you want smaller capsules, check those websites and get a product with less than 200 EPA, then the capsule will be smaller. You can order them directly, and you don't need me for that. If you dare, you can also buy liquid fish oil. The liquid fish oil from Carlson's laboratory and Xymogen is just excellent.

IN MY OFFICE, for my family, my patients and for myself, I have Super Omega Ultra-Pure, the best concentrated fish oil, with high grade omega-3 (each capsule with 500mg of EPA and 320mg of DHA), highly purified, IFOS certified, specially designed by a laboratory recognized by the Academy of Anti-Aging and according to my specifications. (Why would I take anything else?). I take one or two capsules twice a day.

The Role of Supplements in Healing

Whether we are very healthy or we are affected by a medical condition, our body needs a daily supply of vitamins and minerals. We might get all that we need through our food. Or we might not.

Nutritional supplements have become an essential ingredient in the management of pain, arthritis, injuries, and inflammation. Experience shows their importance in the healing protocol of multiple conditions. No food group or meal preparation can contain all of the vitamins and minerals that a person needs. Modern industrial farming techniques – over-cropping of the land, artificial fertilizers, early harvesting, and processing of food – result in fruits and vegetables that don't have all the nutrients they should have. As a result, people need to take vitamins and other supplements to obtain the necessary nutrients to remain healthy. However, during illness and injury, the need for those nutrients is increased. As a result, a deficiency of vitamins or minerals may affect the healing process. Moreover, if a person is on a weight-loss diet, the deficiencies may be more pronounced since typical weight-loss diets usually deprive the body of several vitamins and essential minerals. When vital nutrients are in deficit, the whole process of injury repair slows, prolonging pain and swelling as well as the suffering of affected tissues.

The United States is a country of people who are well-fed but undernourished. In general, although people eat in abundance, they do not get all the vitamins and supplements their bodies need. Some degree of vitamin and mineral deficiency is a common problem among the people of this country, and the need for supplementation is great. As an example, a nationwide food consumption survey in 1977 and 1978 showed that more than 25% of the population was deficient in vitamin B6, vitamin A or vitamin C. The deficiency of vitamins and minerals is most pronounced in several sub-groups of the population. In addition to the chronically ill and the dieters, deficiencies were also found among adolescents, alcohol abusers, drug users, vegans, diabetics, pregnant or lactating women, the elderly, and the poor. The consumption of empty calories, like processed food and restaurant food, is another risk factor for malnutrition. The problem is even worse when more than one of these factors is present.

Most of the time, nutrient deficiencies are only marginal, causing no significant signs or symptoms and giving no evidence of organic disease. Yet, these deficiencies adversely affect the body's ability to maintain health in the face of biological and psychological stressors. Numerous biological changes are now known to be associated with marginal deficiencies. These include increased susceptibility to infection, the promotion of degenerative tissue changes, and the slower healing of injured or degenerated tissues. With aging, the need for certain nutrients increases but, unfortunately, the ability to absorb these nutrients decreases. This phenomenon contributes to the susceptibility of the elderly to many chronic diseases. Some of those chronic diseases happen to people in their mature age. Just ask around: many people you know have already been diagnosed with deficiencies of vitamin B, vitamin A, calcium, iron, omega-3s, and others. Deficiencies of important nutrients have an immediate and direct consequence on cartilage, musculoskeletal, and neurological structures.

To sum it up, it is necessary to correct nutritional deficiencies for people living in the United States. There are two ways to do so – by nutrient repletion and nutrient therapy. Nutrient repletion is accomplished by improving the diet. A varied diet, rich in nutrients and poor in "anti-nutrients," is the first step in correcting these deficiencies. This is the diet we call the Jupiter Institute Omega Diet, a diet that should keep people in the "omega-3/antioxidant" state (that I also call "omega-3/good-eicosanoids-antioxidant" state), instead of the "omega-6/free-radical" state (that I also call "omega-6/bad-eicosanoids-free-radicals" state).

Sometimes, however, an improved diet is not sufficient to result in adequate nutrition repletion. A patient may fail to follow the diet over the long term, perhaps because of a lack of motivation, knowledge, or means. When dietary recommendations are not adequate to correct the nutritional deficiencies, nutrient therapy is required. Nutrient therapy means taking nutrient pills, often at dosages well above the recommended dietary allowance, to prevent or treat nutritional deficiencies. This is accomplished through the ingestion of vitamins, minerals, and supplements, also known as micronutrients, in the form of tablets and capsules. While thousands of articles support the use of micronutrients, most publications agree that liberal consumption without guidance is irresponsible and dangerous and may do more harm than good. Nutrient therapy is not a matter of taking a few vitamins because you read that they are good for you, but rather of seeking guidance to find which supplements are most needed. I don't want you to get the idea that if you just take a particular vitamin that you will be fine. If you suffer from chronic pain, arthritis, injuries, neck and back pain or neuropathies, taking vitamins and supplements is NOT the solution, but part of a sound program. So, please don't make the mistake of thinking that a handful of pills will fix your problem. That is the passive-pill-taker attitude that rarely works in the eradication of pain conditions. Instead, assume the active attitude of incorporating the various therapies and lifestyle changes we encourage. Taking supplements without considering the other treatments may not yield any improvement; the use of nutritional supplements is just one of several simultaneous therapies that you will need to follow.

However, you need to be very cautious when taking vitamins. Read on.

Vitamins

The vitamins with the greatest therapeutic effect for arthritis are the ones with active antioxidant properties: vitamin A, vitamin C, vitamin E, and some of the B-vitamins. Vitamins B1, B6, and B12 play an important role in the functioning of the nerves and are important additives in the treatment of painful neuropathies. Additionally, vitamin B12 nourishes bone marrow, which prevents anemia. Overall, B-vitamins are known to relieve headaches: vitamin B6, in particular, is known to fight pain. Supplementing the diet with B-vitamins is recommended for anyone who is struggling with pain and injuries. It is usually recommended to take supplements containing all the B-vitamins (B-complex) since they are more effective when the entire complex is taken together. The combination of B-complex with vitamin A, vitamin C, and vitamin E is the core of most nutritional supplement programs. However, excessive amounts of B-complex or dubious brands may cause adverse reactions. The same is true of poor-quality B-vitamins. Vitamin C and vitamin E have powerful antioxidant and anti-inflammatory effects, but they must be taken in correct amounts to be effective. It is unwise to overdo a good thing. Vitamin C helps in tissue repair and injury healing. Vitamin E protects tissues against damage caused by free radicals and improves nerve function. Vitamin E is also known to protect omega-3 fatty acids against free radical attacks.

But it is also true that you can overdose on vitamins and minerals: large doses and excessive doses of vitamins can cause problems, and even some standard doses may interfere with certain prescription medicines. Some people may experience adverse effects from too much calcium or iron. Yes, taking excessive amounts of vitamins can adversely affect people's health. If you think that more is better, you are wrong: many vitamins can cause serious or life-threatening side effects if taken in large doses.

Studies show that taking excessive amounts of vitamins can be risky and counterproductive. Doing this for just a few days may not cause a problem. However, when an individual who suffers from an ailment, or who is debilitated by age and inflammatory or degenerative conditions, takes excessive amounts of vitamins (especially those of poor quality), unpredictable adverse effects can occur. The old saying "the more the better" does not go for vitamins. Mega-doses of vitamins or supplements can be dangerous.

Cautions

Because high levels of vitamin A can be toxic, it is safer to take mixed carotenes that convert into vitamin A in the body. B-vitamins, mainly B3 (niacin), B5 (pantothenic acid), and vitamin B6 (pyridoxine) play a role in the maintenance of multiple tissues, but excessive intake can cause adverse reactions.

Vitamin D and folic acid are two vitamins that, although essential for the structure of tissues, cause adverse reactions when taken in excess. The problem when buying vitamins is that although there are hundreds of brands, most products do not contain what the label says. Many brands of vitamin C have no vitamin C at all in the tablet. Many bottles of vitamin B and vitamin E contain only a fraction of what the label says. Unaware of this, a person may take four or five vitamin tablets a day, but their minimal nutritional content provides no benefits. Some dubious brands may even have impurities that can cause immuno-allergic reactions.

To make matters worse, many supplements are contaminated with unwanted chemicals and even toxins, that add toxicity to our already toxic-affected bodies. In these cases, saving a few dollars every month by buying cheap vitamins may adversely affect our health.

Many of the vitamins you find over-the-counter and in health food stores are not even made in this country, making me wonder "but where were they made?" An answer I was never able to get despite inquiries, emails, and phone calls, that always brings me to the next question: "Why don't you want me to know where they were made?" "Is it because they were made in a non-safe, nonhygienic, toxin-ridden place?... Is that why?" That is the only possible explanation I can figure.

A typical finding is a label that makes people believe the product was made in the USA, giving a false sense of safety. But when you look closely you read "manufactured for XYZ company, USA," or "distributed by ABC Company, USA." As you can see, in both cases the label does not say where and by whom the product was made, so I ask again "Why don't you want me to know? What are you hiding?"

See? Those vitamins may be unsafe or unreliable.

As you can see, taking vitamins is not for the misinformed.

And you can also see that certain questions arise:

Which vitamins are safe then?

Which brands? Where to buy them?

How much is too much?

Reliable Vitamins?

You already got the message: I don't trust any vitamin brand from health food stores, pharmacies, or supermarkets. Thousands of reports of serious adverse events associated with vitamins and supplements are streaming into the FDA from consumers and health-care providers. Symptoms include headaches, signs of heart, kidney, or liver problems, skin disorders, aches, allergic reactions, fatigue, nausea, pains, and vomiting. Moreover, the reports described more than 10,300 serious outcomes (some included more than one), including 115 deaths and more than 2,100 hospitalizations, 1,000 serious injuries or illnesses, 900 emergency-room visits, and some 4,000 other important medical events.

There are numerous side effects caused by vitamins, whether taken in excess or not, and reports show that many multivitamin products contain minerals such as calcium, iron, magnesium, potassium, metals, and zinc, that can cause side effects such as tooth staining, increased urination, stomach bleeding, uneven heart rate, confusion, and muscle weakness or limp feeling.

Studies also show that many labels are not reliable and often manipulate information.

THIS IS WHAT I RECOMMEND:

As I wrote earlier, the vitamins and supplements I recommend are the ones produced by laboratories affiliated with the American Academy of Anti-Aging Medicine and the American Society of Naturopathic Physicians.

Because of reliability and quality, I only recommend products from those laboratories. I just don't trust any other laboratory, over-the-counter products, beautiful websites, health food stores or else, and you should not trust them either. I here give the name and website of those excellent laboratories, so you can buy them directly. They are more expensive, but these are the kind of products you don't want to save money on. (Attention: don't buy all of them, just choose ONE product).

Laboratory	Web site	Multivitamin Product
Douglas	www.douglaslabs.com	Ultra-Preventive
Metagenics	www.metagenics.com	PhytoMulti, Wellness Essentials
NuMedica	www.numedica.com	MultiMedica, Foundation Essentials
Nu-Vitals	www.jupiterinstitute.com	Medi-Naturals, DETOX-Vitamins
Ortho Molecular	www.orthomolecularProducts.com	AlphaBase
Prothera	www.protherainc.com	Multi-Vitamin Complex, Multi-Thera 1
Protocol For Life	www.protocolforlife.com	True Balance
Pure Encapsulations	www.pureencapsulations.com	ONE Multivitamins
Thorne Research	www.thorne.com	Basic Nutrients
Vital Nutrients	www.vitalnutrients.net	Multi-Nutrients
Xymogen	www.xymogen.com	Active Essentials, Active Nutrients

In my office, we use our choice of multivitamin: Medi-Naturals. It is designed for us by one of the above laboratories. For those who need stronger or detox-assisting vitamins we use DETOX-Vitamins. These are the ones most of our patients take.

Reminder

As a minimum, every morning you should take a good fish-oil capsule and a good multivitamin. That is for those who are healthy. However, if you have any sort of inflammatory condition, you should take double or triple that amount since the metabolic requirements are much higher. Consider taking one of each three times a day, or two of each twice a day, until you get better.

Cartilage Building Supplements

Glucosamine

Glucosamine is a supplement that provides raw material to rebuild damaged cartilage. It is not as fast-acting as NSAIDs; it is rather slow. Instead of just eliminating the symptoms, it works by healing the injured tissues that are the root cause of those symptoms. It also decreases the activity of the enzymes that attack the cartilage, helping to restore the eroded cartilage. People taking high-quality glucosamine can decrease the loss of cartilage in the joints and on many occasions even gain new cartilage. Glucosamine eases osteoarthritis pain by normalizing cartilage metabolism and promoting its healing. The most recommended type of glucosamine is glucosamine sulfate. Glucosamine chloride, another variety, is much less effective and should only be used by those individuals with an allergy to sulfur. Many books and publications support glucosamine as an effective medication for arthritis, pain, and inflammation.

As mentioned above, the beneficial effects of glucosamine are slow to appear but long in duration. It takes 6-8 weeks before the benefits of glucosamine can be felt. While those taking NSAIDs such as Ibuprofen and Naprosyn see the drug's effect disappear after one to three days. Those who have been taking glucosamine for any amount of time find its effect lasting from 100 to 120 days after the glucosamine has been interrupted.

Caution: most glucosamine preparations are unreliable and may even contain impurities, so only certain brands are recommended. Many of the brands found in grocery stores and pharmacies do not contain what the labels say, or they contain the wrong type of glucosamine. Some brands bought by mail from unreliable sources are also of poor quality. One study shows that 80% of the store brands are unreliable. Consumers of glucosamine, vitamins, and supplements should be aware of misleading marketing strategies that may cause them to purchase a poor-quality product. We recommend that people avoid cheap store brands or fancy marketing labels. It is acceptable to save on paper towels and laundry detergent, but it is not safe to save on a product that is taken by mouth every day. It is not smart to buy cheap glucosamine and other supplements.

DON'T take Glucosamine alone, take it in combination. See further down.

Chondroitin

Chondroitin is a glycan compound required for the formation of cartilage proteins. It seems to protect joints from breaking down and its activity helps injured cartilage. It inhibits the action of destructive enzymes in the joint. Many publications describe chondroitin as a cartilage protector that works by stimulating the production of healthy cartilage, and by inhibiting the adverse action of eicosanoids. In all, chondroitin decreases inflammation and promotes cartilage repair in the arthritic joint. The recommended dose is 600mg twice a day or 400mg three times a day.

I am not a strong believer in chondroitin. I think you can do without it.

Some publications assert that chondroitin is not absorbed in the digestive tract, that it is useless to take it, and that only injections of chondroitin are effective in decreasing pain and inflammation. However, whether it can be proven or not, some people claim that it is effective.

Do what you feel is right.

AKBA, sent from Mother Nature

AKBA stands for Acetyl- Keto-beta-Boswellic Acid, a naturally occurring pentacyclic compound isolated from the gum resin exudate from the stem of the tree Boswellia serrata (frankincense). This means that AKBA is an extract of Boswellia, a plant with incredible anti-inflammatory effects.

Boswellia Serrata has been used in folk medicines for centuries. It is collected by performing an incision in the trunk of the tree and then collecting the resin that is then stored in a specially made bamboo basket for removal of the oil content and getting the resin solidified. After processing, this oleo gum-resin contains 30-50% of Boswellia serrata but also some unwanted contaminants. The process of decontamination and concentration continues until a more purified product is obtained: a purified boswellic acid rich in the bio-active and anti-inflammatory AKBA. Its medicinal properties are also effective in osteoarthritis, inflammatory conditions, wound healing, asthma, and even in some cancerous diseases. Extracts of Boswellia Serrata have been clinically studied in multiple centers.

Some laboratories and writers call this same product "5-LOXIN Boswellia Serrata" or "Indian Frankincense," but these are all the same thing.

This product works better when you combine it with other products designed for the same objective, for example, COMBINED WITH PHYTOCHEMICALS AND TURMERIC. As I wrote earlier, many of my patients take "Joint Aid," that combines AKBA with these two products, achieving nice relief.

As I wrote earlier, combining products with Boswellia, antioxidants, turmeric, fish oil, and glucosamine, and taking them twice a day, provides a very interesting relief from pain, stiffness, and inflammation.

Collagen

Collagen is a long-chain amino acid and the most abundant protein in the body. It is found exclusively in animal tissue, especially bones and connective tissue, and it is responsible for giving skin its elasticity, hair its strength, and it holds muscle, tendons, joints, and ligaments firmly attached yet flexible. Imagine it as an elastic cement that holds all your bones, muscles, and organs together but allowing them to move.

Over time, with age, dietary and bowel factors, the body's natural collagen production declines, making us lose elasticity and flexibility in joints, muscles, and related structures. That is bad news for our cartilage, ligaments, tendons, and for walking, exercises, and daily activities.

Bio-Cell collagen, a product we use in our office and you can buy in health food stores, provides some raw material to help reconstruct and repair whatever lesion you might have. It is a good helper and works better when combined with the above supplements, rest, the diet I mention, and the alternative medicine therapies.

Devil's Claw

This is a plant product with anti-inflammatory properties. It is used to relieve the symptoms of arthritis. Its origin is the plant Harpagophytum procumbens, a desert plant found in Kalahari, Madagascar, and Namibia. For centuries, natives of the Kalahari and Namib deserts have dried and chopped up the roots of the plant for use in remedies to treat joint problems, pain, and indigestion and to apply to sores and other skin problems. Historically, devil's claw has been used to treat pain, fever, liver disease, kidney problems, and malaria. Today, it is used to fight inflammation, relieve arthritis, pain, and headache, and to treat low back pain. It also relieves neck pain.

It is best taken combined with other supplements that may increase its beneficial effects.

Phytochemicals

Phytochemicals are, as the name says, chemicals extracted from plants, and some of them carry particular beneficial effects. Such is the case of the anthocyanins, that are a type of phytochemicals with strong antioxidant power. They are extracted from colorful plants and fruits, that provide a wide range of health benefits.

All brightly colored fruits and vegetables contain antioxidants that are important compounds for the protection of our bodies.

The dark-colored fruits and vegetables are rich in anthocyanins, that give a great beneficial effect in any inflammatory condition. They are found in high concentrations in blackcurrants, blackberries, acai, maqui berry, dark grapes, and blueberries, as well as in red cabbage, plums, red onions, cranberries, pomegranate, beets, elderberries, and cherries. In addition to acting as antioxidants and fighting free radicals, anthocyanins may offer anti-inflammatory, anti-viral, and anti-cancer benefits. They also have a strong anti-inflammatory effect (on whatever is inflamed, hurt or wounded in the body), antimicrobial, and neuroprotective effects. Without a doubt, they are needed for proper management of arthritis, wounds, injuries, and inflammation.

They will work better if you take them combined with Turmeric and Boswellia/AKBA in the same capsule.

It makes sense.

If you are fighting arthritis, it makes even more sense to take at the same time: glucosamine, Boswellia, phytochemicals, and curcumin.

Turmeric (Curcumin)

Turmeric is a plant product similar to ginger and is obtained from the plant Curcuma longa. The turmeric plant is a perennial herb that is native to Asia. It is cultivated widely in China and India for its medicinal value. Its anti-inflammatory properties are known throughout the world. It has been used in India for centuries.

Curcumin is a key chemical in turmeric and is known to reduce inflammation, pain, and stiffness related to arthritis and rheumatoid arthritis. It is also beneficial for muscle aches, but it provides many other benefits: it possesses anti-arthritic activity, it is an excellent antioxidant, it is a liver and bone helper, it improves immune systems and helps fight infections, and reduces pain and inflammation.

And curcumin works even better when combined with other anti-inflammatory and healing products.

Use the Cooking-a-Chicken Principle when taking care of your joints, ligaments, and your muscles. Too little and too few spices and the chicken will be tasteless. Too much of too many spices and the poor chicken will taste bad. Too little of some spices and too much of the others will not be good either.

Use the right spices and the right amount and the chicken will come out great.

See? No guessing here. You have to follow the advice of those who have studied the problem and know the right combination.

What combination? The Glucosamine, Turmeric, phytochemicals, and Boswellia combination.

Many books and publications claim that the combination of glucosamine with chondroitin provides great success in the treatment of pain and osteoarthritis. Some authors, such as Dr. Jason Theodosakis, affirm that together glucosamine and chondroitin can halt, reverse and even cure arthritis. What is important about glucosamine and chondroitin together is that, unlike NSAIDs, they do promote healing of the damaged joint, albeit quite slowly. They alter joint structure favorably and interfere with the progression of disease. Numerous clinical trials have evaluated this combination and have demonstrated these benefits. Overall, the combination of glucosamine and chondroitin has a positive structural effect on the joints that makes it very effective in the treatment of osteoarthritis and joint pain. Similar to glucosamine, much of the chondroitin and the combined glucosamine/chondroitin products sold on the market today present the same challenges with purity, integrity, and effectiveness. This lack of consistency is so alarming that the Journal of Rheumatology evaluated these products with regard to quality, purity, and concentration of ingredients. The result of this study showed that only 8% of the glucosamine and chondroitin products provide what the label says while more than 90% are unreliable. The unreliable brands not only provide products with lower quality and potency, but they most likely contain impurities that may cause adverse reactions. Only a handful of the over 200 brands of glucosamine and chondroitin are acceptable. We recommend that you first check the label to make sure the product says "Made in the USA" or "Manufactured by XXX, U. S. A." Then, as mentioned before, consult a reliable professional – your physician, chiropractor or local health-food store manager – for guidance. You can also visit our website for guidance regarding vitamins and supplements.

Here are some products we recommend:

Laboratory	Web site	Products name
Douglas Labs	www.douglaslabs.com	Glucosamine plus; joint-tendon-ligament; oswellia-turmeric complex (with Boswellia, curcumin and devil's claw)
Metagenics	www.metagenics.com	Collagenics
NuMedica	www.numedica.com	Joint Replete (for glucosamine and chondroitin); take with CurcuCalm (to get Boswellia, curcumin and bilberry) or with salicin-B (nice product with Boswellia, berries, turmeric)
Nu-Vitals	www.jupiterinstitute.com	Joint-Aid, Collagen-Plus
Ortho Molecular	www.orthomolecularproducts.com	Chondro-Flex
Prothera	www.protherainc.com	glucosamine/chondroitin; arthroThera (with glucosamine, chondroitin, devil's claw, and bromelain); joint support formula (a nice product that contains glucosamine, chondroitin, MSM and Bio-Cell collagen).
Protocol For Life	www.protocolforlife.com	Glucosamine & Chondroitin with MSM
Pure Encapsulations	www.pureencapsulations.com	Glucosamine, chondroitin with MSM; Boswellia AKBA; Joint Complex (with Boswellia, MSM, turmeric); joint optimizer; and ligament

Thorne Research ...... www.thorne.com............ Restore (a nice product that provides Bio-Cell Collagen, glucosamine turmeric, devil's claw)

AR-ENCAP (Nice product with Glucosamine, Boswellia, Devil's Claw, Curcumin, MSM)

Vital Nutrients .... www.vitalnutrients.net............ glucosamine & chondroitin; Joint Ease (that contains curcumin and Boswellia).

Xymogen............... www.xymogen.com .... saloxin (containing Boswellia, berries), synovx DJD (with MSM, glucosamine and chondroitin)

Some of these products are excellent, and provide both relief and healing. Those with salicin, Boswellia, devil's claw and curcumin bring you decreased inflammation, while glucosamine and collagen work on healing and reconstruction.

My advice: choose just two products of the same laboratory. Don't mix.

IN MY OFFICE, and for my patients, I use two products the above laboratories design for me:

Collagen-Plus...a very effective combination of glucosamine with Bio-Cell Collagen and purified MSM, and Joint-Aid...a combination of white willow bark (for natural salicin), 50mg of AKBA, turmeric extract and berries with great anthocyanins

If you are struggling with any of the problems mentioned in this book, don't have the illusion that by just taking the above products you will do well. You won't. You should take the products, rest, especially rest the affected area, adopt an omega-3 lifestyle, eat the right way, review the alternative therapies I describe, consult a professional within conventional medicine or alternative therapies. Plus, take your fish oil and the multivitamins, as these are the basic supplements.

SAM-e

SAM-e (S-Adenosylmethionine) is a sulfur compound used by the body to regenerate cells and reduce pain and osteoarthritis. It somehow decreases inflammation. SAM-e is often recommended for treating inflammation, arthritis, and other painful conditions. It is believed to improve joint mobility. Some clinical studies show that SAM-e may relieve some cases of osteoarthritis and might be good therapy for relief from pain and swelling. The usual dose is 300-400mg three or four times a day.

MSM

MSM (methylsulfonylmethane) is naturally produced in the body, but levels decrease with age and degenerative illnesses. Some publications assert that products with MSM decrease inflammation, relieve pain and spasm, and improve cellular function at the site of injury. The sulfur in MSM is thought to work as a kind of biological "cement" to help repair damaged tissue. Other publications deny these statements saying that MSM has shown no clear benefits. These publications state that there are no human studies to show that MSM is effective in joint repair. Our position in this argument is that it may provide benefits to many. Only recognized brands, however, are recommended. The recommended dose is usually 1,000-1,500mg a day in divided doses.

I don't trust websites, I don't trust statements of "doctors" I don't know, I don't trust nice labels or attractive names like "organic," and "natural."

I often go to health food stores to review their products. If I find some products of interest, I then do a little research to check their origin.

Make sure the product is "made in the USA" or "manufactured by XYZ company" in the USA. If it says, "manufactured for distribution by XYZ," or "distributed by XYZ," then don't buy it and alert your friends and relatives. Until proven otherwise, it WAS NOT MADE IN OUR USA.

Unreliable products, purchased out of convenience or for their cheap price, may not only be ineffective but may cause adverse reactions and even allergies. Companies dedicated to providing high-quality brands regularly test their products using national protocols. They also employ manufacturing techniques that avoid the use of contaminants and solvents and control the quality of the ingredients. Only a few companies provide products of good quality. Remember you are taking these products every day for healing, so you need to use a good product. As with cars and furniture, cheap brands give you unreliable products.

The general public needs to be aware that many of the manufacturers of glucosamine, chondroitin, vitamins, and minerals are based in foreign countries that may not have governmental agencies such as the U.S. Food and Drug Administration that vouch for the safety and efficacy of products of this kind. Many of the foreign suppliers not only provide poor quality supplements, but they also have problems with the hygiene of their workers and the plant. Since they are untouchable by American authorities, they succeed in supplying our market with inferior and sometimes unsafe products. Some authors suggest that 80-90% of the supplements sold in pharmacies, grocery stores, and even health food stores should be avoided. We recommend you check with your physician, chiropractor, other medical professionals, or the manager at your local health food store to determine the best brands.

For the treatment of - neck and back pain, chronic osteoarthritis, injuries, sprains, neuropathies, pinched nerves, arthritis, sciatica, tendinitis, bursitis, inflamed ligaments, and muscular pain. All the above products are very good, but, again, should not be your sole approach. They should be part of the whole treatment. Taking some NSAIDs, for a short time, is recommended as well.

Whenever you can, consult with your doctor for possible adverse reactions or unwanted side effects.

If you are already taking several products, keep in mind that you can get stomach irritation, so protect yourself with some over-the-counter Zantac or Pepcid and visit your doctor if needed. If you are taking any form of blood thinners, just stop where you are and see your doctor.

Points to keep in mind.

Remember, taking vitamins and supplements could be useless if:

1. That is all you do to improve your condition and you don't care about the other six points of our program: diet change, medical care, physical therapy, chiropractic treatment, acupuncture, and exercise.

2. You take cheap, unreliable brands that give you uncertain amounts of the active ingredient. Only buy supplements from reliable sources that clearly state, "Made in the USA," and don't be swayed by fancy marketing.

3. You take incorrect amounts. If you underdose, you are missing out on the nutritional benefit that is needed to heal your condition; if you overdose, you run the risk of toxicity.

4. The pills are outdated. Check the expiration date.

5. You are taking the wrong nutrients for your condition. An example of this is taking lots of B-complex and vitamin C for degenerative knee disease, but not taking glucosamine.

INTERCHAPTER REMARK: The supplements I describe are very effective in managing the ailments presented in this book. Both doctors and patients need to remember to use them properly as a daily part of the therapy. These products will enhance healing and improve repair.

Combining the above supplements with alternative therapies described in previous chapters is an excellent idea: they might improve and heal your problem, relieve pain, and change your lifestyle.

Food Sensitivity and Gut Dysbiosis

Now, that is a mystery. What does this food subject have to do with all the joint and neuromuscular problems I wrote about?

Well, this indeed is a very important topic, and you got some hints when you were reading earlier chapters. Here is the problem: toxins and inflammatory particles from the intestine can spread through the blood and lodge themselves right there where you are hurting. They can contribute and magnify the inflammation and they can interfere with the healing.

The gut makes a difference.

If the gut is sick (even if you have no symptoms) with a condition called DYSBIOSIS, then your pain control management, your repair process, and your healing will be impaired. This gut of yours, that is, your intestines or bowels, will be at peace or at war depending on the foods you eat.

Intestinal inflammation, dysbiosis, leaky gut, and bad health

Welcome to the fantastic world of your intestines. Yes, we are far away from your joints and neck and back, but for many people, this is where their inflammation begins.

Down there, behind your bellybutton, many yards of intestine work every day to nourish your body. The small intestine is full of food (digested and undigested), enzymes, and water, while the large intestine contains undigested food particles...and the many pounds of bacteria needed to digest and process it. That's not all: gasses, fermentation byproducts, and toxins coexist in your gut. All that and more are kept in your gut by the thick and firm intestinal wall and, fortunately enough, what happens in the bowels stays in the bowels (and goes down the toilet).

Nevertheless, certain factors and events may create abnormalities in this contained system and things may end up...well...not contained.

Can you imagine intestinal particles leaking from the wall of the gut and into your bloodstream and then spreading into your tissues? It sounds horrific, and it is, but it's not as rare as you might think.

Keep in mind that the intestines are full of the bacterial flora, that we now call with a new fancy name: "microbiome." This flora, or microbiome, represents the combination of trillions of bacteria, viruses, yeast, protozoa, and even parasites living, swimming, and eating together in peace and harmony...or so it is supposed to be. However, after thousands of years of harvesting, gathering, hunting, and farming, the human diet has changed. That change has been prevalent since World War II, and extremely so over the last fifty years, and humans now live in a world full of gastronomic choices and tasty opportunities. There are all kinds of delicacies within our grasp and we're free to eat and drink whatever we want. Thus, many people guide themselves by their palate and taste buds when they decide what to eat next. However, the trillions and trillions of intestinal bacteria most of the time do not agree with this freedom, and neither do the genes inside the billions of intestinal cells. In the opinion of these bacteria and cells, your diet should be restricted to foods they know and can easily digest, and if they don't get their way, they will get irritated. Also, foods with chemicals (processed foods and drinks), foods contaminated with toxins, and foods high in omega-6, irritates the cells and the bacterial flora even more. Even food that you think of as being "healthy" can be contaminated with new types of grains, pesticides, fungicides, hormones, antibiotics, heavy metals, chemicals of all kinds, colorings, flavorings, artificial sweeteners, even plastic particles. Can you imagine all these intruders in your home? No wonder the microbiome gets upset. This irritation upsets the peace and harmony among bacteria and other microbes, and a civil war begins in the gut. Like any war, there is a lot of collateral damage.

As the wrong diet continues, the gut flora is in trouble: irritation (in every sense of the word) causes the different species of gut flora to attack each other, leaving the battlefield littered with corpses. The dead bacteria, and the products created by their decomposition, cause inflammation as the body tries to quell the uprising on both sides and sweep up the mess. Inflammation-causing molecules and white blood cells are sent to the area to clean, fight, and rebuild, but it's not an easy battle. Soon enough, the fight between bacteria and white blood cells spreads through the gut, leaving more dead bodies, that trigger the incoming of even more inflammatory molecules. As this messy situation gets worse and begins to build on itself, it becomes full-on dysbiosis. "Dys-" meaning "bad" and "bio" referring to the living bacteria and other cells inside of you. Dysbiosis is a total imbalance of the microbial environment inside your body: too many bad bacteria, not enough good bacteria. It is an abnormal situation, full of inflammation, dead bacteria, dead white blood cells, broken cells, toxins, inflammatory molecules, and frequent overgrowth of bad bacteria.

Yes, this dysbiosis is caused by the food that a person eats, and it means more than a stomachache. Eventually, a point is reached where the inflammation molecules of the dysbiosis cannot be contained by the walls of the gut and begin to leak into the bloodstream, spreading through the body. This is not good...but why does this happen? Why the drastic reaction resulting in containment failure? The answer lies in your genes, and what your great-great-grandparents ate for dinner.

For centuries before refrigeration and industrial agriculture, humans ate only the food sourced within a few miles of their home: local grains, local fruits, vegetables, local meat, etc. Their intestinal microbiome grew accustomed to these foods, and the genes of the bacteria would reflect this. The gene coding of the bacterial flora gets passed from parent to child, and the same foods would be eaten every day by the whole family, from generation to generation, and the gut bacteria lived in peace with the local nourishment. Japanese people traditionally ate rice, pickled vegetables, and fish, Moroccans enjoyed grilled meat and simple breads, and so on. It would have been practically impossible for a Japanese villager to eat a Mexican taco al pastor, or for a Moroccan to sit down with a big bowl of Japanese fried rice, but this has changed. All kinds of foods have penetrated every market in every country, allowing consumers to dine on food that doesn't match what their ancestors ate. It's only natural; Scandinavians want to eat Chinese food, Koreans find American cheeseburgers to be exotic and tasty, and Americans can easily take advantage of the rich melting pot by eating hummus, sushi, falafel, tofu, and other dishes. Millions of people want to enjoy all kinds of gastronomic adventures but those adventures often end up in misfortune...and metabolic disasters.

However, these factors don't affect everybody equally. Depending on their genetic background and the health and status of their bacterial flora, some people will not get or will not be affected by dysbiosis, some will get only mild symptoms, while others will have their entire equilibrium thrown into chaos. There is no way to predict who will be affected or how.

Some people can enjoy donuts, chimichangas, oatmeal, pickled herring, and cream cheese and will never get dysbiosis or bad health, but others will.

Some people are "yeast abusers," consuming lots of bread, cheese, wine, and beer and suffering from a terrible dysbiosis, but others do the same with no problem and they laugh and enjoy.

One person might eat too much meat and meat products and develop gut disorders but have a friend who eats even a heavier meat-product diet and remains healthy.

Other people are carbohydrate abusers and get dysbiosis because of that. Others don't.

Some have horrible food sensitivities and others don't.

We see many people consuming all kinds of bad foods, fast foods, etc., and not getting sick and we wonder what protects them, and what makes others get dysbiosis.

What we know is that the following determine whether or not the person gets food sensitivities and if they develop dysbiosis:

a) The genetic background of the person.
b) The type of flora the person has.
c) Previous exposures to wrong foods, toxins, and chemicals.

One way or another, getting the food sensitivity test is very necessary, so you can withdraw from the foods that hurt you.

Withdrawing from foods that were not present in our ancestor's diet (that don't match with our genes) is also necessary. Like French and Swedish people should probably avoid eating enchiladas or Thai food.

You should also avoid a diet heavy in omega-6 since it is the most common factor negatively affecting intestinal health.

At any rate, irritation, inflammation, and illness go together as phases of the same process. In the beginning, except for some gas and bloating here and there or occasional diarrhea, it is mainly asymptomatic. The afflicted person is totally unaware: it is essentially silent, hence, the name Silent Bowel Illness (SBI).

To summarize so far, your diet and lifestyle can cause SBI and dysbiosis. Dysbiosis leads to the leakage of toxins and inflammatory molecules into the bloodstream. This, in turn, will affect your joints, muscles, brain, liver, and all the painful and injured areas. Besides, those toxins can wreak havoc to the metabolism and cause many more problems: weight gain, obesity, diabetes, tumors, high cholesterol, vascular disease, allergic reactions, immune disorders, etc.

If no action is taken, the disease enters the advanced stages. Too many dead germs and dead cells add toxicity to your inner environment. Then the dysbiosis reaches the point of not being silent anymore. Symptoms include indigestion, bloating, constipation, diarrhea, gas, cramps, food intolerance, etc. These symptoms typically get lumped together as Irritable Bowel Syndrome (IBS), but that's not the end of the story.

All the processes and turbulence of dysbiosis will eventually cause the wall of the intestine to become inflamed and weak, and the cells of the intestinal wall start to separate, allowing particles from the gut to pass into the bloodstream. Food particles, feces particles, toxins, inflammation molecules, pieces of bacteria...all kinds of things leak through the wall of the intestine, into the blood, and begin to travel around the body. This is known as "increased bowel permeability" or "intestinal hyperpermeability," or simply "leaky gut."

Someone has to clean up the mess, and so the leaking inflammation particles and waste products come into contact with the liver, our main detoxification organ. It does a good job for a while, but one liver can only do so much, and as the leakage continues the liver cells get overwhelmed and start to get sick. As the liver loses its health, the detoxification process declines and the body starts accumulating toxins, causing a deadly cycle. Nothing good will happen after that. All the inflamed parts of the body affected by arthritis, pain, or injuries will be unable to detoxify properly. Tissue repair and healing will be adversely affected. Moreover, at this stage other medical disorders start to appear, all related to the same process.

Your Gut and Dysbiosis

Let's review this problem with a little more detail. As I wrote above, all those great gastronomic choices we have, with all kinds of delicacies, drinks, and foods, are capable of irritating our gut. If we additionally eat food with chemicals (processed foods and drinks), foods contaminated with toxins, foods not ethnically correct, processed carbs, and bad fats, then the intestine becomes even more irritated.

If the person has food sensitivities or is a carb or wheat abuser, the intestinal cells and the flora will become even more irritated and even aggressive.

SBI - After the initial phase of Silent Bowel Irritation, this gut irritation and bacterial flora restlessness end up causing inflammation and then things get worse. As the battle between food particles, bacteria, and the intestinal wall continues, inflammatory molecules enter the battlefield, and shortly after, the white blood cells arrive. The result is more dead germs and more dead cells, that adds toxicity to the environment. This advanced state of Silent Bowel Irritation and inflammation, combined with alteration and overgrowth of bacterial flora is now an advanced state of Dysbiosis and might not be that silent anymore. Some of the symptoms are indigestion, bloating, constipation, diarrhea, gas, cramps, gastritis, food intolerance, colitis, etc. Irritable Bowel Syndrome, also known as IBS is a typical symptom.

There are other causes of leaky gut: alcohol excess, viruses, medications, toxins in foods, stress, gluten, foods contaminated with heavy metals, gut infections, parasites, so keep all those factors in mind. Some people may have more than one factor at the same time. If Martin, a common middle-class American, has a lot of stress, abuses alcohol, and eats foods he is highly sensitive to, he may get a bad case of dysbiosis and leaky gut from those three factors.

Some individuals are more affected in their immune system. The leaking particles attack and annoy the immune system, driving it mad. In this very slow and mostly silent process, the immune system reacts producing antibodies that then go and attack distant organs, including joints, nerves, and muscles. The presence of antibodies precedes by years the development of disease. In other words, first, the person gets the antibodies that can be detected in a blood test, and much later, years later, the disease of that organ develops.

As I wrote above, the leaking waste products also attack the liver, our main detoxification organ. As the liver loses its health, the detox process declines and the body starts accumulating toxins. With a faulty immune system and an unhealthy liver, I can assure you that nothing good is going to happen to that person.

Why would you need to know all this?

Because you need to know that the inflammation of the gut leaks and spreads through the body and affects important areas and organs.

The inflammatory and toxic particles will attack your joints, your aching muscles, your painful nerves, your pain areas, injured areas, and surgical site areas.

Hence, if you eat bad food (with omega-6s, with acidity, with the free-radicals it generates, with the absence of omega-3, its lack of antioxidants, and its poor nutrient value) and FOODS YOU ARE SENSITIVE TO, you will be getting dysbiosis.

If you eat foods you are not supposed to according to your genes (the Nutrigenomic rule) you may get dysbiosis.

Dysbiosis is a very serious condition

The leaking particles can cause all kinds of disorders. Here is a brief list of those medical problems:

- Atherosclerosis-neurotransmitter imbalance (causing anxiety disorder, depression, cognitive decline, brain fog), fatigue, skin diseases, Lupus, rheumatoid arthritis, and cancer

- Infectious diseases, immune and autoimmune disorders, liver disease, and hormonal decline

- Weight gain and obesity, including resistance to weight loss efforts, diabetes, and high cholesterol

- Vascular disorders

There are more health disorders to talk about, and there is a lot more that can be said about dysbiosis, but that is not the main goal of this book and I don't want to digress into that topic.

Just type "dysbiosis" on the Internet and you will get lots of information. Read it. Study it as if your health depends on it.

An example. Mary Sue is 42 years old, overweight, has chronic low back pain (at times intense), and a bad shoulder with pain and stiffness. She comes to see me because the usual medications, anti-inflammatories, and physical therapy are not helping. "Could you send me to a specialist so I can get a shot?" she suggests.

Mary Sue consumes dairy, wheat, and eggs (without knowing she is sensitive to them). She has stress from her job and a difficult daughter. She has irritable bowel (with troubling constipation). Her parents are both French, but she enjoys fish tacos, burritos, salsa, and Chinese food, "Yes, this is what I like to eat and I don't want to change." She works in a store and usually eats one or two donuts at lunchtime with her sugary, creamy iced latte. Her blood test shows high cholesterol, high glucose, and a positive Lupus (ANA) test.

Do you see the picture? Do you see how her dysbiosis is hurting her and giving her medical conditions and a general health decline?

Do you think all she needs is a shot?

Will I fix her with some pills?

So, this is what I do. I first send her for X-rays and I give her some short reading material about what I wrote over the last few pages, "Read this and study it, Mary Sue, and check the Internet for those keywords." By the time she comes back she already has some ideas. After the food sensitivity test and dietary adjustment, an anti-inflammatory program starts (with all the components I described in the chapters above). I teach her how to eat a healthy diet. I guide her through food choices and meal preparation. That's the beginning. Then we initiate a gut healing program, detoxification, her hormones, and thyroid are checked, and we discuss conventional and alternative medical therapies.

Food Sensitivity

You might ask yourself why this subject is important. What could be the metabolic importance of having a few allergies to some foods like clams or peanuts? The answer, however, is of enormous magnitude: 90% of the time they relate to dysbiosis.

Even if you are doing your best, and you are eating just like I tell you to eat and avoiding all the bad foods I wrote about, you can still get bowel and whole-body inflammation because of unknown food sensitivity.

Some of my patients tested positive for salmon, tuna, lettuce, broccoli, bananas, and walnuts.

I am sensitive to spinach, apples, and almonds.

Some patients are sensitive to beef, chicken, turkey, lamb, eggs, and all vegetables. Others are sensitive to oats, gluten, all fish and all dairy, but others are not.

And this is NOT food allergy; this is different.

FOOD SENSITIVITIES are silent. You don't feel the food sensitivity and you are not aware of it. The reactions don't come fast and are so silent that you may never know you are suffering from them. Just like that. You don't know you are getting sick because the symptoms are very slow and very misleading.

Food sensitivities are slow immune-reactions triggered by food particles that leaked through the gut. These food particles tease and annoy the immune system forming food-globulin complexes that hurt the metabolism anywhere in the body. As unpredictable as nature itself, these metabolic attacks may occur in any organ and there is no way to predict who will be affected or in what way.

There is also no way to know which foods are affecting a person unless you do the food sensitivity test.

HOW does it happen? Well, part of the reason you already know. Some food particles irritate the lining of the intestine and trigger an inflammatory process that is complicated by incoming white blood cells. As I described above, the clash affects the balance of the bacterial flora and results in dead bacteria, dead white blood cells, and the accumulation of toxins. This means that the food reaction triggers dysbiosis, which in turn creates tiny holes in the wall of the gut through which particles of all kinds pass and go into the bloodstream. They leak through the intestinal cells, hence the name "leaky gut." Not every person has this problem, but those who do have it suffer a variety of chronic diseases because food particles should not be leaking into the bloodstream: it's abnormal.

And again, once these particles are in the bloodstream they are recognized as hostile foreign particles and attacked by the globulins of our immune system. These globulins, that are the "attack-proteins," are called immunoglobulins or simply "IG." They attack those food particles and form a food-globulin complex (like a hand grabbing an apple). These attack-proteins are very abnormal and "thorny" and end up hurting organs and systems of the body causing inflammation and disease. Some immunoglobulins are modified to specifically attack certain food particles, but in the mix-up, some of those "attacking-globulins," known now as antibodies, confuse some organ cells as the enemy and attacks them. This complex effect over the immune system is the root of inflammation, auto-antibodies, and most autoimmune disorders. Any organ can pay the price, liver, muscles, skin, brain, pancreas, joints, nerves, etc.

Nevertheless, all this process happens silently and very slowly. Nothing tells the person that his dinner of two nights ago or that the same breakfast he's been eating for the last 20 years is causing an adverse effect: this micro-storm gives no signs. The effect is very slow and it may take days or weeks to cause medical problems. The person doesn't know it is happening.

As you can see, triggers can be different, but the messy process of dysbiosis is similar in most cases. Hence, we now have a better understanding of the problem. This bowel illness doesn't stop there; it continues and causes an overgrowth of bacteria (worsening dysbiosis) and malabsorption of nutrients that brings about further disastrous metabolic complications.

What Kind of Food?

It can be anything. Apples, almonds, grapes, peanuts, orange, bread, milk, eggs, lentils, yeast products, ketchup, yogurt, chocolate, raisins, tomato products, beef, pork, salami, grouper, soy, cream cheese, banana, corn. It could be any food. The type of food varies with every person, and there is no way to know until a Food Sensitivity Test is done. The FOOD SENSITIVITY TEST is the best way to find out.

"Could this mean that certain foods that I eat, although healthy for some, and recommended by nutritionists, could be like a slow-acting food-toxin for me?" Yep!

Symptoms of Food Sensitivity

The adverse effects might be caused directly by the food particles, or indirectly by annoying the immune system. They may also be caused by the leakage of toxins and inflammatory molecules.

- Respiratory symptoms–cough, sneezing, wheezing, asthma, snoring, sleep disorders, bronchitis, clearing throat often, nasal congestion, sinusitis, hearing loss, sore throat, itchy ears, canker sore, swollen tongue, runny nose.

- Eyes–watery eyes, itchy eyes, blurred vision.

- Immune system–catching colds and infections easily, yeast (fungal) infections, autoimmune disorders, Sjogren's.

- Neurological–poor coordination, headache, migraine, depression, memory problems, mental fatigue, intellectual difficulties, confusion, insomnia, poor concentration, autism, Attention Deficit Disorder (ADD), learning disabilities.

- Skin–eczema, psoriasis, dermatitis, acne, hives, rosacea, rashes, hair loss, cracked nails, excessive sweat, dandruff.

- Metabolism–weight gain, obesity, water retention, cravings, food addictions, binge eating.

- Emotions–mood swings, anxiety, fear, irritability, anger, nervousness, hyperactivity, depression.

- Energy–body fatigue, sluggishness, apathy, lethargy, restlessness, severe tiredness.

- Musculoskeletal–stiff muscles, Lupus, arthritis, stiff joints, tendinitis, Rheumatoid Arthritis, pain in joints, weak muscles, osteoporosis, fibromyalgia.

- Malabsorption–vitamin deficiency, iron deficiency, anemia, calcium deficiency, nutritional diseases caused by lack of vitamins and mineral absorption.

- Digestive system–irritable bowel syndrome (IBS), diarrhea, constipation, liver disease, bloating, heartburn, belching, stomach pain, stomach ulcer, indigestion, esophageal reflux.

"What will happen if I ignore the symptoms?"

"Your disease will get worse!"

Repair

Here are some basic ideas for you regarding the repair of an inflamed gut. Obviously, it is essential to keep your bowels healthy. There are several steps you can take towards maintaining a happy, functioning intestinal microbiome and improve dysbiosis:

1. Remove trigger foods from your diet, such as wheat, processed foods, bad fats. Stay away from the omega-6 lifestyle while adopting a healthy diet full of omega-3 and antioxidants, like a Mediterranean diet.

2. You may need to avoid dairy products as well and perhaps eggs, according to your food sensitivity test. However, it might be OK for you to consume wheat. Meanwhile, some other products, like beans, seafood, gluten, etc. might be hurting you without you knowing, that takes us to #3.

3. Get the food sensitivity test.

4. Don't eat foods your genes are not made for. Eat according to your genetic line. That is the Nutrigenomic rule.

5. Detoxify your gut: learn about different gut detoxification programs (I outline a few of them later on.) and start reversing the existing damage.

6. Heal the gut with functional foods, supplements, and a dietary program designed to decrease dysbiosis, provide liver support,

introduce probiotics and essential gut nutrients, and improve digestion and overall bowel health.

7. Prepare for the future and have a plan for improving the health of your gut in the long-term.

These are some general ideas and should be complemented with the more detailed "gut restoration program" that follows.

Unfortunately, there is no quick cure for this condition. I wish it was as easy as taking a pill twice a day for a week. You need to have an understanding of what is going on, where the problems are, and how you are going to heal yourself. It requires your active participation.

Fat

Some kinds of fat can cause dysbiosis, while some fats may prevent it. You have probably heard it before: some fats are bad; some fats are good.

There is now considerable evidence that a diet high in saturated fat is capable of disrupting the bowel harmony, cause gut inflammation, dysbiosis, and even promote the leakage of toxins from the gut into the bloodstream.

As I explained earlier, and I will explain in the Nutrition Chapter, through leakage, GUT INFLAMMATION IS EXPORTED TO ALL TISSUES AND ORGANS OF THE BODY, wreaking havoc in the whole metabolism and attacking any structure or gland of our anatomy.

Now that you understand the importance of having a healthy gut, I am going to explain a more comprehensive gut repair management program:

Gut Restoration Program

The ten basic rules of healing the gut are known as the "10 Rs" of management:

1. Relax your adrenal glands, (they have a strong adverse impact in the gut). Explore the vast world of stress management and relaxation techniques and choose the ones you like. Read about these subjects and explore the amazing field of adaptogens.

2. Retreat from bad foods, the wrong ways of eating, bad habits, and avoiding the food groups I described and will describe later on in this book.

3. Review your family background to eat according to the Nutrigenomics principle

4. Recognize that a Mediterranean Diet is the best way of eating; acidic foods mixed with alkaline foods with plenty of omega-3's and antioxidants.

5. Remove bad bacteria, toxins, heavy metals, and unwanted waste from your gut, through detoxification.

6. Relieve the liver from its toxic overload and improve its functions and bile flow

7. Remember food sensitivities. If you have persisting pain, significant arthritis, or any inflammatory condition then get the food sensitivity test.

8. Repair the gut with the necessary functional foods and supplements

9. Replace stomach acid and enzymes if needed

10. Re-inoculate the gut with friendly bacteria by taking probiotics and prebiotics.

THAT'S RIGHT. This is not "take the blue pill twice a day for a week" and you are done. The program requires your understanding of what is going on, where the problems are, and how you are going to heal yourself. It requires your participation.

It is not a three-week vacation; it is a path.

Retreat from Trigger Foods: Dietary Changes

You cannot treat dysbiosis by taking a morning pill for a week, or by "being good with a diet" for two to three weeks. Healing this condition requires taking a path, a long path. A path for good health.

Adjustment in the diet should be the first step. But where do you start to decrease dysbiosis?

Would it be enough to just stop eating wheat, gluten, dairy, and soy? Maybe.

But maybe not.

What about beans, eggs, seafood, mango? ...And coffee, chocolate, and nuts? Would they cause dysbiosis, too? Should you stop eating them?

Perhaps you should.

Perhaps you shouldn't.

The dietary roots of dysbiosis vary from person to person, and many people with this disorder are not sensitive to wheat, gluten, or dairy, but rather get an adverse reaction from chocolate, seafood, or nuts. Only a test called the FOOD SENSITIVITY TEST can tell you which foods you are sensitive to.

INTERCHAPTER REMARK: As you learned, a sick gut spreads toxins daily, that contributes to inflammation and poor healing. Fixing the gut, then, is a necessity. Keep in mind that stress can hurt the gut causing dysbiosis and triggering hormones that promote inflammation. If you are also eating foods you are strongly sensitive to, your inflammatory condition may get much worse and might trigger medical diseases of all kinds.

Now you have a better understanding of the whole picture of inflammation and pain and your mind and body are more ready to accept the beneficial effects of alternative therapies. So now we enter the phase of reviewing those modalities. A few things are still needed, like an emphasis on NUTRITION, that I describe in the Nutrition chapter, and the effects of hormones, thyroid, adrenal gland, toxins and sleep in the successful management of neuromuscular, arthritic and painful conditions.

Therapies

Acupuncture

Acupuncture is a powerful medical technique that helps strengthen the immune system, reduce inflammation, control pain, and improve the quality of life. Acupuncture is highly effective in the healing of injuries and the treatment of multiple painful conditions. Because it affects a person's inner bioenergetics, those who receive acupuncture not only heal physically but quite often experience new and profound states of peace, clarity, and harmony. It has been determined that the human body is a bioenergetic system. When this system is disturbed, pain or illness sets in. Acupuncture treatment restores energetic balance by stimulating the body's natural ability to heal itself without the use of drugs or surgery.

History

Acupuncture is one of the oldest known forms of medicine. It was developed in China over 3,000 years ago, where it was used to maintain health and treat disease. Acupuncture was brought to Europe in the late 17th century and from there it has spread to other countries, including the United States. When China opened its doors in the 1970s, Americans were able to gain more direct exposure to this healing technique. Although the American public quickly became enthusiastic about acupuncture's potential for the treatment of pain and disease, American physicians were reluctant to endorse it. Even now, many American doctors refuse to accept it as a viable form of medical care. There are two reasons for this attitude. First, it has been difficult for some doctors to accept the underlying principle of acupuncture: that health and disease are- directly related to the flow of energy (Qi) through the body's energetic channels (meridians). Energy medicine, although gaining popularity in Western cultures today, is not described in classic anatomy books. Secondly, attempts by American physicians to replicate the Chinese technique by practicing acupuncture themselves proved mostly unsuccessful. For many Western doctors, acupuncture is still too new, too nontraditional, and too difficult to understand and practice. Nevertheless, the medical establishment's initial skepticism began to moderate in the early 1980s. Numerous articles in medical journals and books on acupuncture demonstrate its effectiveness, including its success in the treatment of pain conditions. Currently, acupuncture is used to treat hundreds of millions of people around the world for almost every disease. It is documented that more than 15 million Americans have received acupuncture, mainly for pain control. Since pain is the number-one symptom affecting people with arthritis, acupuncture has been used to treat many kinds of arthritis, including osteoarthritis, fibromyalgia, and rheumatoid arthritis. Acupuncture is now being endorsed by the National Institutes of Health, by the White House Commission on Complementary and Alternative Medicine, and by many American medical organizations.

How it Works

A person's life force or energy, called Qi (pronounced chi), does not remain stationary but flows constantly through channels in the body, much like rivers of water. These rivers of Qi are called meridians, and they connect inside the body to each other and with the deep organs. Acupuncture is performed using hair-thin needles that puncture the skin at specific places called acupuncture points.

The stimulation caused by the needle affects the flow of energy to a particular organ or area of the body and can modify and correct the flow of Qi through a particular meridian. The needle works like a valve controlling the flow of water through a pipe. There are many meridian systems in acupuncture, and each is accessed for different reasons. Also, there are about 360 basic acupuncture points on the surface of the body that have specific names and functions. Additionally, there are several hundred "trigger points" that can also be stimulated with the needles. All of these meridians, acupuncture points, and trigger points are interconnected by approximately 70 additional channels, forming a complex web of energetic activity. Using this knowledge, a skilled acupuncturist can open or close the valves of energy at the acupuncture points. They can decrease excess flow in high-energy areas while increasing the flow of healing energy to low-pressure areas. The meridians are, however, invisible and do not correlate with the familiar anatomical charts of Western medicine. In Chinese medicine, illness is a manifestation of the relationship between a patient's constitutional makeup and the stimulus of the environment. All illnesses and symptoms result from imbalances in quantity, distribution, and flow of the vital energy called Qi. A suffering or damaged area accumulates blood, fluids and Qi becomes stagnant. Chinese medicine specifies that there must be movement of Qi, blood, and fluids if a sick organ is to heal and return to balance. Where there are pain and injury, the flow is blocked. This blockage prevents that area from receiving oxygen-rich blood, among other things that aid healing. Acupuncture improves the flow and facilitates healing by eliminating the obstruction and relieving pressure in the area. To define the movement, excesses, deficiencies, and distribution of Qi in the body, the Chinese apply the concept of yin and yang.

Yin and yang represent the expression of a dynamic equilibrium between excess and deficiency of Qi. While a yin condition is passive, inferior, chronic, cold, and poorly defined, a yang condition will be bright, superior, active, hot, and acute. A yang illness may present with a fever, heat, and severe pain. According to Chinese medicine, the balance of yin and yang within an individual must be in harmony. Qi must flow in the proper direction, allowing the yin and yang to be in equilibrium. Acupuncturists first identify the balance of yin and yang, diagnosing the pattern and type of disharmony in a particular individual. Once the diagnosis is made, the acupuncturist searches for the appropriate meridians and acupuncture points on those meridians that control the flow of Qi to the problem area. Then, they insert the needles that, like valves, decrease or increase the energy flow and bring balance to the affected area.

Technique

Acupuncture needles used to be made of gold or silver, but nowadays they are made of stainless steel and are sterilized and individually packed. They are used to puncture the skin at acupuncture points, and sometimes rotated or moved for greater efficacy. Electric stimuli are frequently used in combination with acupuncture. In these cases, short cable wires are connected to low-intensity units to deliver a fixed current to the acupuncture points and provide greater stimulation. On other occasions, acupuncture is performed together with Moxa burning, in which a dry paste of the chopped leaves of mugwort (Artemisia vulgaris) is attached to the needles and lit. This procedure heats the handle of the needle, which transmits heat to the acupuncture points, augmenting the effectiveness of the treatment. All of these procedures are relatively painless. On average, patients require between three and six acupuncture treatments to begin getting relief; although, the number of sessions will vary. Long-standing and complex chronic conditions might need one or two treatments a week for several weeks. New conditions may get relief after one or two sessions.

Acupuncture for Pain, Arthritis, and Injuries

Acupuncture is highly effective in treating both acute and chronic pain and injuries, and can be used alone or as a part of a comprehensive program.

The list of conditions effectively treated with acupuncture is extensive and includes:

- Acute arthritis
- Cancer pain
- Carpal tunnel syndrome
- Chronic arthritis
- Degenerative disc disease
- Fibromyalgia
- Headaches
- Joint pain
- Muscular injuries
- Myofascial pain
- Neck and back pain
- Neuropathy
- Pinched nerve
- Postherpetic neuralgia
- Sciatica
- Sports injuries
- Strain injuries
- Tennis elbow
- Trigeminal neuralgia
- Whiplash injuries

The advantages of integrating acupuncture into a comprehensive pain management program are numerous. In some cases, acupuncture by itself may resolve the pain while in others it will just reduce it. But in both cases, it will assist the patient and the doctor to more successfully care for a medical condition. Whether for healing or for facilitating healing, acupuncture's role in medicine is enormous. Arthritis is something that acupuncturists commonly treat. There are several types of arthritis, and Chinese medicine classifies them according to their symptoms. The "wind" type moves from one joint to the next, the "damp" type is the swollen type, the "cold" type is cold to touch, the "hot" type is swollen and hot, and the "bony" type is the late-stage type. These different types of arthritis require different acupuncture treatments and respond differently to the treatment. Although the response may vary from case to case, acupuncture provides many arthritic pain sufferers with an alternative or addition to modern arthritis therapy. Acupuncture can result in the powerful relief of pain, injury, and arthritis. "But acupuncture doesn't work!" I have heard this kind of comment on numerous occasions from people who have had a particular medical condition for many, many years. One patient, specifically, had been suffering from arthritis in her left hip for more than 25 years. She said after her second acupuncture session, "Oh, Doctor Nuchovich, I tried it, but acupuncture just doesn't work." People expect from acupuncture the same immediate relief they can get with pills. This is an incorrect conclusion based on misinformation. If a joint has been degenerating for over 20 years and consistently swollen, there is no way that one or two sessions of acupuncture can reverse it. Taking two Celebrex and one Darvocet, on the other hand, will provide fast relief, but no real healing. Acupuncture and pills are completely different – one is a healing technique while the other is simply a cover-up for symptoms. Acupuncture addresses the imbalance causing the pain; pills just mask the pain. Understand that it takes time for the body to erase years of abnormalities, and have patience with the healing process.

Conditions Effectively Treated with Acupuncture.

Respiratory problems:
- Allergies
- Asthma
- Bronchitis
- Hay fever
- Rhinitis
- Sinusitis

Neurological problems:
- Facial pain
- Fatigue
- Memory problems
- Paralysis
- Stroke

Hearing problems:
- Hearing disorders
- Tinnitus

Emotional problems:
- Anxiety
- Depression
- Insomnia
- Nervousness

Digestive problems:
- Abdominal pain
- Chronic diarrhea
- Colitis
- Constipation
- Gastritis
- Indigestion
- Irritable Bowel Syndrome (IBS)
- Nausea

Gynecological problems:
- Cramps
- Dysfunctional bleeding
- Hot flashes
- Infertility
- Menopause
- PMS

Other conditions:
- Addiction (smoking, alcohol, drugs)
- Chronic fatigue
- Gout
- Heel pain
- Impotence
- Incontinence
- Pain control
- Stress reduction
- Urinary disorder
- Weight control

It has been demonstrated through many books, studies, and publications that acupuncture is an effective adjunct to conventional medical treatments and can be successfully employed alone or as part of a multidisciplinary medical approach. Acupuncture has also been used in spinal cord injuries and has been found to contribute to significant neurological and functional recoveries.

How to Find an Acupuncturist

Acupuncturists who are licensed and credentialed by the state are more likely to provide better care than those who are not. Although credentials do not ensure competency, they do indicate that the practitioner has met certain standards to treat patients. However, a certificate on the wall is no guarantee of expertise. We recommend selecting practitioners who have had formal training, rather than those who simply attended a few courses and seminars. Be sure the doctor has completed a recognized acupuncture training program. Traditional Chinese Medicine (TCM) acupuncturists claim that many doctors who practice acupuncture do not have adequate training. They recommend finding a therapist who has many years of experience and who is trained in TCM.

Oriental acupuncturists, born and trained in the Far East, are considered the best.

Do not necessarily use the first acupuncturist you find; instead, search for acupuncturists in your area. When you find them, inquire about their background, their training, and their experience before you consider treatment. If possible, arrange to meet with them before you commit to a session. Acupuncture is recognized and recommended by the following organizations: The National Institutes of Health, The National Center for Complementary and Alternative Medicine (a subdivision of the U.S. Department of Health and Human Services), The White House Commission on Complementary and Alternative Medicine, Harvard Medical School, The University of Maryland and numerous colleges and universities throughout the country. The Arthritis Foundation and pain organizations also recognize acupuncture as a major treatment modality. Additional recommendations come from Spaulding Rehabilitation Hospital (Boston), Albert Einstein College of Medicine (New York), University of Massachusetts, Columbia University (New York), University of Arizona, and many scientific publications and books. A final note: Acupuncture offers the promise of treatment that in some cases will reduce or eliminate the need for medications and in others will ameliorate conditions for that Western medicine is unsuccessful or incomplete. Acupuncture, as a modality, is widely acknowledged as a safe procedure. In the hands of a well-trained practitioner, complications are very rare.

Chiropractic Care

Chiropractic care is perhaps the most popular alternative medicine treatment in the United States. Chiropractic care treats diseases by moving and adjusting the bones of the spine and other structures. These manipulations are based on the belief that diseases are caused by pressure, especially of vertebrae and discs, on the nerves. Chiropractors do not use drugs, injections, or surgery in their practice. They also believe that the body responds to stressful conditions in a way that affects the nervous, immune, and metabolic systems simultaneously. Working on the spine, for instance, may provide benefits to organs and metabolic systems throughout the body. Chiropractic treatment is a wonderful technique that provides enormous relief in such conditions as arthritis, pain, and injuries. Criticized by physicians who were too stubborn to investigate it, or perhaps too afraid to accept it, chiropractic treatment has survived the challenges of our modern medical society. It has proven itself as a technique that provides relief and improves the quality of life, and it has saved numerous people from unnecessary surgery.

There are more than 60,000 chiropractors in the United States. According to recent surveys, there has been a significant increase in the use of chiropractic health care by the general population. Chiropractors typically train for eight years before entering into private practice. There is an undergraduate program, a post-graduate professional college study program as well as a clinical internship. The areas of science and clinical studies are those pertinent to the total health care of humans including anatomy, physiology, diagnosis, nutrition, pathology, radiology, and therapeutics. Chiropractors have been recognized as providing exceptional care for back pain, headaches, neck pain, nerve disorders, and other spinal related conditions. Also, chiropractors have been proponents of recognizing the capacity and integrity of body and mind to deal with stress and disease. They have collectively criticized the overuse and abuse of drugs, injections, and surgery.

Chiropractic care seeks to restore normal physiologic function and thereby improve the health of the individual. The principle of treatment is based on the idea that misalignment of the vertebrae, called subluxation, causes many diseases and that chiropractic realignment of the spine is the cure. Chiropractors are trained in the highly effective technique of "unblocking" the spine, relieving its dysfunction, and improving the bioelectrical conductivity of the nervous system. Chiropractic adjustments aim to restore proper spinal motion, thereby directly influencing spine-related disorders. Several publications suggest that adjustment to the spine also has the potential to influence neural (nerve) integrity, which positively affects dysfunctional organs. For more than a century, chiropractors have advocated that an optimally functioning nervous system is necessary for good health. The significance of the nervous system and its influence on the body's ability to adapt to the environment is becoming increasingly relevant as research advances. Moreover, there is a growing awareness of the need to consider prevention and health maintenance rather than waiting for disease to happen. Chiropractors typically understand this important concept, although many medical doctors do not. This is why chiropractic care is becoming a mainstream treatment for tens of millions of Americans who are seeking better health and drug-free relief.

Conditions for which Chiropractic Treatment is Recommended

- Arm pain
- Arthritis
- Asthma
- Back pain
- Bursitis
- Colitis
- Cramps -numbness -tingling (paresthesias)
- Degenerative disc disease -hip pain
- Injuries
- Joint subluxation
- Menstrual cramps
- Muscle tears
- Neck pain
- Neuralgia (nerve pain)
- Neuropathy
- Nutritional disorders
- Pinched nerve
- Respiratory disease
- Sciatica -scoliosis -shoulder pain
- Tendinitis
- Tinnitus
- TMJ (temporomandibular joint) problems

Technique

Although chiropractors take the patient's medical history and perform a standard physical examination, it is the examination of the spine and muscle system that makes the chiropractic approach different from that of other health care practitioners. A careful spinal examination and analysis will be performed to detect any structural abnormalities. In some cases, spinal X-rays may be necessary. The spinal examination, when analyzed with the skill and experience of a chiropractor, greatly aids in the identification of problem areas in the musculoskeletal system, that may be contributing to the ailment. Evaluation is followed by manipulation of one or more spinal areas, and particular attention is paid to the areas of the spine where a spinal dysfunction (subluxation) has been detected. The adjustment is usually given by hand. It consists of placing the patient on a precisely designed adjustment table and then applying pressure to the areas of the spine that are out of alignment.

Chiropractors employ a wide variety of treatment methods. The experience and knowledge of the chiropractor will determine the type of manipulation and the frequency of subsequent manipulations.

Counseling

In addition to spinal manipulation, many chiropractors give nutritional advice. They also counsel on posture, on the types of sports and exercises that are best, and even on good sleeping habits. Chiropractors may recommend rehabilitative exercises and cervical support pillows. On many occasions, the treatment is complemented with physical therapy and massage to augment the healing benefits. Counseling patients in areas such as nutrition, proper exercise, diet, lifestyle changes, and general health matters demonstrates the chiropractic concern regarding the "whole person." The effectiveness of chiropractic treatment is proven by studies that demonstrate that chiropractic patients are more satisfied with their chiropractic care than with medical treatment. Chiropractic care will continue to grow in the 21st century, and the benefits of this unique health-enhancing approach to rehabilitation will reach new levels of public awareness.

Nutritional Supplements

There can't be any doubt about the multiple benefits they provide. They have been used for decades and some have been used for centuries. I address them in the Supplements chapter.

Nutrition Therapy

An incredibly important topic, that I address in the Inflammation and Nutrition chapters.

Acupressure

Acupressure is an alternative medicine technique similar in principle to acupuncture. It is based on the concept of manipulation of the life energy that flows through the body in canals called "meridians." Arthritis, illnesses, painful conditions, and injuries disrupt the normal flow of energy through the body. This often causes disruption and blockages in the flow of energy through the meridians, creating areas of high tension that impairs the body's ability to heal itself. The practitioner exercises manual pressure (no needles) on what are called "the acupressure points" and attempt to revive, block, or unblock the affected meridians.

As the flow of energy improves, the body regains its balance and health is improved.

Acupressure was developed in Asia over 4,000 years ago. It uses the power and sensitivity of the hand to gradually press key healing points, that stimulate the body's natural self-curative abilities. It is effective in the relief of stress-related ailments, pain, nerve pain, muscle pain, joint pain, stiffness, back and neck pain, and is ideal for the release of tension, increased circulation and reduced pain. Some medical studies suggest it may be effective at helping manage motion sickness, nausea, and vomiting, for helping neck and lower back pain, tension headaches, and stomachache.

I think that this therapy goes beyond just knowing the technique. If the practitioner has "good energy" and somehow can transmit it, the treatment can be very beneficial.

In the hands of an expert practitioner, acupressure points have also been employed to increase arousal, decrease sexual tension and reportedly aid in alleviating sexual dysfunction, including infertility, decreased sexual desire, premature ejaculation, and impotence.

Other benefits provided by this therapy are improvement in anxiety, carpal tunnel, colic, and hiccups.

As much as it is recommended by many, some publications affirm that its results and effectiveness are unreliable and that many of the claims are biased.

My opinion is that, as with other techniques, some people may benefit from it while others may not. Since it is not an invasive technique, a patient facing any of the problems outlined above should consider giving it a try.

My advice to you: if after you have seen your doctor and found that nothing major is happening and you have a chance to try acupressure; try it.

Shiatsu

This is a form of Chinese acupressure modified by Japanese therapists. It is based on traditional Chinese medicine and on the similar acupuncture points that are along the energy channels called meridians. The shiatsu therapist uses massage and then applies his or her thumbs to those points, encouraging the energy flow. The technique also uses joint stretching and manipulation as well as mobilization and deep massage. Hence, it is a therapy based on acupressure but being modified and more complete.

Like in acupuncture and acupressure, the theory behind shiatsu is that our bodies are made up of flowing energy, called Qi, that can become blocked and cause high pressure, pain, and suffering. Shiatsu finger pressure and massage help remove the blockages by realigning meridian points, improving energy flow, and thus balance the Qi and ease body and mind. When one balances Qi or vital energy, healing occurs in the body. The nervous and immune systems are both stimulated by applying pressure to the meridians, providing relief for both body and mind. Shiatsu also restores the circulatory system, improving blood flow throughout the body.

Many reports state that this form of therapy offers no medical benefits and affirm that it is useless. However, in my opinion, Shiatsu is a non-invasive therapy that may help reduce stress, decrease pain, and contribute to overall well-being. It can be used in the treatment of a wide range of medical, musculoskeletal, and emotional conditions, like muscle stiffness, muscle injuries, low back pain, neck pain, neuropathies, joint disorders, shoulder pain, headaches, indigestion, and can even stimulate the nervous system and relieve anxiety, stress, insomnia, mental fatigue. It may even be beneficial for PMS and bowel disorders.

Shiatsu and Asian Bodywork Therapists (ABT) are located throughout the United States, often in the vicinity of a school. The highest credential for Shiatsu and ABT is the national certification exam for Asian Bodywork Therapy administered by the National Certification Commission for Acupuncture and Oriental Medicine (NCCAOM). Practitioners who pass this exam become a Diplomate of ABT. The website for NCCAOM (https://www.nccaom.org) also has a Find a Practitioner page.

Reflexology

Reflexology is an alternative medicine technique involving the application of pressure to the feet and hands with specific thumb, finger, and hand motions without the use of oil or lotion. It is based on the concept that certain zones and reflex areas of the hands and feet correspond to areas of the body, and therefore, manipulation of those areas would bring improvement to the related ailing areas. This idea is not widely accepted and many call this type of therapy an unproven modality without a scientific background. Concerns have been raised by medical professionals that treating potentially serious illnesses with reflexology, which has no proven efficacy, could delay the seeking of appropriate medical treatment.

However, many others describe its benefits as remarkable.

Interestingly this technique started many centuries ago both in China and Egypt and that several tribes of Native American Indians practiced it as well. Nevertheless, it only became popular in this country in the mid-'70s.

There is no consensus among reflexologists on how reflexology is supposed to work; a unifying theme is that areas on the foot correspond to areas of the body and that by manipulating these, one can improve health by improving the energy flow.

Reflexologists divide the body into ten equal vertical zones, five on the right and five on the left.

Addressing muscle pains, headaches, poor circulation, fatigue, pain, arthritis, digestion problems, the technician searches for sensitivity or tenderness in certain areas of the foot, which usually indicates bodily weaknesses or imbalances within a corresponding organ or anatomic area. With repeated practice of applying pressure and manipulating nerve endings, a reflexologist can help to clear any channels of blocked energy through moving the flow of blood, nutrients, and nerve impulses to ultimately improve overall health and balance.

Reflexology can help in allergies, rhinitis, back pain, colic, constipation, gastritis, fatigue, cough, indigestion, insomnia, stress, PMS, IBS, hay fever, asthma, pain, arthritis, impotence, bladder disorders, and sinusitis. Reflexology may reduce pain and psychological symptoms, such as anxiety and depression, and enhance relaxation and sleep. Studies also show that reflexology may have benefits in palliative care of people with cancer.

It can be used alone, but it works better when combined with other forms of therapy. Practitioners of reflexology include chiropractors, physical therapists, and massage therapists, among others.

Craniosacral Therapy

Craniosacral Therapy is a very gentle form of alternative medicine designed to release tensions deep in the body to relieve pain and dysfunction. It was developed by Osteopathic Physician John E. Upledger, an academic professor of biomechanics, after years of clinical testing and research on variations of the old cranial osteopathy techniques.

Using a very soft and light touch practitioners release restrictions in the soft tissues that surround the central nervous system. The technique uses very light touches to torso, spine and pelvic bones that, as they say, modulates the flow of the cerebrospinal fluid

Many consider it a useless form of therapy, stating that there is no scientific basis for any of the practitioners' claims that the technique is really helpful and that all positive claims are biased or come just from the benefits of temporary relaxation.

We know that the central nervous system is heavily influenced by the craniosacral system, which includes the membranes and fluid that surround, protect, and nourish the brain and spinal cord. As we live our life, our body endures stresses and strains and also occasionally injuries. Frequently, these changes can cause body tissues to tighten and distort the craniosacral system, bringing on ill-effects to nerves, brain, and spinal cord, creating distortions and tensions in these structures. These distortions and tensions can result in restrictions in the functions of cranial nerves and the brain itself and can create a barrier to the healthy performance of the central nervous system, and potentially every other system it interacts with. Left on its own, this dysfunction may end up affecting the pituitary and pineal glands, with all the possible hormonal imbalance that may result.

Fortunately, such restrictions can be evaluated, detected, and even corrected using simple methods of touch. With a light touch, the CST practitioner uses his or her hands to evaluate the craniosacral system by gently feeling various locations of the body to test for the ease of motion and rhythm of the cerebrospinal fluid pulsing around the brain and spinal cord. Soft-touch techniques are then used to release restrictions in any tissues influencing the craniosacral system.

Craniosacral Therapy can be a very useful modality alone or combined with conventional medical care or other forms of alternative medicine. It has been useful in a wide variety of health problems and it claims that clinical improvement occurs thanks to the reestablishment of proper motion of all tissues that influence the craniosacral system

By normalizing the environment around the brain and spinal cord and enhancing the body's ability to self-correct, Craniosacral Therapy uses hands-on methods to alleviate a wide variety of dysfunctions, from chronic pain and sports injuries to stroke and neurological impairment.

This technique claims to be effective in treating:

- ADD
- Autism
- Brain and Spinal Cord Injuries
- Chronic Fatigue
- Chronic Neck and Back Pain
- Concussions
- Fibromyalgia
- Headaches
- Infant and Childhood Disorders
- Learning disabilities
- Migraines
- Motor-Coordination Impairments
- Orthopedic Problems.
- Post-Traumatic Stress Disorder
- Scoliosis
- Stress and Tension-Related Disorders
- TMJ Syndrome
- Traumatic Brain Injuries

Should you try it? My answer is yes, but do what I did. Make a list of the practitioners in your area, then go and try one and then another until you find the one you connect with.

Yes: it is the same story with craniosacral therapists, chiropractors, acupuncturists, yoga studios, reflexologists, and with all alternative medicine practitioners. Not all of them are good. You will have to try a few until you find the one that is good, effective, and congenial. But, isn't this the same problem with medical doctors, attorneys, architects, and other professionals? Alternative practitioners are just humans, too. Not all of them are good and congenial. Go meet some and find one you like.

Myofascial Release

This form of therapy is a gentle treatment performed directly on the skin. It enables the therapist to accurately detect fascial restrictions and apply the appropriate amount of sustained pressure to facilitate the release of the fascia.

It is a therapy you need to try. It is a safe and very effective hands-on technique that involves a form of deep localized massage that applies gentle sustained pressure into the fascia and connective tissue to eliminate restriction and pain and restore motion.

The fascia is a thin, tough, elastic sheet of connective tissue that wraps most structures within the human body, it extends like a layer between skin and muscles and also penetrates deep into limbs and the body separating muscles and surrounding organs. It covers nerves, veins, arteries, and even essential organs. It is one continuous structure that exists from head to toe without interruption. Each part of the entire body is connected to every other part by the fascia.

This fascia plays an important role in the support and function of our bodies since it surrounds and attaches to all structures. In the normal healthy state, the fascia is relaxed and wavy in configuration. It can stretch and move without restriction.

When one experiences physical trauma, injury, scarring, a sprain, or inflammation, either caused by daily activities, sports injuries, trauma, inflammatory responses, surgical procedures, etc., the lesions can create restrictions in this fascia, called Myofascial restrictions. These can produce tension and pressure on sensitive structures, causing spasms, pain, inflammation, and restricted motions. These restrictions will NOT show up in regular X-rays, myelograms, CAT scans or, MRIs. The fascia then loses its pliability and becomes tight, restricted, and a source of tension to the rest of the body.

The Myofascial pain that occurs can have different sources. It can be generated from the skeletal muscle or connective tissues that are attached to the fascia. It can be generated from damaged myofascial tissue itself, or it can be related to tension in the affected organ. In either case, the restriction or contraction inhibits blood flow to the affected structures, thus accentuating the contraction process further unless the area is treated. The specific technique of release to different parts of the body varies, but generally includes gentle application of pressure or sustained low-load stretch to the affected area. During myofascial release therapy, the therapist locates myofascial areas that feel stiff and fixed instead of elastic and movable under light manual pressure. These areas, though not always near what feels like the source of pain, are thought to restrict muscle and joint movements, that contribute to widespread muscle pain. The therapist will begin massaging and stretching the areas that feel rigid with light manual pressure, that stretches and loosens up restricted movements. The therapist then aids the tissue and supportive sheath in releasing pressure and tightness. The process is repeated multiple times on the same trigger point and other trigger points until the therapist feels the tension is fully released. During a typical Myofascial Release session, the therapist uses a multitude of techniques designed to decrease stiffness and improve flexibility, strength, and movements.

When I tried it, it felt just like that. The therapist massaged the affected areas, sinking her fingers in specific points where she did deep stretching through pressure, releasing the restricted areas. She loosened up problem areas and my low back, hips, and thighs felt a lot better. The effect was beneficial and lasting.

A high percentage of people suffering from pain, arthritis, lack of motion, stiffness, and neuropathy may be having fascial problems, but are not diagnosed.

Many different types of health professionals can provide myofascial release therapy, including appropriately trained osteopathic physicians, chiropractors, physical or occupational therapists, massage therapists, or sports medicine/injury specialists.

Myofascial therapy can be given alone but is best when combined with other forms of therapy. It can enhance the benefits provided by other treatments like acupuncture, chiropractic manipulation, massage, acupressure, and physical therapy, especially if the treatment is given simultaneously by a professional. Myofascial release therapy can also improve skeletal and muscular alignment before surgery, or during rehabilitation, and even help athletes achieve better alignment before sports competitions.

Myofascial release therapy may be helpful for back pain, for treating myofascial pain syndrome, which is a chronic pain disorder caused by sensitivity and tightness of tissues and muscles throughout the body. The pain usually originates from specific points within the fascia, called "trigger points."

Myofascial release focuses on reducing pain by easing the tension and tightness at the trigger points.

It shows beneficial effects for headaches, neck and back pain, fibromyalgia, repetitive strain injuries, sports injuries, muscular imbalances, muscular pain, pelvic misalignment, neuropathies, muscle weakness secondary to chronic neuropathy.

Contraindications: osteoporosis, fresh injuries, burns, aneurysm, healing fractures, deep vein thrombosis, and taking blood thinners.

Massage

Dynamic moving compression of the body and limbs is the fundamental medium of massage. There are many kinds of massage, some are therapeutic, some are not. Sure, a good massage is always welcome, even if it is just for comfort, relaxation, or something else, but here I will address the ones used for managing arthritis, pain, and injuries. A little warning, if the injury is fresh, let's say a torn muscle or sprained joint that happened a day or two earlier, don't massage it, leave it alone, rest that limb as much as you can, and follow my Introduction to Inflammation, and Nutrition chapters. You can also use acupuncture alone or with electrical stimuli, to help the tissue fibers reattach and heal. If the wound is fresh, after surgery or trauma, don't massage.

Massage Therapy is a hands-on manipulation of soft tissues of the body, muscles, and joint structures for medical purposes like aiding in healing, improving pain control, aiding in digestion and breathing, enhancing well-being, assisting in blood and lymphatic flow, decreasing inflammation and aiding in injury relief. Professional massage therapy may also alleviate mental problems, immune dysfunction, stress, and insomnia. Other indications include back pain, headaches, arthritis, sprains, stress, fatigue, gastrointestinal disorders, restless legs, and more.

Since massage is not attached to specific medical or integrative care protocol, practitioners in different countries have no regulations controlling them and are therefore able to expand, vary, and modify their skills at will. Hence, we now have close to a hundred different types of massage and of course, each one claims to be the best. Over the last forty to fifty years, with the increment in travel, communication, and creativity, many types of massage became popular, including variations practiced by certain ethnic groups or popular in just certain countries. The mechanism of action may differ according to the massage technique of the different cultures around the world, although the basic principle is similar. In addition to all this, there are different kinds of massage therapists (nurses, physical therapists, plain therapists, chiropractors, etc.), different kinds of massage (as I describe here), different places to get massages (offices, home centers, clinics, home visits, spas, oriental studios, doctor's offices, resorts, hotels, athletic clubs, hair salons, etc.) and in all kinds of different settings. Some add exotic furniture, music, and special aromas to enhance the effects.

Recently, my daughter was in Cambodia and got a "Cambodian massage." She described it as a combination of regular massage with chiropractic manipulation and shiatsu. The therapist cracked her back efficiently. My daughter felt great for several days. Interesting.

The best way to use massage for medical-healing purposes is:

a) To see a therapist proficient in different kinds of techniques, who will be able to apply variations of his/her massage according to your particular problem. If the therapist is good at combining the massage with some acupressure, myofascial release, or other therapies, that is the therapist you want to use.

b) To combine this therapy with other therapies, like chiropractor's manipulation, nutrition, adrenal management, anti-inflammatories, sauna, detoxification, etc.

Deep Tissue Massage

Used for chronic muscular tension and injuries. It uses slow motions, direct deep pressure, and friction. It is a very specific type of massage treatment in which the therapist uses knuckles and elbows to manipulate muscle tissue as far down to the bone as possible. It is a bit invasive and not for everyone. This modality can be helpful to the following people: athletes who are considerably harder on their bodies than the average person, people who are undergoing physical therapy to aid in the breakdown process of scar tissue, or anyone who has very dense tissue and needs this kind of therapy. It is especially helpful for chronically tense and contracted areas such as stiff necks, low back tightness, stiff and sore shoulders. Indications include chronic pain, chronic stiffness, recovery from sports injuries, postural disorders, fibromyalgia, and chronic muscle tensions.

Deep tissue massage uses many of the same movements and techniques as Swedish massage, but the pressure will generally be more intense. It is also a more focused type of massage, as the therapist works to release chronic muscle tension or "knots" (also known as "adhesions"). In individuals who suffered chronic muscle injuries, there are usually adhesions (bands of tender fibers) between muscles, tendons, and ligaments, that can block circulation, lymphatic flow, and can cause pain and inflammation. Deep tissue massage works by physically breaking down these adhesions to relieve pain and restore normal movement. To do this, the massage therapist uses direct deep pressure or friction applied across the muscles and deep structures that often triggers some discomfort and pain. This soreness is an inevitable part of the therapy.

Swedish Massage

Uses slow and long gliding motions, with rather superficial friction. Motions are in the direction of the blood flow. It is mainly used to provide relaxation, improve muscle function, and relieve muscle tension and it is excellent for stress management. This technique is frequently found in hotels and spas, and the therapists frequently use fragrant oils, baby oils, and combined aromatherapy. Beneficial effects are enhanced with additional acupressure or shiatsu.

But Swedish massage therapy goes beyond relaxation. Swedish massage is exceptionally beneficial for increasing the level of oxygen in the blood, decreasing muscle toxins, improving circulation and flexibility while easing tension. Studies show that it may decrease the levels of the stress hormone cortisol, and it can boost the immune system.

A Swedish massage can be slow and gentle, or vigorous and bracing, depending on the therapist's style and what he or she is trying to achieve. The therapist lubricates the skin with massage oil, sometimes aromatic, and performs various massage strokes and soft compressions, releasing tension and gradually relaxing the muscles. The massage type may vary according to whether you are in a spa, hotel, professional massage center, or at a physical therapy center getting a massage for specific medical conditions.

Lymphatic Drainage
Used for inflammation, detoxification, edema, and neuropathies. The therapist applies special strokes and pressure to encourage lymphatic flow. With an increase of lymph flow, immune function is increased, and harmful substances are removed from the tissues and neutralized in the lymph nodes. It is said that this technique stimulates increased production of lymphocytes, thus enhancing immune function.

This technique can also be applied to people who are suffering from a lack of energy, fatigue, and inflammation. Continued applications of lymphatic drainage, while the person is healing from injuries and limb inflammation due to arthritis, can help to enhance the tissue regeneration process by keeping the tissue as healthy as possible.

The use of lymphatic drainage has another application: detoxification. In this contaminated world where we live, the accumulation of toxins in our tissues affects body energy, hormones, and general health. Using this technique alone or at the same time as other forms of full body massage, may help mobilize and eliminate some of these toxins aiding in the process of detoxification. This improves general health, decreases fatigue, and immune dysfunction.

Contraindications: acute inflammation, tumors, thrombosis, active heart disease, infection, and cellulitis.

Oriental Massage

Uses motions and pressure combinations according to different Asian techniques.

One variation is the Chinese Massage, which uses specific rubbing, grasping, and kneading on specific points to relieve muscle tension and balance yin and yang to improve the bio-energy (Qi). Tibetan Massage is performed on the spine, abdomen, head, and neck and seeks to regulate the pressure between organs and brain, improving breathing, digestion, and bowel function; it also aims to improve mental conditions, stress, provide relaxation and improve sleep.

Neuromuscular Massage

A form of deep massage applied to individual muscles attempting to reduce knots and release trigger points. It consists of alternating levels of concentrated pressure on the areas of muscle spasm. The massage therapy pressure is usually applied with the fingers, knuckles, or elbow. The therapist applies even more pressure than in other types of massage. It is used in cases of pain, neuropathies, nerve entrapments, and gait disorders.

This is a more modern form of massage therapy, based on understanding how the neuromuscular system functions.

It uses a very detailed and strong massage of muscles, tendons, ligaments, connective tissue, etc., using thumbs, fingertips, elbows, and forearms. Tense muscles often form bands of muscle fibers even tighter than the rest. These are areas of hypertonicity and ischemia. Searching thoroughly, the practitioners can feel bands of tight muscle fibers; the areas that are in the most trouble. These are found and treated until they release.

European Massage

Very similar to Swedish massage, European massage uses gliding strokes combined with rubbing and percussion. Movements are slow and soft. It's probably the most commonly known massage therapy style, providing a simple, relaxing technique with fantastic benefits for overall well-being. Primarily defined by the style of stroke applied, European massage has five basic styles of sliding and gliding type strokes, like the one called "effleurage" which is a fancy French word meaning "to skim" or "light touch" and consists of stroking with varying pressure. The friction technique uses deep muscular stimulation by using rolling and compression movements. The main purpose of this light, skimming touch is to warm up the muscles and encourage the veins and lymphatic system to return blood to the heart. Then there is "petrissage" which is a kneading motion using circular movements, wringing, and light squeezing. These movements are slightly deeper with some applied pressure designed to compress the underlying muscles. Tapotement (another French reference meaning to tap or drum) is a technique that uses rhythmic movements like beating and tapping specific to European massage and most easily recognized by its rhythmic application with the edge or a cupped hand and sometimes with just the tips of the fingers. On occasion, the therapist will use vibration, done by hand, or by using an electrical vibrator to facilitate relaxation.

Thai Massage

This is an ancient healing system thought to have been developed by Buddhist monks in Thailand 2,500 years ago.

It combines acupressure, Indian Ayurvedic principles, and assisted yoga postures. Traditional Thai massage uses no oils or lotions and the recipient remains clothed during the session. It uses passive stretching and gentle pressure along the body's energy lines to increase flexibility, relieve muscle and joint tension, and balance the body's energy systems.

There is constant body contact between the giver and receiver, but rather than rubbing on muscles, the body is compressed, pulled, stretched, and rocked.

Thai massage typically works with compression – rhythmic pressing movements directed into muscle tissues by either the hand or fingers. Thai massage usually takes place on a futon mat on the floor, with the client wearing loose or stretchy clothing like yoga gear.

The therapist Is also on the mat and moves your body into various stretches and positions, without any work on your part. This is why it is sometimes called "lazy man's yoga." Thai massage can be both relaxing and energizing, so it is a good choice if you want to be active after your massage.

The therapist uses a variety of different techniques on clients, who are either laying face up, laying face down, seated, or on their side.

Gyrotonics

Now, here we are getting into something different. You may need to search "Gyrotonics" on YouTube to see what it is.

Gyrotonics is an original and unique movement method that addresses the entire person, decreasing stiffness, opening energy pathways, stimulating the nervous system, increasing range of motion, and improving strength. The Gyrotonic Method is practiced in groups or private classes under the instruction of a qualified Gyrotonic Trainer. A specialized line of wooden equipment, consisting of weights and pulleys, is used to facilitate natural movements, provide resistance and elongate muscles, while the instructor guides the patient through circular and fluid exercises that stretch and strengthen skeletal muscles, tendons and ligaments. Those wooden machines carry rotational discs and weighted pulleys, facilitating the movements and allowing the exerciser to improve joint and muscle functions using flowing, circular movements with arms, legs, hips, and shoulders. Exercises start with movements at the base of the spine and progress to the arms, neck, and shoulders. Pulleys with straps are attached to your feet as your legs are stretched and strengthened, while at the same time encouraging movement in the abdominal muscles. Then later on your shoulders are strapped the same way while arms and torso exercises follow. Special attention is focused on spinal motions to increase mobility and stability of the spine and pelvis.

I have tried Gyrotonics and still attend the sessions every so often. After my last back and hip injuries (from a soccer match I knew I should not have participated in), I was able to control pain with some of the therapies I mention in this book, but running and jogging became prohibitive. It was thanks to Gyrotonics that I was able to return to the field and I was able to run again.

I urge you to check gyrotonic.com.

Gyrotonics was developed based on principles of yoga, Tai chi, dance, swimming, and gymnastics. The repetitive circular movements are designed to increase muscular capacity, correct imbalances, deformities, and enhance overall body mechanics.

This therapy is ideal for individuals with neuropathy, back pain, disc diseases, neck pain, scoliosis, hip disorders, and it is recommended for dancers, golfers, soccer players, athletes, individuals who need rehabilitation. It improves posture, spinal flexibility, hip dysfunction, stiffness, and shoulder problems.

With Gyrotonic exercises, each movement flows into the next, allowing the joints to move through a natural range of motion without jarring or compression. These carefully crafted sequences create balance, efficiency, strength, and flexibility.

Reiki

Reiki is an ancient Japanese form of natural healing that focuses on energy. It consists of the therapist laying their hands on the patient. There is no massaging or rubbing. The therapist first lays the hands on the head of the patient for a few minutes and then moves them down the body all the way to the toes. It is based on the concept of modulating the inner energy, or Qi, that flows through the body. This is indeed interesting, as we can see there are several types of therapies based on the same concept of "the energy flowing through channels in our body." Western medicine does not accept this idea; however, western medicine is just a few centuries old while the idea of flowing energy, Qi, is several thousand years old.

Reiki treats the whole person including body, emotions, mind, and spirit creating many beneficial effects that include relaxation and feelings of peace, security, and well-being. It is a simple, natural, and safe method of spiritual healing and self-improvement that everyone can use. It has been effective in helping virtually every known illness and malady and always creates a beneficial effect. It also works in conjunction with all other medical or therapeutic techniques to relieve side effects and promote recovery.

Special Exercises

Tai chi and yoga represent a class of exercise that differs from the classic "stretching-flexibility-strengthening" programs currently employed by conventional medicine. They bring many benefits and are highly recommended for the appropriate patient. Both yoga and Tai chi originated in South Asia; they are highly successful complementary therapies with centuries of knowledge and proficiency behind them. Both incorporate a mind-body approach to the rehabilitation of disorders like pain, injury, arthritis, and multiple neuromuscular disorders. They are also extremely effective for reducing stress. Yoga and Tai chi include movement in slow motion, body positions, meditation, and breathing techniques – but they are far more than that. When done properly, they affect the energy of the body and mind. Indeed, yoga and Tai chi are like icebergs: they are a lot deeper than they appear. To enjoy the benefits of yoga and Tai chi, you must understand them and accept their principles. As a first step, you need to accept a difficult concept to visualize and comprehend: your bio-electricity is not like a battery driving your heart, but rather like a flow of vital forces that run through your body like a river. Most people are oblivious to it, but it is there, flowing like water through your limbs, skin, and organs. Tai chi and yoga, in their different ways, exert an influence on this flow of energy, providing strong and highly favorable effects. They offer additional benefits to each of the Jupiter Institute Pain Program therapies that we describe in this book. Both require careful instruction.

The following exercise programs, Yoga, Tai chi, and Qigong, were designed to provide significant metabolic improvement to those who practice them. This improvement can translate into enjoying a state of well-being, the prevention of health complications, or helping whatever therapy the person utilizing. These three exercises bring on all kinds of benefits, but they should not be the main therapy for medical conditions. They are assistants, aides, and supporters of the main therapy, but regardless of what you may read on certain websites and publications, they cannot be the only therapy. The main medical problem affecting the patient can be a limb problem (arthritis, sprain, etc.), a neurological, respiratory, or digestive disorder, and the treatment might be medical and/or alternative medicine combined. Then any of these three exercise modalities can be used to help manage the condition. They will make the disorder more manageable and they might even accelerate the healing while providing more comfort and well-being. They will make your body, soul, and mind stronger and better adapted to confront whatever is ailing you. Use these exercises wisely and with common sense. They are NOT for acute problems or very recent injuries or surgeries.

Yoga

Like it or not, when we focus on pain management yoga is controversial. Beyond all those wonderful yoga studios, books, and websites, too many articles have been written about injuries caused by this modality. That is the reason why I didn't include it in my first book. I needed to give it some thought, read more about it, and then perhaps have the guts to try it.

Yoga is neither a religion nor just a series of postures. It is a philosophy of life and a powerful system of self-awareness that uses low-impact activity. The motions and positions that are so typical of yoga represent just a portion of this otherwise very complex mind-body program. Yoga's capacity to increase good health and well-being is well-documented, with numerous books and journals attesting to its medical benefits. For many people, yoga has proven to be a safe and effective way to alleviate many forms of neck and back pain. Yoga can provide several healing benefits for people with various types of strain. It can also help in the healing of injured muscles and in decreasing the recovery time after an injury. Studies have shown that yoga may provide a treatment option for patients with osteoarthritis by decreasing pain and disability. More than 75 trials have been published about yoga in major medical journals. These studies have shown that yoga is a safe and effective way to increase physical activity and muscular strength, improve flexibility, and promote relaxation. It increases body energy and decreases aches and pains. Yoga is a meditative form of exercise that stretches and strengthens muscles, increases range of motion, improves circulation, empowers the natural power of the human body, and significantly enhances the quality of life. There are many styles of yoga – from gentle to athletic – practiced today. Beginners should always stick with gentle styles of yoga. Yoga teaches the basic concept of mind-body unity: if the body is sick and suffering, mental health will be affected, and if the mind is stressed and agitated, the health of the body will be compromised. Hence, the integrated healing of mind and body is the main goal in the practice of yoga.

Background. Yoga originated in India some 5,000 years ago, which makes it perhaps the oldest mind-body health program known to man. It combines philosophical ideas, spiritual concepts about bio-energy, and physical exercises that were taken from observation, experience, and immense knowledge. Yoga was developed as a way to access, build, and nurture our natural energies. It was created also as a philosophical compilation of techniques, positions, and motions that provide spiritual advancement and a practical way of self-improvement. Various schools of yoga emphasize different techniques, but they all teach a methodical practice of breathing, meditation, contemplation, physical postures, mental concentration, and a path to awakening spiritual awareness.

Practice. Many hospitals across our nation provide yoga classes for multiple purposes. Cedars Sinai Medical Center in Los Angeles encourages yoga as a way to improve cardiovascular disease, decrease blood pressure, and improve blood sugar control. They use yoga for their cardiac rehabilitation patients. Stress reduction and relief from fatigue are two of the many benefits of yoga. Some centers offer yoga as a way to improve fertility; others offer it for people suffering from pain or recovering from injury. Researchers at the UCLA Medical Center in Los Angeles found that just four weeks of regular yoga sessions significantly reduced the frequency and severity of chronic pain. Today's yoga participants are young and old, flexible and stiff, slim and overweight, men and women. They are everyday people who are just like you, but who want to treat their bodies well and cure their ailments without pills, doctors, or side effects. Yoga is especially good for people with arthritis and pain because these conditions tend to reduce confidence and self-esteem while yoga increases them. Multiple publications have reported that yoga improves strength and flexibility, decreases stress and anxiety, and is an excellent tool for pain management. A study at the Western Virginia School of Medicine analyzed the effect of yoga therapy for lower back pain and found that patients practicing yoga experience a reduction in pain intensity, functional disability, and they use less pain medication.

Some of the Beneficial Clinical Effects of Yoga:

- Cardiovascular: decreased heartbeat and blood pressure
- Musculoskeletal: increased strength, flexibility and range of motion of joints, and improved balance
- Joints: relief for stiff, damaged and arthritic joints
- Mind and Nervous System: enhanced alertness, memory, concentration and focus, less fatigue and stress, greater relaxation and lower emotional tension
- Lungs: more efficient breathing and blood oxygenation
- Digestion: better digestion and less constipation
- Pain: reduction in pain and improvement in painful conditions through beneficial stimulation of the pain center (the part of the brain responsible for sending messages to areas of the body)

A word of warning. Although practicing yoga brings many benefits, the number of injuries caused by this exercise is increasing. Doctors and physiotherapists are reporting an upsurge in the number of inexperienced students injuring themselves after straining to get into difficult positions. This may be due to improperly trained instructors and over-motivated, eager-to-perform students. Yoga injuries are mainly caused by strain and over-stretching of ligaments, tendons, nerves, and muscles. It is recommended to join only yoga centers in which the instructors are fully trained, certified, and proficient; learning from poorly trained instructors at sports centers is strongly discouraged. Find a qualified instructor, and avoid pushing your body too fast or too hard to reach positions that you are not accustomed to. Progressing slowly while reducing the need to compete are both extremely important in yoga.

The opportunity came about when once again my passion for soccer left me in pain. After many years of soccer and basketball, with all the running, physical contact and falls, nature finally caught up with me, and my years of joint abuse led me to develop knee pain and back problems in the lower lumbar area. Therefore, as I was getting treatment from a chiropractor friend of mine and an acupuncturist, I thought it was time to open my mind, read more about yoga, and even try it. The experience opened my mind even more and now I must accept the beneficial effects these classes had. My knee and back got considerably better, and it is time for me to acknowledge this already well-recognized modality of therapy. Hence this chapter.

Yoga is definitively an optional therapeutic modality for those suffering from pain and arthritis.

However, it is not for every pain, and it isn't for every arthritis. Yoga is good, yes, but it is not for everyone.

Besides, as I am starting to understand, it is not just a therapy but a mind-body healing practice. Let me make this point a little clearer. Yoga is not a therapy for arthritis, injures or inflammation, or for recent sprains, tears, trauma, post-surgery, or any acute neuromuscular disorder. Rather, yoga, just like Tai chi and Qigong, are helpers and aids in the final (not early) steps of recovery.

It will help you to understand yoga better if you accept a more modern approach regarding the roots of pain and joint disorders.

Pain, distress, and emotional processing centers of the brain are affected by the neurological impulses coming from the problem areas. Some of this cascade of events involves the stress reaction that might start an adrenal-cortisol cascade bringing a whole variety of adverse events arising from adrenal dysfunction. Directly or indirectly an imbalance in neurotransmitters may follow, pushing the individual to further mood changes, metabolic distress, and other physiologic misfortunes. The adverse effect of combined adrenal disorder and brain chemical imbalance promotes a surge of free radicals and inflammatory molecules that hurts the problem area and the body as a whole. And there you have it. The presence of the mind-body connections will involve a complexity of metabolic and hormonal reactions that are going to make the arthritic joint, the pain or injury area even worse. Although this complexity sounds discouraging, it opens the gate for the beneficial effects of yoga, that might not be able to heal the injury itself but may improve some of the biological, hormonal and neurological phenomena associated with it, therefore providing a substantial contribution to the healing process. Also, yoga improves the brain chemical (neurotransmitter) balance and ameliorates the adrenal reaction, that brings on beneficial effects on inflammation and free radical control.

A recent review by Duke University examined the effects of yoga in different joint diseases and found it effective in the treatment of pain and osteoarthritis. In this research study, it was found that when performed correctly yoga can improve painful joints, decrease stiffness and swelling, increase mobility, and relieve general discomfort.

Performed correctly, some of the yoga poses are even more beneficial. Combining poses, breathing, relaxation, and meditation distracts your mind from pain, stretches your muscles and tendons, reduces the body's tension, brings on relaxation, and improves circulation.

Paths

There are four paths in yoga, each with a different purpose. "Bhakti" yoga is the way of love and devotion to the Divine. "Jnana" yoga is dedicated to the search for knowledge about life. "Karma" yoga is dedicated to encouraging students to find union with the Supreme or Divine spirit through selfless actions. And "Hatha" yoga is the system with the "asanas" or postures and is the one most familiar in our western society. It is the one we know and see in magazines, TV, books, etc.

Some of the positions, or poses "asanas," provide extra benefits. The Butterfly pose, sitting and bringing the soles of the feet together and knees wide open, while keeping the back straight, is beneficial for hip pain. The Supported Warrior pose, standing and placing hands against the wall like pushing it, then relaxing and taking slow deep breaths, is beneficial for knee pain. The Cobra pose is good for back pain and some other poses may be good for shoulders and elbows as well. The "Balasana," child's posture, relaxes the back and promotes healing of back injuries. The posterior stretch, sitting and bending over to grab the ankles, stimulates the abdomen and the digestive system. Keeping and holding the pose called "half spinal twist" and then focusing on deep breathing, relaxes the lower spinal area. But there are over 1,000 poses "asanas" in yoga, ranging from simple postures to more difficult ones, all designed to help body organs to function more efficiently, clear the mind, favor healing processes and promote a state of well-being. In class, the asanas are held for a certain length of time, combined with deep slow breathing, allowing the mind to focus, promoting relaxation and calmness while stretching muscles and tendons.

Today, with consistent and dedicated practice, individuals can appreciate reduced stress, improved health and energy, feelings of well-being, and the healing or amelioration of diseases in the body.

You may like yoga or you may not, and you may or may not accept it, but I tell you that if it wasn't a good exercise-therapy modality, it wouldn't have been so accepted and now practiced worldwide.

These pages bring you just a short introduction to yoga and I encourage you to explore the many books, publications, and websites on the matter.

Styles

There are many styles in Hatha Yoga, although they all focus on the main principles of postures, breathing, coordination, alignment, and meditation. Sivananda Yoga, developed by Vishnu-Devananda, is the largest yoga school and follows a combination of breathing, postures, and relaxation. Anusara Yoga, more modern, promotes spiritual orientation.

Bikram Yoga is a series of asanas practiced in a room heated to 105 degrees temperature, where the heat allows better stretching of muscle and tendons while the sweat detoxifies the body. Ashtanga Yoga is the Power Yoga and it is a physically demanding exercise designed to provide a serious workout. Iyengar Yoga focuses on alignment while Kripalu Yoga is a variant of classic Hatha Yoga with accentuated focus on meditation and a higher level of consciousness. Vini Yoga is a gentler form of yoga, with emphasis on coordination and more simple asanas. Kundalini Yoga is more modern and focuses on a controlled release of energy (be careful with this one; some of its yoga poses, when performed too often or incorrectly, have been associated with some mental adverse effects, like headaches, confusion, anxiety, depression, etc. Never start with Kundalini unless you are well-informed).

Even in Hatha Yoga, the most popular one, we find variations like Gentle Hatha, Yin Yoga, Organic Vinyasa, Restorative Yoga, and others, providing the student with a variety of options to choose the one he or she feels more comfortable with.

Before you start, find out WHAT STYLE of yoga you will be attending, and have it explained to you by the owner or instructor of the studio.

Starting Yoga

Read about it first. There is a ton of information on the Internet.

Don't just throw yourself into yoga but rather search among the studios in your area. Visit them and talk to the instructors. Find out what type of yoga they offer and what styles are offered in their different classes.

The combination of positions, that we call poses or "asanas," combined with breathing practices, known as "pranayama," are generically called "Hatha Yoga." It is the most popular in the U.S., and it is the one you want to start with.

Choose a Beginning class of Gentle Yoga and discuss with the instructor your physical limitations, your areas of pain, or your health conditions to find out whether your chosen class is adequate. Ask about appropriate clothing.

The beginners' class will combine students with varied experience and flexibility. You will be following the guidance of your teacher while enjoying the three main components: positions, or poses "asanas," breathing techniques, and phases of relaxation. Some classes will also include music, chanting, and meditation. The integration of relaxation and meditation allows for stress relief, reduction of mind and body tension, spiritual awakening, and disengagement from daily worries. These are the essential components of the practice of yoga.

Dim light, candlelight, and incense are elements frequently used to help students tune into the session and disengage from daily stress and concerns.

Arrive early. Don't interrupt an ongoing class.

Again, if you have not been exercising, and you have significant joint problems, pain, or injuries, or you know you are rather stiff, familiarize yourself with the studio and do research on the Internet BEFORE you start. Joining the wrong class, trying to achieve difficult poses, and pushing your body too hard may end up causing severe discomfort and even injuries.

It is important to know that yoga is not competitive. Different students will follow the asanas according to their abilities and limitations. Don't force yourself to be like experienced students. The old saying "no pain, no gain" should not be applied here. Listen to your body, avoid pain, and be gentle. Don't go beyond your limitations. Look at what other students are doing for guidance but not for "showing that you can do it too." If the pose is too difficult or complicated or one or more of your joints is hurting, then don't do it, just sit, relax and wait till the next pose; just like I do.

BUT WAIT! – Not every published study agrees with the benefit of yoga for pain and arthritis. Some data from the National Institutes of Health questions the validity of many studies and claims they were not done correctly. Despite all those wonderful websites and books, some scientific studies show no improvement in pain and arthritis using this technique. We do agree that yoga improves well-being and brings on cardiovascular, metabolic, and neurological benefits, but when we address specifically the problem of pain and arthritis the opinions and the research studies are divided and the jury is out.

Also, there have been so many injuries related to yoga that many publications caution against it. Like it or not, the fact is that yoga can have negative side effects. Some of them are injuries to back, neck, knees and shoulders, exhaustion from the efforts, the strain of the asanas, and other adversities. You can find on the Internet several websites describing the dangers of yoga and you should review them as well. Whether you blame it on the instructor or the misinformed and unprepared fragile student, the fact remains that yoga has caused all kinds of injuries in thousands of persons...and you could be one of them.

Don't use yoga if you have a fresh injury, acute disease, or you are sick. Don't use it for new injuries, sprains, or new joint diseases. You should not use it if you have active inflammation, infection, recent surgery, or recent fracture.

Several articles recommend that the physically demanding postures of yoga should be avoided in those suffering acute diseases. Yoga meditation, while very beneficial, can be adverse in individuals with a psychiatric background since it has been described as causing mood changes, hallucinations, mania, depression, and even panic attacks. Individuals with osteoporosis or debilitated muscles or tendons can suffer fractures of delicate bones, ruptured muscles, strains, and even aggravated pain. Having written this, I will leave it up to you to decide whether to try it or not.

Tai chi

Tai chi is a form of exercise originally developed in China as a form of self-defense. Although it was initially designed as a form of martial arts training, it has evolved into a sequence of movements practiced in slow motion that bring on improvements in health and physical conditioning. The graceful form of this exercise is now used for stress reduction and better management of a variety of health complications.

Tai chi is a gentle exercise program that is part of traditional Chinese medicine. Derived from the martial arts, Tai chi is composed of slow, coordinated movements, meditation, and deep breathing, that help correct imbalances in joints, nerves, and muscles and enhance physical and psycho-emotional health. Practicing it encourages positive biological and psychological effects for people of all ages. Many studies, journals, and books state that Tai chi improves neuromuscular function, lessens the pain of arthritis and fibromyalgia, and enhances flexibility and strength. Additionally, Tai chi is an excellent complementary therapy for a wide range of conditions, including gout, heart disease, hypertension, headaches, sleep disorders, anxiety, depression, stress, and even asthma.

History

The principles of Tai chi were born from a blending of Chinese martial arts with the philosophical ideas of Taoism. Tai chi is a combination of two antagonistic ideas: the sophistication of martial arts, that attempts to overpower and hurt the enemy, and the Taoist principles of gentleness and yielding. This synthesis was originated some eight centuries ago by a Taoist priest who used his fundamental wisdom of self-defense and philosophy to create the soft, slow movement of a non-combative martial art. This ancient form of movement is still a daily routine for millions of people across China. It was introduced to the United States in the early 1970s and has since grown in popularity. The idea behind this wonderful exercise is that the energy of the human body, Qi, flows in the body through many channels. When Qi flows properly, the body, mind, and spirit are in balance, and health is maintained. The slow movements of Tai chi facilitate the flow of this essential bio-energy through the body. Tai chi movements emphasize the importance of weight transference, which is an essential component of good balance. Through gentle and fluid movement, it improves posture, coordination, and gait.

Tai chi in Motion

Movement: slow, gentle movements, full of grace and coordination that look like both a dance and a slow-motion Chinese martial arts fight.

It involves a series of movements performed in a slow, focused manner and accompanied by deep breathing. It is a low impact exercise and puts minimal stress on muscles and joints, making it generally safe for all ages and fitness levels.

To understand Tai chi, we have to accept the concept of the yin, yang, and Qi, that relate to the energy forces within the human body.

Yin is a feminine force, negative, receptive, and dark, while yang is a masculine and more positive force, more creative and brighter. These two forces have to live in balance and harmony inside of us if we want to enjoy good health and be stable in body and mind, but forces outside our body can create an imbalance in them and hurt their harmony. This lack of harmony and the health conditions we encounter affect the flow of energy, the Qi, within us, bringing on numerous medical complaints. The continuous and connected movements of Tai chi seek to re-establish the harmony of yin and yang and facilitate the flow of Qi. This Qi is our life force. Only the living are imbued with Qi. A lack of flow of Qi leaves a person sluggish, tired, achy, or ill. With an abundance of Qi, the person feels vibrant, alive, energetic, and alert to the possibilities of life. Tai chi movements are a way to develop and increase this Qi and to bring harmony to yin and yang.

Tai chi has also been called the perfect exercise, although it is more than a simple exercise because of its philosophy and impact on health. Tai chi combines deep diaphragmatic breathing, dance-like movements, and poses, it can be a remarkably potent workout for people of many ages. It's accessible to everyone, regardless of age or fitness level. Its slow and fluid movements improve the body's alignment, posture, strength, flexibility, coordination, balance, and stamina.

I have taken Tai chi classes and found a positive effect on flexibility, energy, mental clarity, and recovery after exercise. As occidental and pragmatic as I am, it is not easy for me to comprehend all this yin, yang and Qi, however, I did feel the benefit. On many occasions, I still interrupt my jogging to perform some of the dance-like movements of this wonderful exercise. You don't need to totally understand Tai chi to enjoy its benefits. Go ahead and try it.

Benefits. In China, it is believed that Tai chi can delay aging and prolong life, increase flexibility, strengthen muscles and tendons, and aid in the treatment of heart disease, high blood pressure, arthritis, digestive disorders, skin diseases, depression, cancer, and many other illnesses. Tai chi has been found to improve both physical and psychosocial health and to improve practitioners' balance, leg strength, cardiovascular endurance, pulse rate, muscular flexibility, immune system response, sleep habits, happiness, sense of self-worth, and the ability to concentrate and multitask during cognitive tests. And last, but not least, Tai chi is a great helper in the management of pain, arthritis, old injuries (not fresh or acute ones), inflammation, and rehabilitation. Whether you are using only conventional medicine or alternative medicine or both (which is what I advise) adding Tai chi will help you get better sooner.

Qigong

This ancient Chinese system of "energy medicine in motion," consists of exercises and meditations that stimulate the flow of Qi, our life energy. It was created by ancient masters who understood how certain movements and postures could balance the body, mind, and spirit by interconnecting yin, yang, and the flow of our Qi.

Take a look at some of those exercises on YouTube.

The practice of Qigong increases and balances our life force, the Qi. It works directly on the body's meridian system, where the Qi flows, stimulating and nourishing the internal organs and making the energetic communication between them more efficient. By increasing the effectiveness of all body systems, Qigong helps build Qi, providing more energy to the metabolism and assisting the body in its fight against illnesses. To have good health and better recovery, a person needs to have sufficient Qi flowing freely throughout the body and internal organs.

Many athletes enjoy Qigong because it improves strength, stamina, coordination, and other skills necessary for peak performance. As a spiritual art, rooted in Taoism (Daoism), it deepens awareness of self and nature and creates a feeling of harmony, tranquility, and peace.

Qigong is a combination of meditation and gentle exercises composed of movements that are repeated several times, often stretching the body, increasing fluid movement, and building awareness of how the body moves through space.

It is a holistic system of coordinated body postures and movements, breathing, and meditation rooted in old Chinese medicine, martial arts, and philosophy.

Some practitioners claim it's not an exercise but rather a form of meditation and breathing in motion. Incorrect postures result in decreased or blocked energy flow, the unnecessary expenditure of energy, a decrease in body energy, and greater susceptibility to injury or illness. Most people breathe in a non-optimal way, therefore one of the highlights of this practice is adopting a new breathing technique. As we make progress in these two fields, we embrace new gentle movements. That is essentially the practice of this art.

Qigong is not a substitute for proper medical care; however, its practice confers multiple health benefits. Some of the indications are stress, disease prevention, hypertension (that might even allow a reduction in medications), aiding in the management of chronic illnesses, asthma, pain, chronic fatigue, head problems (brain fog, headaches, depression, anxiety), digestive disorders (like constipation, IBS, indigestion, gastritis), arthritis, painful conditions, and injuries (not in an acute phase).

Feldenkrais

This is an interesting approach to human movement, employing exercises designed to improve flexibility, posture, coordination, management of chronic back pain, as well as improving neurological and psychological problems. Some of the movements are done by the therapist, as a manipulative technique, some are done by the patient.

The Feldenkrais Method is based on the principles of physics and biomechanics, an empirical understanding of human physiology, and the connection between mind and body. It relieves muscle tension and can be very beneficial for hip and back pains. Practitioners use gentle movement to increase and ease the range of motion of affected joints, improving flexibility, coordination, stiffness, and pain. It is effective in easing stress and tension as well.

The Feldenkrais system is used for more than just relieving symptoms but also to train the nervous system to find new pathways around areas of damage. It focuses on enhancing the communication between the brain and body. It has demonstrated success in the rehabilitation of stroke victims and others suffering from neurological injuries, like brain tumors, head injuries, multiple sclerosis, and ataxia, that cause disordered movement or a lack of coordination. Patients with pain and dysfunction due to orthopedic problems may find this modality very helpful.

People who experience severe movement difficulties because of injury, surgery, or neurological processes, high performers in the arts or athletes who want to improve their skills or maintain their competitive edge and individuals who want to stay vital and active, or are dealing with persistent aches, pains, and stiffness may find a great deal of improvement with this modality.

My advice? If you have any of the above problems and there is a center near you, try it.

Exercise

Physical activity is essential to the success of the management of all the conditions we mention in this book and for the recovery of injuries, arthritis, painful disorders, and most inflammatory conditions. Our program encourages exercise.

But don't just throw yourself in the water recklessly, as many people do, and like I used to do myself.

Our Jupiter Institute recommends certain rules regarding exercise:

a) According to your condition, and what you are dealing with, you should consult one, two or even three experts to learn which exercises are good for you, how to do them, when to do them, and especially, which ones not to do.

Examples: if your knees or hips are not good and you have adrenal dysfunction, you should not spend 45 minutes on the treadmill. If your lumbar discs are not good, the usual abdominal exercises could make them worse. If you have a shoulder problem, why would you lift weights? If your hormones and your adrenals are low, and you are gaining weight, spending two hours in the gym will make things worse.

Ask some of the many experts I mention in this book. Ask a chiropractor, a physical therapist, an acupuncturist, a Gyrotonic expert, etc.

b) You must like your exercise routine and avoid exercise you don't enjoy.

c) Certainly, if you dislike an exercise your cortisol level will rise and this will undermine your health.

d) It should warm your body and bring on a good sweat.

e) Sweating detoxifies your body. Heating your body improves the vascular system.

f) The routine should be practiced regularly.

g) If you want it to be effective, they should cause no harm or risk of injury.

General Guidelines About Exercise

The benefits of exercise are well-documented in many books and publications. Although professional guidance is recommended in many patients, in most instances, exercise is going to be performed after minimal instruction.

Increased physical activity and exercise are known to provide multiple benefits to people with arthritis and all the health problems we mentioned, including improved cardiovascular conditioning, blood pressure control, improved lung function, increased muscular tone, boosting metabolism, and increased fat and glucose burning. However, I must emphasize, exercise does not produce weight loss but is rather a tool in weight loss management.

AS LONG AS THE TYPE of injury, surgery, lesion or whatever condition you might have does not contraindicate exercise, then the effects of exercise are multiple, and the general benefits are:

1. Exercise improves strength and flexibility.

2. It decreases stiffness and pain.

3. It improves balance and muscle endurance.

4. It improves the cardiovascular and pulmonary systems.

5. It promotes relaxation and stress reduction.

6. It improves insulin sensitivity, sexual function, sleep, and even resistance to diseases.

7. It improves blood pressure and hypertension management.

8. It assists in controlling weight and obesity management. It boosts metabolism, helping burn fat and glucose. It raises good HDL.

9. It improves mental alertness and sleep patterns.

And at the level of the joints, the benefits are:

10. Exercise improves the biomechanics of the joint.

11. It improves the flow of the joint fluids.

12. It strengthens the muscles, tendons, and ligaments of the joints.

13. It keeps the joints healthy and more functional.

14. It improves the blood flow to the areas affected by arthritis, injury, and inflammation.

Arthritis

Many doctors and patients think exercise is counterproductive for an arthritic joint. They believe that when a joint is swollen, tender, or stiff, that exercise will make it worse. Nevertheless, plenty of studies and personal experiences vouch for the tremendous benefit of exercise in the arthritic joint. Study after study has shown that exercise movements have healing power and they are good medicine for arthritis.

There is no doubt that appropriate rest helps reduce joint inflammation, however, it is also a fact that excessive rest is deleterious to health. Research shows that excessive rest can reduce fitness and cause muscle wasting, tendon and ligament weakness, contraction, and even degeneration of the joint cartilage. Given this effect, it is paradoxical for physicians to recommend rest for chronic arthritis and painful conditions. Rest may worsen the conditions and decrease the functional capacity of the limb.

With an appropriate exercise program and the good guidance of a Physical Therapist, arthritic patients can safely improve their strength and enhance their functional capacity. Increasing the strength in the muscle improves the performance of many everyday activities and relieves physical and psychological discomfort.

Helping the Muscles

As we review the multiple benefits and indications of exercise, we also need to take into account the effect on the muscular tissue. Exercise increases muscular activity, demanding more supply of oxygen, glucose, nutrients, minerals, and vitamins. Proper nutrition is mandatory if one wants to satisfy the requirements of muscular activities with water, protein, and carbohydrates. The recommended foods that satisfy the muscular demands are included in the composition of our meal replacements. However, we usually recommend taking extra protein, water, and sometimes a cup of clear broth after vigorous exercise. Patients who are "big exercisers," need closer supervision regarding possible injuries, mineral imbalance, adequate protein intake, and proper hydration, etc.

Recommendations.

Despite the current recommendations from books and publications, patients suffering from pain, arthritis, and injuries should not just engage in any type of exercise that they choose. Let me rephrase it: exercise is very important for the arthritic patient and for those who have minor spinal disc disorders, but the key is that they should not do just any exercise. As good as exercise may be, it can further damage a joint, ligament, or tendon that is already hurting. The wrong type of exercise can irritate a bursa even more or worsen bursitis, it could trigger tendinitis, and may worsen chondromalacia. Also, the wrong type of stretching may further strain or sprain a ligament or muscle that is already hurt.

Moreover, a bad disc or swollen cartilage may get worse if the person does an inappropriate exercise. Furthermore, individuals who are overweight may aggravate hip and back conditions if they engage in jogging or even long walks, and a whiplash injury may get worse if they go to the gym.

Make up your mind, Doc, should I do exercise or not?

The answer is to do the right type of exercise and with the right frequency and intensity. However, it is difficult for the average person to choose which exercises to do, and how often or how intense. As a general rule neither medical doctors, internists, or family physicians know much about this, and therefore they try to guess. Books on the other hand give a person too many explanations and the person ends up not knowing what to do. The solution is to ask the two professionals who know best about exercises: Chiropractors and Physical Therapists. If you know a Gyrotonic specialist, Tai chi teacher, or myofascial release specialist, you can ask them too. But do not ask anyone else! No other professionals know as much about neuromuscular anatomy, joint physiology, body mechanics, human biophysics, and healing techniques as these professionals. They will advise and guide you in regards to which exercises you should do, how often, and how intense. They will also advise you as to whether stretching or weightlifting are indicated or forbidden.

As much as we encourage exercise, without guidance exercise may cause more harm than good and you need to be aware of it. Bad exercise advice may adversely affect you, therefore, it is important to find a good chiropractor and a good physical therapist. For this, you would have to ask around. Ask doctors, friends, relatives, or neighbors. Do not guide yourself by fancy marketing. Go and inquire.

Through books, you can learn about different types of exercises: flexibility exercises, strengthening exercises, aerobic exercises, and even sports. I don't want to get too deep into the subject because first, it is not the main goal of this publication. Second, I would need a whole book to teach you and show you pictures of exercises and how to do them. Third, I think that exercises need to be taught 1-on-1 by a therapist. Yes, you can use books as a guide, but the indication of which exercise, how many exercises, when to exercise, length of exercise, which exercises not to do and when not to exercise, etc., needs to be taught by someone who knows this field very well and in person.

For example, In the case of the knee: If you have three individuals, Bobby, a slim guy who is a surgeon and plays soccer on weekends, Jeannie, obese and diabetic, a busy landscaper, and Martin, a tall, big guy, hyperlipidemic, hypertensive, overweight and with COPD, who is a 60-year-old man and used to play basketball twice a week until six years ago, but now is a successful businessman and does not do any activities. These three have the same complaint of pain, stiffness, and mild swelling in the left knee. The three of them may need to engage in exercise. Well, their knee may look the same in the three of them. Should the exercise recommendation be the same then? Let's take a look. Bobby's knee is strong and without degeneration, but he has a partial tear in the medial ligament and bursitis next to the patella. Jeannie's ligament and tendon are good, but she has degenerative changes in the cartilage with inflammation and spurs. Martin, on the other hand, has a partially torn meniscus, calcific tendinitis, and effusion. The treatment for these three patients should NOT be the same. The exercise treatment for each one of them should not be the same either, and should be taught in a one-on-one encounter with a therapist, and should not be done by following a general book. As much as I like those exercise books myself, and as much as I read many of them, I still state that there is nothing better than the personal guidance of a therapist.

Research

The beneficial effects of exercise were confirmed by two important studies. The first one was in humans and it did not involve dissection but rather multiple MRIs as part of the evaluation. The thickness of the cartilage of the knee was measured in a group of individuals. Then these individuals were placed in a supervised exercise program that included flexibility, strengthening, and aerobic exercise for several weeks. At the end of the study, the new MRI studies showed that the thickness of the cartilage had increased, meaning that exercise had made the cartilage thicker, which is a significant beneficial change since thicker cartilage improved the physiology of the joint. The other study involved animals and dissection. It showed that in animals, exercise generates thicker cartilage, more lubricating fluids, and a stronger and better functioning joint. In another study, at Wake Forest University, Duke took about 300 elderly people with osteoarthritis of the knee and divided them into three groups. The first group got only health education, the second group performed aerobic walking only, and the third group did strength training only. After 18 months, those who just got health education were in the same shape but the two active groups were feeling better with less pain, less stiffness, and better joint function. These studies succeeded in showing that exercise is beneficial for arthritis.

Similar studies were done at Tufts University at the Center for Physical Activity and Nutrition. In this study, they recruited 46 individuals with crippling arthritis, who experienced pain and stiffness every day. What was very particular about this study is that the therapist went to the home of the patients to instruct and push them to do the exercises. These consisted mainly of stretching, flexibility exercises combined with strengthening exercises. Half of the participants got this active exercise, while the other half, that was the control group, received mainly a small lecture and emotional support. No specialized equipment or tools were used for the exercise. After four months, the difference between the two groups was amazing. The exercise group had a lot less pain and their physical function had greatly improved. Those who exercised were able to walk, go outside, get in and out of their cars, sit, stand, and even climb stairs much easier. They even slept better and their whole quality of life had improved. Those who did not exercise, the ones who got just emotional support, and health education, those who got "someone to listen to them," had very little improvement.

Action

As you read this chapter, you need to understand that nothing will happen by just reading this book. I mention this because I have seen people attending lectures but then not doing anything new about their activities. They think "Hey, I went to the lecture and that is enough," or they say, "Hey, I am trying." But I know they are not. I know that their effort is just attending the lecture and when they get home, they do nothing with what they learned. I know of those who go through financial conferences and do nothing with the financial advice that they learn, and I also know about heart patients that go for two hours of a "seminars and bagels" conference. They listen and they say "Oh, that is very interesting," or "Oh, he is such a good speaker," but they do nothing to change. If you are reading with the intention of changing and improving, this book is your tool.

In cases of vigorous exercise or significant sweating, we recommend replenishing your potassium with fruits, pumpkin seeds, potato with the skin, bananas, and peanuts. For people who are doing exercise regularly, we also recommend the intake of supplements. It is difficult to follow a careful nutrition program that will provide all of the vitamins and minerals that muscles need. Vitamin B could easily become depleted and the same goes for Vitamin C and other vitamins. Taking vitamins will nourish the muscles and protect them against possible damage during exercise.

Types of Exercise

Exercise programs for people with pain, arthritis, and injury should be individualized and planned on a case by case basis. Following a book is not recommended. Rather following the advice from a professional is what is best.

Almost all exercise programs should include some type of low-impact activity to build up muscle strength without adding additional stress to the arthritic joint. Examples of these include swimming, brisk walking, and biking. Exercises should include a program to increase the range of motion and at the same time strengthening the muscles. Combining an exercise program with physical therapy provides the best results in relieving pain and improving function.

There are different types of exercises including range of motion exercises, strengthening exercises, spine exercises, even Ancient Eastern exercises such as yoga, Tai chi, and Qigong. Classic exercise includes going to the gym, biking, brisk walking, and jogging.

Although there are multiple types of exercises, we can easily classify them into four groups: flexibility, strengthening, aerobics, and sports activities.

Flexibility Exercises

Flexibility exercises move the joints and muscles through their full range of motion and gradually increase how far they can move and the ease at which they move. As the joints become more mobile, they can function more effectively with less pain. These exercises help relieve stiffness, and when done properly, they have a beneficial effect on the inflammation process of joints, tendons, and ligaments.

Flexibility exercises decrease stress and lesions in the muscles, improve posture, and provide relief. However, either stretching or stretching with the wrong motion, may cause muscle and ligament injury. Have your therapist instruct you in the proper flexibility exercise techniques.

Strengthening Exercises

Strengthening exercises increase the strength of the muscles that move, protect, and support the joints. These types of exercise improve the muscular wasting and weakness that often accompany painful joints. Strengthening exercises improve muscle mass and muscle function that directly and indirectly improve the physiological function of the joint. The process of increasing the strength of the muscle improves the blood flow to the tissues, providing oxygen and glucose and eliminating the waste products that all have a positive effect on the healing process of injuries, arthritis, and inflammation areas.

Strengthening exercises dramatically improve joint function and decrease pain. Light weights are often used in this phase and they are very helpful. Have your therapist instruct you on the type of strengthening exercises that are best for your condition.

Aerobic Exercises

Aerobic exercises enhance overall fitness by stimulating the lungs and the cardiovascular system. They improve the body's energy balance by energizing joints, muscles, and all tissues in general. The term aerobic means "living with air," and when applied to exercise it means that the person can breathe normally while doing this activity. This is a moderate type of exercise in which the person will be breathing deeper and fuller but without the panting and rapid breathing of fast exercise. During aerobic exercises, the heart and lungs work harder, the person breathes a bit harder and the heart rate is increased.

Sports Activities

Sports activities can be done alone or in groups. They increase muscular activities and make the heart and lungs work a lot harder. In many situations, this may be beneficial but it may be counterproductive too. Sports activities in groups (basketball, soccer, swimming teams, etc.) are not recommended because they may end up pushing the individual to exercise much more than what is allowed for their arthritic joints, injuries, inflammation areas, etc. However, sports activities alone (swimming, jogging, etc.) may provide very important benefits as long as certain parameters are followed. These parameters need to be dictated by a health professional (a physician, a chiropractor or a physical therapist) since it depends on the location of the injury, the number of injuries, or affected joints, the weight of the person, the type of sports activity, etc.

Additional Information

We have found the following books to be an excellent source of information regard exercise:

The Arthritis Foundation's Guide to Good Living with Osteoarthritis. A publication of the Arthritis Foundation.

Arthritis: Your Complete Exercise Guide, by Neil Gordon, MD.

Exercise Beats Arthritis, by Valerie Sayce and Ian Frazer.

We also recommend some other very practical books that are listed in the Reference section of this book. You can get all these books in your local library or your favorite bookstore.

Tailoring Your Exercise Program

A "one–type–fits-all" approach does not work for people with arthritis, injuries, or pain. As I described above, according to your condition, occupation, or personal taste, an exercise program needs to be tailored to you by your Physical Therapist or your chiropractor. Medical doctors are not well-versed in this field and a gym instructor is not a good guide either. Work with your therapist and have them explain to you which exercise program is more appropriate for you. A carefully tailored exercise program, especially when combined with physical therapy offers tremendous help with the improvement of function and the relief of pain and stiffness for those who suffer injuries and arthritis.

Exercise is an important step in the recovery so don't just do any exercise but follow instructions. Consult with your Physical Therapist and chiropractor to find the right exercise. Some of the books we mention on our website (www.jupiterinstitute.com) are excellent sources of information regarding exercises

Precautions

As you engage in exercise activities you should use these following precautions:

1. Make sure you do not have any medical conditions that may worsen with inappropriate exercises. Talk to your doctor. A medical evaluation may be needed.

2. Do not perform exercises either too intensively, or too frequently in the first few weeks of the program. Start slowly.

3. Choose forms of exercise that minimize the stress to painful, inflamed, or damaged joints, or muscles.

4. Know to stop when the pain increases. Pain is a warning that you are causing damage to your body. The old clichés that "the more it hurts, the better it is for you," and "no pain, no gain" are not true and are dangerous misconceptions.

5. Do not exercise if your physician indicates that you have active cardiopulmonary disease, infectious or febrile illness, or severe vascular disorder. If you are currently ill, talk to your doctor before doing any type of exercise.

6. Don't overdo...you are here for the long run and you don't want to abuse your body too early.

7. Never exercise to show off, it is not a good idea.

8. Do not do a type of exercise that others like. Do an exercise that you like and enjoy. Choose exercises and activities that appeal to you.

9. Competitive exercises are not good for arthritis. They add extra strain to tissues and joints. Attempting to perform as well as others do may end up pushing your muscles, ligaments, joints, and tendons to levels of function for which they are not prepared.

10. Respect gravity. If you suffer from low back pain, hip trouble, or even a knee disorder, jogging and long-distance walking may cause more harm. If you are obese, the gravity effect may be even worse.

11. No alcohol or meals before exercise. Do not exercise too close to bedtime or the energizing effect may keep you awake.

12. Don't push yourself beyond your limit or you may end up hurting yourself even more. If a movement hurts, stop, and evaluate what has happened. Again, do not follow the dubious cliché "no pain – no gain."

13. Do not do stretching if you don't know how to do it well. Don't improvise and don't think that you know. Ask your therapist how and when to stretch or you may end up hurting your ligaments, tendons, and muscles.

14. Respect your pain. Exercise but don't overdo it. Adjust your activity level to avoid excessive pain. Learn to recognize when your pain tells you that you are abusing your joints. If you get increasing or sudden pain, chances are that you may be doing too much or you may be doing inappropriate exercise.

15. Warming-up is an important phase of exercising. If you don't know how to warm-up properly, ask your therapist.

16. Swimming and water activities are excellent for people with arthritis, inflammation, and injuries.

17. Do not exercise if your joints are severely inflamed. When joints, muscles, and tendons hurt, or they are swollen and very tender, exercise could worsen these conditions. Consult with your doctor or therapist if this occurs.

18. Going to a gym may or may not be a good idea. On one hand, it provides you with the means and tools for good exercises, like exercise mats, weights, machines, stationary bikes, rowing machines, etc., but on the other hand, it might encourage you to engage in exercise that you should avoid.

19. The length of your exercise session may vary depending upon your available time but even if you have only 10-15 minutes to exercise, remember that doing something is far better than doing nothing.

20. Try to exercise all parts of your body. You can achieve this by combining the treadmill with some floor exercises or the stationary bike with some weights. Some gyms offer you exercise stations where you combine the exercise of different parts of your body. Don't forget your abdominal and back exercises.

I don't advise push-ups. They cause excessive strain on joints and muscles; don't do them, they may hurt you.

Warming-up

It is a good idea to warm up your body before you start doing exercises for your specific problem area. Arthritic joints and injured muscles or tendons can stiffen up very easily, particularly if you have not done any exercise for a while. Warming-up is a gentle way of starting to move and it helps to get joints and muscles ready for exercise. Once muscles start working, blood flow increases, and tissues get better prepared for exercise. You should not do stretching at this stage as doing these in cold tissues, may cause micro-tears and damage. In general, don't do stretching without the counseling of your therapist as it may cause more harm than good. Starting the warming-up phase can be done sitting or standing. Then, doing a full repetition of each, do a series of the following: raising arms over shoulders, flexing the arms, raising shoulders without raising the arms, a gentle clap of the hands forward, raising one knee and then the other, rotating the body to the right and then to the left, slowly bending forward and then backward, mid-level squatting. On the floor, sit up and bracing your knees, lay down flat and raise one leg and then the other. Do all these exercises in very slow motion and causing only minimal stretching. You can also do a slow military march moving your arms in circles while doing front circles or side circles. Again, do all these very slowly, while taking deep slow breaths, and forcing the air out of your lungs in the exhalation phase.

Additional Therapies

There is another group of therapies that may have very beneficial effects in individuals struggling with the conditions I mention in this book.

Relaxation Techniques

Research over the past 30 years has shown that pain and many neuromuscular disorders are influenced by emotional and social factors. These need to be addressed along with the physical causes of pain if the individual wants to achieve adequate levels of comfort.

It is well-known that chronic stress is one factor that contributes to chronic pain and it is also known that relaxation techniques can bring on relief.

Pain of any kind and persisting degenerative arthritis increases muscle tension, that in turn distresses the neuromuscular system and creates more pain. When muscles are tense, they tighten and increase pressure on the nerves and other tissues as well as the pain sites, which can make the pain worse. Sometimes it is the other way around, where the distressed nerve is the culprit of pain and inflammation. Whatever is the primary cause, however, relaxation can help break the pain-tension cycle when combined with other forms of therapy.

Relaxation calms the mind and recharges the body. It is particularly important for people who live with pain. It also reduces stress hormones in the blood, relaxes the muscles, and elevates the sense of well-being. Using these techniques regularly can lead to long-term changes in your body to counteract the harmful effects of stress.

Choose whatever relaxes you: watching a movie, music, prayer, gardening, going for a walk, talking with a friend on the phone, etc. Here are some other techniques you might try:

Deep Breathing

Make yourself comfortable, loosen any tight clothing. Breathe deeply, so that your abdomen expands and contracts like a balloon with each breath. Listen to your breathing. Relax your stomach muscles. Inhale to a count of four, hold for a count of four, exhale to a count of four, then hold to a count of four. Repeat for ten cycles. As you breathe out, imagine your tensions are being breathed away. Every time you breathe in, imagine you are breathing in peace

Guided Imagery

Using imagery with relaxation helps to distract your mind from stressful thoughts. Breathe slowly and deeply. Take deep, slow, full breaths. Think about your special place - your favorite place in the whole world. A place you can go to escape everything. It can be a real place or a made-up spot. Imagine yourself lying comfortably in your own special spot. You feel completely at home there. For example, imagine a tranquil scene in which you feel comfortable, safe, and relaxed. Include colors, sounds, smells, and feelings. Do this five to ten minutes each day. Do a little Internet search about this technique if you find it is helping you.

Self-talk

Talking to yourself may help you change how you think about your painful condition. It may also help you analyze which therapies are more effective and visualize the root of your distress.

Mindfulness Meditation

This technique is gaining more and more importance nowadays as people are realizing the adverse effects of stress. The first step involves choosing a quiet and comfortable place where you can lie down. You don't want to be distracted. After you are comfortable turn your awareness to your body. Mentally examine your body for any areas where there may be tension, and see if you can consciously release or soften those areas of the body so that you can be totally relaxed. Next, focus your awareness only on your body and let everything else drop away. Then with your mind, you turn your attention to each part of your body, one at a time, and you focus more and more on the affected areas, concentrating on your thoughts for healing.

Detoxification

The adverse effects of outside toxins (environmental) and inside toxins (from dysbiosis) are well-known and I address them in different parts of this book. I have one of the following chapters fully dedicated to this annoying problem and to detoxification. Suffice it to say that detoxification is important to all individuals affected by the conditions I address in this book.

Detoxification interacts with all the other therapies I mention here, facilitating them, allowing them to work better, lowering the inflammatory process, and making the condition more manageable.

Homeopathy

This therapy uses plants, liquid concentrates and minerals to achieve relief from many painful disorders and illnesses. Those who practice it use tiny amounts of natural substances, with the belief that the body can cure itself by stimulating the healing process. However, some authors state that those homeopathic preparations are not effective for treating any condition, and large-scale studies have found homeopathy to be no more effective than a placebo, indicating that any positive effects that follow treatment are due to factors such as normal recovery from illness. I talked to many individuals who underwent this kind of treatment and most of them described significant relief from whatever was affecting them.

According to the American Institute of Homeopathy: Homeopathy is holistic because it treats the person as a whole, rather than focusing on a diseased part or a labeled sickness. Homeopathy is natural because its remedies are produced according to the U.S. FDA-recognized Homeopathic Pharmacopoeia of the United States from natural sources, whether vegetable, mineral, or animal in nature.

INTERCHAPTER REMARK: Alternative therapies are fantastic modalities that help people heal and repair affected areas of the body as well as the whole body and soul. Combining them with the right supplements and proper nutrition enhances their effects.

Nutrition

You might hear the words "inflammation" and "omega-3" in the same sentence when talking about nutrition, but how do they correlate? Omega-3 and omega-6 are compounds absorbed from foods that play a major role in the inflammatory response. They are used by the cells that produce eicosanoids, the "Attack!" and "Heal!" enzymes. The omega-3 eicosanoids promote anti-inflammation, encourage the decrease in swelling, and push for repair. The omega-6 eicosanoids produce a strong inflammatory response, promoting swelling and focusing on attacking invaders, and hindering repair.

The role of omega fatty acids in inflammation

If omega-6 eicosanoids predominate, then the inflammatory response can be overwhelming, causing pain and swelling to persist. Aspirin and other anti-inflammatory drugs reduce inflammation and pain by intervening in this process. They block the enzymes that cause cells to produce omega-6 eicosanoids. Don't be fooled; because of the risks associated with long-term use, these drugs should only be used for a short course while the necessary lifestyle changes are implemented. The best way to control this process is through diet, controlling how much omega-3 and omega-6 are in your body. While we cannot control the process of inflammation, we can exercise some influence over it, and right there is your first hint. If your diet is overwhelmingly rich in omega-6, you are encouraging those cells to continue your inflammation. Conversely, eating foods rich in omega-3 may lower inflammation and heal faster.

Eicosanoids & the Omegas

Every tissue in the body contain eicosanoids, including cartilage, bone, ligaments, arteries, the heart, and other internal organs. They are complex molecules that coordinate the tissue's metabolic function, interacting with hormones, minerals, and nutrients to assure that cells have the proper function, adequate energy supply, and good waste elimination. They are very important for good health. When a healthy person eats well and has good metabolism, eicosanoids exhibit "good behavior" in the tissues. As regulators of cellular function, the eicosanoids' good behavior helps tissues work well, repair themselves, and fix the daily wear-and-tear.

However, if a person is not healthy due to poor dietary habits, a hormonal imbalance, obesity, diabetes, frequent exposure to mental and emotional stress, and/or over-consumption of sugars, bad fats, carbohydrates, alcohol, tobacco, and caffeine, eicosanoids will behave "badly" in the body. This bad behavior causes cell damage, interferes with repair, causes inflammation, and hurts the local tissues.

This gives rise to multiple problems in the body, although the symptoms and warnings might be slow at the onset, and you may not have any clue about what is going on. It might take years for someone to find out that their joints or arteries are ill or that certain organs are suffering as a result of their diet. Healthy people have a proper balance of good and bad eicosanoids, working against each other in balance. Cells are doing what they're supposed to, bodily functions are working well, and the person feels comfortable. However, numerous agents in diet and the environment are capable of breaking this healthy balance by increasing the number of bad eicosanoids. When this happens, disease occurs, which adversely affects the organs and tissues of the body.

What do omega-3 and omega-6 have to do with eicosanoids? The cells that create inflammation-controlling eicosanoids do so with the help of the omega-3 and omega-6 that you consume.

Omega-6 is found in high levels in what I call the "typical American diet" – fried food, fast food, and the badly-fed (no grass) meat and animal products typically found in grocery stores. Since omega-6 stimulates the production of bad eicosanoids, this diet easily upsets the good-bad eicosanoid balance. Bottom line: a diet containing excessive omega-6 is bad for your health. It creates an imbalance that promotes inflammation, heart disease, osteoarthritis, diabetes, strokes, and even cancer.

A point to remember: There is a strong relationship between dietary style and eicosanoid behavior. Moreover, there is a strong association between your general lifestyle and the good or bad behavior of your eicosanoids. Even if you are a good person, you work hard to support your family, and everybody loves you, if you suffer an injury or joint disorder, and you have significant stress, you eat a typical American diet, and you abuse carbs, alcohol, and bad fats, your eicosanoids will turn bad on you and hinder the repair of whatever injury or joint problem you have.

Foods containing omega-3 are good for the body. They counteract the bad effects of omega-6 fatty acids, mitigating all the adverse effects described above: preventing heart disease, improving the function of the brain, immune system and bowels, decreasing fatigue, headaches, arthritis, and lowering the risk of cancer. Countries with the highest life expectancy and the lowest incidences of chronic disease often have diets high in omega-3. Oily fish (such as sardines, mackerel, herring) and certain nuts, fruits, and seeds are all very concentrated sources of omega-3...and all are lacking in the typical American diet.

Fats, Oils and the Production of Eicosanoids

There are many types of dietary fat, and many ways of classifying them: animal fats, vegetable fats, frying fats, cooked fats, natural fats, man-made fats, hydrogenated fats, saturated and unsaturated fats, processed fats, trans fats...the list goes on. It's easy to get confused and difficult to remember which are good for you and which are not. For simplicity's sake, I am dividing fats and oils into two categories: those that provide omega-3 fats and those that provide omega-6 fats. To reiterate, omega-3 fats are good for your health, generating good eicosanoids, while excessive amounts of omega-6 fats are detrimental to healthy cellular function. As you will see, however, it is the ratio of omega-3 and omega-6 in each oil that determines its overall effect in the body. Even further, it is best to make each teaspoon count, as all oils are high in calories.

One easy way of adding omega-3 and tilting the eicosanoid balance in your favor is by taking concentrated, purified, high-quality fish oil supplements. You can find a list of types and brands later on.

In summary: Omega-6 is bad! People who end up with high levels of omega-6 in their body, whether it's a result of diet, lifestyle, or environment, are in what I call an "omega-6/bad eicosanoid/free-radical/pro-inflammatory" state or, more simply, "The Omega-6 Lifestyle." This lifestyle is the opposite of what you should strive for; it's pretty bad for your health, your disease prevention, and your healing. Those living The Omega-6 Lifestyle become ill more easily, get injured more frequently, and take longer to recover, and their inflammation will take longer to heal. Since their immune system is strained, even a regular cold or flu can be severe and last for weeks

People in The Omega-6 Lifestyle will get into trouble sooner or later...much sooner than later. Since their disease develops slowly – sometimes very slowly – they will not see symptoms until the disease is much advanced. At that point, the damage to the tissues and organs has been done. They won't find out what bad shape their joints are in until they are already in the full swing of arthritis. Often, they'll suffer from fatigue, headache, neuropathies, and bowel problems without even knowing that their bodies are sick. Some get diabetes, heart problems, and cancer. Every case is different, but most of the sufferers share a common trait: a lack of knowledge. They do not know or refuse to accept the idea that their nutrition and lifestyle are directly related to the onset of their diseases, and some will never know what killed them.

There is, of course, an alternate path. People who live what I call the "omega-3/good-eicosanoid/antioxidant/anti-inflammatory state," or simply "a healthy lifestyle," or "omega-3 lifestyle," reap the benefits. They will be rewarded with faster healing and better health, fewer sick days, and more time doing what they love. Additionally, the onset of many common diseases of aging, such as hypertension and arthritis, will be delayed or prevented altogether. It is not necessary to eat solely foods rich in omega-3 to reach this state; just eat more of them while consuming fewer omega-6 foods.

The amount of omega-3 in the average American diet is quite low at approximately 5%. Many millions of Americans don't even achieve that dismal percentage, which results in a very poor omega-6/omega-3 ratio of approximately 20:1 to 30:1. The ideal ratio necessary to achieve a healthy lifestyle is in the range of 3:1 to 4:1. To attain this, most people need to increase their omega-3 intake by 25-30% while substantially decreasing their intake of omega-6s. Diets like our Jupiter Institute Omega Diet, help people withdraw from the omega-6/bad eicosanoid/ free-radical state and achieve the omega-3/good eicosanoid/ antioxidant state, a much healthier lifestyle. The transition to an omega-3/good eicosanoid/antioxidant state decreases inflammation, damage, and provides the internal environment necessary for healing and repair. Let me highly recommend this diet for anyone struggling with pain, arthritis, or injuries.

And let me emphasize as well that starting your day with raw vegetables, high-quality olive oil and the best omega-3 fish oil you can get makes a lot of sense. You are fighting inflammation and helping your body.

Nutrition and Joint Damage
Poor nutrition (promoting a deficiency of nutrients and vitamins, and the presence of free radicals and anti-nutrients) prevents the repair process from progressing normally. The collagen first becomes

less structured, and later becomes abnormal and deficient in important components. This process triggers an inflammatory reaction in which injured cells pour their enzymes into the intercellular space, damaging the tissue and producing a flow of proteins, eicosanoids, and inflammatory cells. As the degeneration and inflammation progress, the proteins and fibers that make the cartilage a strong tissue begin to weaken and dissolve. This process leaves areas that are damaged, scarred, partially ulcerated, and irregular like a street full of bumps and holes that needs repair. As the joint tries to work under these conditions, usage creates friction and heat, which triggers additional swelling and pain, that spreads to the tendons and ligaments. The body responds to this cartilage breakdown by sending calcium in an attempt to fortify and stabilize the joint. Unfortunately, this natural response results in calcium deposits, that grow and become spurs. Joint stiffness and enlargement follow. The process could still be stopped and reversed, but when the causes that created it are not addressed (and the patient concedes to Celebrex, Ibuprofen, etc., a pat on the back and no further treatment), the degeneration continues and degenerative osteoarthritis ensues. A key issue to remember is that cartilage needs nutrients to keep it healthy and strong.

Nutrition plays an important role in daily cartilage repair. If the cartilage is supplied with nutrition that provides good eicosanoids, fresh antioxidants, proteins, and adequate vitamins, it will remain healthy cartilage, quick to repair itself. If the cartilage is fed with nutrition that provides bad eicosanoids, free radicals, and poor vitamin content, the health of the cartilage will become compromised. Daily wear and tear that is not repaired is the first step in joint degeneration.

Message: what you eat makes a difference. If you eat the anti-nutrients way (waffles, pancakes, fast food, chips, milk, cottage cheese, cream cheese, donuts, mac-n-cheese, boxed juices, BBQ ribs, fried food, etc.), instead of what I recommend in the next chapters, then you are hurting yourself.

The dietary lifestyle of a person has a significant impact on the evolution of injuries, arthritis, painful areas, and even in surgical areas, wounds, and many medical conditions (bronchitis, pneumonia, heart disease, fractures, etc.).

Diet has a major impact on arthritis, pain, and inflammation, both as a cause and an aggravator of these ailments.

A nutritionally balanced approach to food such as that offered by the Jupiter Institute Omega Diet may improve how a person feels and will likely help to control the inflammatory process, often with unexpected side benefits like overall well-being, lower blood pressure, improved cholesterol, etc. Understanding why and how this anti-inflammatory diet works is an important step in appreciating the value of our program.

One of the best medicines for treating the inflammation of arthritis and injuries can be found not in the drugstore, BUT IN THE GROCERY STORE: THE PROPER FOOD.

But nourishing your body properly is not just having a salad with every meal with some olive oil on top or to follow some of those false Mediterranean dishes from supermarket magazines. It goes way beyond that.

Many authorities agree that what we choose to put into our bodies can either strengthen or weaken us, making us more or less healthy while increasing or decreasing the symptoms of disease. Nutrition is known to affect the inflammation process.

Following dietary guidelines to improve arthritis, inflammation, and pain, has multiple advantages. Some of those benefits include an improvement in the immune system's ability to fight infections and cancer, and improvements in both the cardiovascular system and glucose metabolism, decreasing the risks of heart attacks, diabetes, and stroke.

I call those dietary guidelines by different names: like "Mediterranean Diet," "Jupiter Institute Omega Diet," "Omega-3 Lifestyle Diet," and "Anti-inflammatory Diet," but in the end, they are more or less the same. Whatever the name I use or anyone else uses, just remember the basic concept: good food is good, bad food is bad, and there is no way around it. I am going to teach a few key issues regarding friendly and unfriendly foods that may trigger or relieve inflammation and pain.

Our Dietary Program Consists of Two Parts

1) Avoidance teaches you how to eliminate inflammation-causing foods, including foods with omega-6s and those that trigger free radicals.
2) The Jupiter Institute Omega Diet, that tells you what foods help you reduce free radicals, and what foods help you increase your intake of antioxidants and omega-3s.
   It sounds simple, but it is a bit more complicated than that.

The Avoidance Plan

Certain foods have a direct and toxic effect on inflammation and pain. Some of these foods provoke an allergic reaction while others act as toxic biochemical aggressors. There is evidence that particles of the foods listed below can cross the intestinal membrane, enter the bloodstream, form immune complexes, and then cause immuno-allergic injury in the tissues. By removing offending foods from the diet, people with painful conditions can avoid this adverse consequence and experience significant improvement in their symptoms.

Foods that Cause Arthritis, Inflammation, and Pain:

- Chocolate
- Corn
- Dairy products
- Egg yolks
- Green and wax beans
- Milk
- Nightshade vegetables (like eggplant, green and red pepper, and tomatoes
- Nuts (mainly peanuts and sunflower seeds)
- Processed fruit juice
- Red meat
- Sugar
- Wheat and wheat flour
- Yeast and foods made with yeast

Our recommendation to avoid the above foods is based on numerous observations and reports of suffering people who removed these foods from their diet and found that their symptoms decreased while their quality of life improved. Wheat is a well-known trigger of arthritic conditions by provoking an allergic reaction to gluten. Gluten triggers an immuno-allergic type of response that can lead to inflammation and swelling. Milk has been found to cause a variety of allergic reactions that cause inflammation and worsen arthritis. The nightshade vegetables are strongly and consistently linked to arthritis. They contain chemicals that not only promote inflammation but also increase pain and interfere with the repair of damaged joints. This does not happen in all individuals, BUT IT DOES happen in some, so I want you to take this into account as you make your decisions.

As you can see, certain foods and snacks contain two, three and even four offenders, like chocolate with peanuts, that also contains milk and sugar: like mac-n-cheese, a cheese sandwich, or a delicious breakfast with a corn muffin, scramble eggs, hash brown potatoes, orange juice and a delightful glass of milk. Also, lunch with bread, cheese, beer, and a salad with tomato and peppers.

Do you think I am kidding? Some people with arthritis, pain, and inflammation start the day without regard for their own health issues, and without knowing that they are just making it worse. They do it because "that's the standard," "everybody does it," etc.

Again, not many people get these immuno-allergic reactions, but those who do and suffer from pain and arthritis should stay away from the above foods and see how they feel. Give it a 100-day trial.

In the same way, not every person is affected by immunotoxins such as wheat, milk, chocolate, and sugar, but we recommend that those who suffer from pain, arthritis, and other inflammatory disorders stay away from these foods. Or, again, at least try 100 days without them and then see. Several weeks or months later you can resume eating one or two of these products to see if the symptoms reappear. If they do not, they may be consumed infrequently and in small amounts.

Acid Versus Alkaline

Arthritis sufferers commonly have a high level of acidity, which is a fertile ground for inflammatory conditions. Acidity can be decreased by reducing the intake of acid-forming foods—such as these below—and switching to the Jupiter Institute Omega Diet.

Acid-forming Foods

- Alcohol
- Beef
- Candy bars
- Cocoa
- Coffee
- Corn products (all)
- Flour products (all)
- Fried foods (all)
- Margarine
- Packaged snacks, chips
- Peanut butter
- Peanuts
- Pecans
- Sugar
- Sugary drinks & soft drinks
- Sweets
- Vinegar

Moreover, some authors state that acidic food makes arthritis, inflammation, pain, and recovery from injuries more difficult and that an anti-acid diet, known as an alkaline diet, is beneficial. I studied this and it makes sense. Acidic foods are pro-inflammatory, create more waste, and trigger the omega-6 system, while alkaline foods are more anti-inflammatory. Therefore I recommend people follow the principles of an alkaline diet when they prepare food at home or when eating out. One way or another, alkaline diets seem healthier and more beneficial for metabolism. It is also known to be very beneficial for the bones. An acidic diet causes osteoporosis while an alkaline diet reverses bone wasting and helps strengthen osteoporotic bones.

Dr. Nuchovich's Alkaline Diet

Message: To make your diet more alkaline, "alkalize," or "alkalinize" your meals: neutralize the acidity of some foods with alkaline foods.

The following list tells you how foods react in your metabolism.

Very Alkaline:

- lemons
- watermelons

Alkaline:

- asparagus
- cantaloupe
- cayenne
- dates
- figs
- grapes
- juicing (vegetable or fruit)
- kelp
- kiwi
- limes
- mango
- melons
- papaya
- parsley
- passion fruit
- pears
- pineapple
- raisins
- seaweed
- sweet potato
- watercress

Moderately Alkaline:

- apples
- alfalfa sprouts
- apple cider vinegar
- apricots
- arugula
- avocados
- ripe banana
- beets
- bell peppers
- broccoli
- currants
- cabbage
- carob
- carrots
- cauliflower
- corn
- daikon
- garlic
- ginger
- grapefruit
- green beans
- guavas
- herbs
- kale
- lettuce
- mustard greens
- nectarine
- oranges
- potatoes
- pumpkin
- peaches
- peas
- raspberries
- sea salt
- strawberries
- squash
- turnips
- watercress

Slightly Alkaline

- almonds
- artichokes
- Brussels sprouts
- cherries
- chestnuts
- cilantro
- coconut
- cucumber
- egg yolk
- eggplant
- goat's milk
- honey
- leeks
- mayonnaise
- mushrooms
- okra
- olive oil
- olives
- onions
- pickles
- quinoa
- radishes
- rice vinegar
- sesame seeds
- soybean
- soy cheese
- soy milk
- spices
- sprouted grains
- tofu
- tomatoes
- whey
- wild rice

Neutral:

- butter
- cow's milk
- cream
- oils

Moderately Acidic:

- barley
- beans (pinto, kidney, garbanzo, adzuki)
- blueberries
- bran
- cereals (unrefined)
- cheeses
- crackers
- cranberries
- curry

- egg white
- egg (whole)
- kasha
- ketchup
- maple syrup
- millet
- molasses
- mustard
- nuts (most)
- oats
- oil (canola)
- pasta
- pastry
- peanuts

- pine nuts
- plums
- popcorn
- potatoes
- prunes
- rice bread
- rice
- pumpkin seeds
- semolina
- shellfish
- sunflower seeds
- soy sauce
- venison
- wheat bread

Very Acidic:

- artificial sweeteners
- beef
- beer
- black tea
- bread (white)
- bread (whole wheat)
- breads
- cakes
- candies
- cereals
- chicken
- chocolate

- coffee
- cookies
- cream of wheat
- factory fruit juices
- flour
- fried foods
- frozen dinners
- flour products (all)
- jam
- jelly
- lamb
- liquor

- lobster
- Mexican food
- pork
- poultry
- rabbit
- seafood
- soft drinks
- sugar
- sugar (brown)
- turkey
- wine
- white fish
- yogurt (sweetened)

Avoid eating acidic meals. Learn to alkalinize your meals using the above classification.

Examples: Alkalize your steak by eating it with sweet potato and salad. Eat your rice with olive oil & ginger. Eat your fish with a tomato pepper salad seasoned with sea salt and lemon juice. A breakfast of coffee, sweetener, bread & jelly, or a dinner of chicken, pasta, and beer are acidic and not recommended. A breakfast of eggs, coffee, cereal is very acidic. A meal of wine, pasta, ragu, bread, and cake is very acidic.

A breakfast of yogurt, fruit juice, bread with cheese and jelly are all acidic; you shouldn't do that. Alkalinize it with fruits or veggies of the alkaline listing.

Apply these principles every time you eat.

The standard American diet, Mexican food, and Cuban food are very acidic and damaging to arteries and the whole metabolism. Learn from other cultures; the old Okinawa diet and many Japanese, Mediterranean and Chinese dishes are alkaline.

Why would you start the day with acidic food like coffee with sugar, yogurt, bread with jelly, cereal, and juice? Why would you splash acid on your suffering areas? Think about it.

However, there are two important points to take into account:

a) I don't recommend a strict alkaline diet but an ALKALIZED DIET, which is different. A pure alkaline diet would deprive you of important foods that your body might need.

Example: a meal of just sweet potato, goat milk, and a salad with watercress, kale, cauliflower, lettuce, and olives, and then some cherries, is very alkaline, but it does NOT give some essential nutrients your body may need. Be careful with this. You better add eggs or chicken to give yourself some protein, or beef, or fish. And you might want to add some rice for energy. See? The idea is not to eat alkaline but to avoid eating just acidic by alkalizing your acidic meal by adding alkaline food. So, do this: choose first your lean protein, then combine it with any combination from the alkaline food list.

Example. Steak and beer or wine with a large salad containing cucumbers, olives, asparagus, cabbage, beets, carrots, and arugula.

b) Apply concepts of nutrigenomics, that establishes that food reacts with your genes. Here we go with another difficult word, nutrigenomics, which means that everybody has to eat according to their genes and their ancestors.

Therefore, avoid food choices that were not present in the foods your parents and grandparents ate; rather, eat according to your genes. Regardless of where you were born. If you are Polish like me, you have no business eating hummus or pineapple. If you are genetically Italian, eat like an Italian, and avoid sushi, turkey, bourbon, corn, etc. If you are Irish or Russian, then tropical fish and tropical fruits are not for you. If you are

Portuguese, eat like a Portuguese; Chinese and Mexican foods are not for you. Are you getting this? Give it considerable thought.

And now, this is a bad cocktail, if you eat food that:

a) does not match your genes (goes against the nutrigenomic law), and

b) is acidic, and

c) belongs to the omega-6 lifestyle (like hot dogs, fast foods, cereal and milk, frozen dinners, etc.).

As I explain throughout this book, this adverse combination "cocktail" will only bring you bad health and will have metabolic and inflammatory consequences on your joints, your injuries, your muscles, and your whole body.

In case you were wondering which kind of food I am talking about when I say it belongs to the "omega-6" lifestyle, here it is. It is the factory-made food, also known as PROCESSED FOODS, and this is the list:

- ✓ All canned, bottled or boxed juices
- ✓ All sugary sodas
- ✓ All wheat products
- ✓ All oat products
- ✓ All processed meats (hot dogs, etc.)
- ✓ All bakery products, like donuts, bagels, cakes, pastry, Danish pastry
- ✓ All sweets, candies, candy bars, all snacks, like pretzels, potato chips, corn chips
- ✓ All cereals
- ✓ All fast foods, all deep-fried foods, most canned foods
- ✓ All crackers and cookies
- ✓ All ready-to-eat dinners, frozen or not
- ✓ Most factory-made dairy products
- ✓ Most cold cuts

Just like I explained in the inflammation chapter.

They are very convenient and very tasty. Are they good? No!

Perhaps you don't have any medical problems, you feel well, you are slim, have no pain, inflammation, injuries, surgical recovery, headaches and you are doing great, so perhaps YOU DON'T NEED any of these food limitations. But if you do have some of the problems I mention in this book...beware of what you eat and drink!!

Eating these kinds of "cocktails" will only bring you bad health.

The Jupiter Institute Omega Diet

The Jupiter Institute Omega Diet is a program designed to improve health and decrease the rate of diseases, particularly diseases known to affect people in the occidental world, such as arteriosclerosis, coronary heart disease, arthritis, vascular disease, and inflammatory diseases. The diet has a positive impact on the relief of osteoarthritis, inflammation, and many painful conditions, and is beneficial for the healing of injuries, traumas, and surgery. The Jupiter Institute Omega Diet is based on the Mediterranean Diet – perhaps the healthiest traditional diet on the planet – with a few important differences. One difference, of course, is that people following this program know why they are eating what they are, unlike the people in the Mediterranean region who eat what they eat simply because of where they live! Another difference is that I have taken the most important points of the Mediterranean Diet and explained, magnified, and encouraged them. These points have significant impacts on health, healing, tissue repair, well-being, and disease prevention. Third, the Jupiter Institute Omega Diet adds certain foods that increase the anti-inflammatory effects of the Mediterranean Diet while limiting or removing pro-inflammatory foods. Fourth, it promotes a more alkaline way of eating, which is much better for healing, encouraging you to eat less of the acid-forming foods. The fifth difference is that I encourage additional intake of fish oil, liquid, or capsules, and I strongly encourage daily consumption of high-quality olive oil, twice a day.

You can call this diet an omega-3 lifestyle, encouraging you to stay away from the adverse omega-6 lifestyle, as I explained at the beginning of the book.

Another key issue in my dietary program is that I also recommend nutritional supplements and vitamins to enhance the healing effect of the Mediterranean Diet, decrease inflammation and arthritis, and promote repair and pain relief. The reason for this is that omega-3 foods are not always readily available and the raw fruits and veggies we may buy don't always contain all the vitamins and minerals we need. As I wrote earlier, I usually recommend purified concentrated fish oil since it is more effective and patients have to take fewer capsules. Therefore, in my program, I use only selected brands of very purified concentrated fish oil and excellent brands of multivitamins, both from laboratories recognized by the American Academy of Anti-Aging Medicine. They are not cheap and they are not available in health food stores, but these are the ones I take and the ones my family and most of my patients take. Sorry, but after learning about how over-the-counter and health food store vitamins and supplements can be contaminated with chemicals and toxins, I don't recommend any other brands.

Just an apple a day will keep the doctor away? Are you sure? In my opinion, an omega, alkalized, Mediterranean diet, and excellent brands of vitamins and fish oil are much more powerful than that apple.

The combination of a healthy diet, nutritional additions, plus avoidance, provides a strong anti-inflammatory and pro-repair effect that assists in the management of injuries, arthritis, pain, and inflammatory conditions. Lastly, I have made our diet practical and easy to follow without the complications of puzzling cuisine and the confusion of strange names. However, before you decide to follow this diet you must know its key ingredients and why it will help you.

DON'T BE MISLED by the magazines you see in supermarkets, enticing you to believe in their false recipes that they give Mediterranean names. There is nothing good in turkey meatballs with creamy Sicilian sauce, or meat lasagna calabrese, or fried eggplants Greek style, or lobster a la Espanola. Just because you use Mediterranean names or add Italian seasoning does not make them good and many of those dishes use food that triggers acidity and omega-6s.

Many restaurants mislead you too.

Therefore, it is essential that you understand the heart of the Mediterranean Diet.

The Mediterranean Diet

In the 1960s, a study called The Seven Country Study analyzed the diets and mortality of over 12,000 men in seven countries: The United States, Finland, Japan, Italy, Greece, Yugoslavia, and the Netherlands. This study was long and complicated and analyzed the causes of diseases and mortality in various age groups in those countries. The review showed that the healthiest participants lived in Japan and Greece. However, when comparing those two countries in greater detail, the Greeks were found to have a much lower rate of heart disease and greater longevity. After analyzing the study and reviewing the Greek lifestyle, it was concluded that in defiance of conventional wisdom the Greeks who participated in the study achieved their low levels of heart disease risk despite endemic poverty, a poor healthcare system, and the consumption of a diet with the highest percentage of fat. The United States, with its great healthcare system, wealth, excellent supermarkets, and wide availability of processed food, take-out restaurants, fast food, and a surplus of eating choices, did very poorly in this study. It also showed much lower longevity and an excessive rate of heart attacks, strokes, and inflammatory conditions. The contrast with the findings in Greece was dramatic. The amazing results of the clinical studies of the Greek population led to a further investigation that extended to other countries of the Mediterranean region. For over 40 years, public health officials have been studying the diets of the Mediterranean. You can research this on the Internet.

The people in Greece have been found to derive the greatest benefits from this type of diet, followed by southern Italy, Spain, and France. The Mediterranean area is bordered by three continents – Europe, Africa, and Asia – and embraces more than a dozen countries. Regions that influence the Mediterranean Diet include Portugal, Southern Spain, Southern France, Southern Italy, Greece, Southern Turkey, Lebanon, Western Syria, Western Israel, Northern Egypt, and the northern regions of Morocco, Libya, and Algeria.

The Important Aspects of the Mediterranean Diet:

- High intakes of fish, olives, olive oil, grains, fresh vegetables, beans, garlic, fresh herbs, and fresh fruits
- Poultry in moderation and red meat occasionally
- An abundance of food from plant sources (fruits, vegetables, beans, grains, and rice)
- Minimally processed, seasonally fresh and locally grown foods
- High consumption of good fat (olive oil, olives, fish, and nuts being the principal sources of fat)
- Low consumption of low-fat cheeses and yogurts (that are used mainly as condiments)
- Fish, poultry, and eggs as the main protein
- Nuts and fresh fruits are a typical daily dessert
- Moderate consumption of wine, especially red wine
- Olives and nuts for appetizers and snacks.

The traditional Mediterranean Diet is affected by regions and seasons. While each Mediterranean country has its customs, they all rely on locally or regionally grown produce, consumed shortly after harvest. Every season provides fresh new vegetables that are often eaten within a few miles of where they were picked. Outdoor markets offer fresh fruits and vegetables and plenty of locally produced olive oil. The consumption of all these products in their freshest state is one of the important features of the local meals. For more detail on the Mediterranean Diet, see the recommended books listed on our website (www.jupiterinstitute.com).

Most of the research shows that adherence to the Mediterranean Diet improves health and longevity, prevents heart and vascular disease, improves arthritis, heals injuries, relieves pain, and even prevents cancer. It also has a powerful anti-inflammatory effect, that has a positive impact on the treatment of arthritis and inflammatory conditions of muscles, tendons, and ligaments. Despite a higher fat intake, people in Mediterranean countries show better overall health and a longer life expectancy. They suffer less from arthritis and pain, and their injuries heal better and with less distress. Their diet has a beneficial effect on fatigue and psychological disorders such as anxiety and depression. The beneficial effect of the Mediterranean Diet on heart disease is dramatic. This diet prevents heart attacks, but if a person has already had one, this diet will prevent or delay the onset of a second heart attack. It can also lower blood pressure and prevent atherosclerosis. Additionally, this diet has a dramatic effect on the joints. It prevents arthritis, and if a person is already suffering from arthritic conditions, it promotes healing and decreases inflammation of the affected joints. The same thing is true with injuries. Injuries, whether from a car accident, surgery or trauma, heal better and faster when following the Mediterranean Diet. The same occurs for those suffering from fatigue, body aches, and psychological disorders such as mood swings, anxiety, depression, and even Alzheimer's disease. Those who are already affected by these conditions do better on this diet and experience a significant reduction of symptoms and an overall improvement in the quality of life. Although the term "Mediterranean Diet" implies that all Mediterranean people eat the same foods, of course, this is not so. The countries of the Mediterranean Sea have different diets, religions, and cultures. Their diets differ in the amount of fat, protein, grains, types of meat, and wine intake. However, extensive studies show that although the diet may vary from country to country, the overall benefit does not change much. Pasta is eaten in some Mediterranean countries, but not in others; sourdough bread or more cheese are eaten in some; lamb in some, not in others; goat in some, in others only fish and poultry. The type and quantity of nuts and vegetables also vary, but these are just variations within the same type of diet. In total, the Mediterranean people who follow this way of eating do not consume vegetable oil or salad dressing, hamburgers, fried food, pizza, martinis, beer, chips, dips, or excessive beef. Unlike people in North America and Northern Europe, they do not consume excessive quantities of saturated fat (from animal products), trans fatty acids (from hydrogenated oils in manufactured and processed food), omega-6 fatty acids (from dairy, corn, meat and bakery products) and processed carbohydrates. However, consumption of omega-3 foods (fish, nuts, and vegetables) and omega-9 foods is high. Instead of having an unhealthy ratio of omega-6 to omega-3 of 20, 30, or even 40 to 1, as in the United States, their ratio is about 3 to 1, which is very good for general health and especially good for preventing cardiovascular disease, arthritis, and even cancer. The effect on the omega fatty acid balance is perhaps the most important factor of the Mediterranean Diet and the one that provides the greatest health benefit. High intake of omega-3 fatty acids from fish, vegetables, and nuts, coupled with the consumption of powerful antioxidants from herbs, fruits, wine, and vegetables puts people in an omega-3/antioxidant state, that provides tremendous health benefits, unlike the omega-6/free-radical state of the American diet, that is toxic, extremely inflammatory and disease-causing.

The Cardiovascular Advantage

Over the last 15 years, many studies have focused on unveiling the metabolic pathways through which the Mediterranean Diet provides its benefits. Among their conclusions is that such a diet:

1) Lowers overall cholesterol levels.

2) Raises levels of HDL (high-density lipoprotein), which is the good cholesterol that provides cardiovascular protection.

3) Lowers levels of LDL (low-density lipoprotein), that is the bad cholesterol that causes heart and vascular disease.

4) Reduces the oxidation of LDL, making it less prone to harden the arteries (atherogenic). This means that even if the LDL is elevated, the Mediterranean Diet protects the coronary and vascular system against its bad effects. In a way, the Mediterranean Diet shields the body against the bad effect of LDL.

5) Lowers the CRP (C-reactive protein), which is a marker of the degree of inflammation in the vascular system. High CRP indicates active inflammation in the blood vessels and indeed throughout the body; it is currently used as a marker to indicate the progression of cardiovascular disease and atherosclerosis. CRP is considered a high-risk factor for heart disease. Research shows that individuals

affected by high levels of CRP are more affected by the devastating effects of atherosclerosis, which includes peripheral vascular disease (lack of circulation in the legs), heart attacks, strokes, and many other conditions. Current cardiovascular preventive practices recommend lowering the levels of CRP. The Mediterranean Diet, as evidenced by publications in many journals and books, offers the beneficial effect of lowering C-reactive protein levels.

6) Reduces the risk of atherosclerosis. The Mediterranean Diet affects the eicosanoid system, increasing the presence and actions of good (anti-inflammatory) eicosanoids, and reducing bad (pro-inflammatory) eicosanoids. The eicosanoids are like super-hormones that control tissue metabolism. As we have noted, good eicosanoids decrease inflammation, increase the healing and repair, and prevent diseases. Bad eicosanoids damage tissue, cause inflammation and pain, and promote arthritis, aches, stiffness, atherosclerosis, and many other major diseases, including immune diseases and metabolic disease. They worsen diabetes, elevate blood pressure, and even promote obesity.

Effects on Inflammation and Pain

The Mediterranean Diet has a potent anti-inflammatory effect, the result of its omega-3 content. Arthritis and joint disease are less common in people following the Mediterranean Diet. When people who are affected by advanced osteoarthritis are placed on this diet, swelling decreases, and spinal stiffness and general healing improves. Painful conditions such as neck, back, and joint pain improve significantly as well. Injury sufferers (from car accidents, trauma, and surgery) heal better when following the Mediterranean Diet, thanks to its beneficial metabolic effect. Sports injuries heal faster too, that is why many trainers use it to treat injured athletes. The anti-inflammatory effect of this diet also protects against coronary atherosclerosis and coronary obstruction, reducing the risk of sudden cardiac death. Other conditions including allergies, asthma, PMS, menstrual cramps, headaches, skin disorders, neuropathy, mood disorders, and irritable bowels also get significant relief from the Mediterranean Diet.

Key Elements of the Mediterranean Diet

Olive oil

For centuries, the nutritional and medicinal benefits of olive oil have been recognized by the people of the Mediterranean region. Recent research has confirmed what the Mediterranean people already knew – that olive oil prevents and heals many diseases, promotes health, and increases longevity. Olive oil is the principal source of fat in the Mediterranean Diet. Because of its chemical structure, olive oil is unrivaled in its value and, thus, the oil best suited for human consumption. It is also extremely well-tolerated by the stomach and intestines, where it exerts a protective function. The excellent digestibility of olive oil promotes the overall absorption of nutrients, especially vitamins and minerals. Olive oil helps sustain human metabolism at a sensible balance and provides the body with good Vitamin E. Studies at university centers showed that olive oil decreases the oxidative state of the LDL, the bad cholesterol, making it less harmful to the vascular system. An even more important finding of these studies is that olive oil decreases the production of arachidonic acid, the father of all bad eicosanoids. The omega-6 foods produce arachidonic acid, that in turn generates the bad eicosanoids responsible for inflammation, disease, and pain. Olive oil reduces the formation of arachidonic acid by inhibiting a specific enzyme called delta-6-desaturase. This action makes olive oil a powerful anti-inflammatory agent that provides benefits at every level of the body. It is especially beneficial in many degenerative inflammatory processes including osteoarthritis, inflammatory arthritis, injuries, and other painful conditions.

Olive oil has been the most distinguished element of Mediterranean cooking for thousands of years. Although Spanish and Italian olive oil dominates international markets, Greek olive oils are excellent products as well. Extra virgin olive oil has a long shelf life and is best for salads and salad dressings. Other types of olive oil can be used for frying, but our recommendation is not to eat fried foods or foods cooked with a lot of olive oil. It is best to consume olive oil in its natural, uncooked state, straight from the bottle drizzled lightly on your food.

Red wine

In studies involving many thousands of participants, red wine consumption has been shown to reduce the risk of death from coronary disease and cancer. Studies also show that red wine, but no other alcoholic beverage, decreases cardiovascular mortality. The habit of moderate consumption of wine has been found to increase longevity. Concerns have been expressed by certain social and religious groups regarding the drinking of wine and a possible association with alcohol abuse, liver disease, and dependency. Nevertheless, studies show that when consumed responsibly, red wine is beneficial for the cardiovascular system and an important component of a healthy lifestyle. The Diet recommends one or two servings of 2-4 ounces each during a meal. Northern Europeans, who became upset with the news of the benefits of wine, performed clinical studies to test whether whiskey, beer, and other alcoholic beverages were as beneficial for the cardiovascular system as red wine. These studies ended in profound defeat, showing that alcoholic beverages other than red wine increase cardiovascular disease. Only red wine has been shown to protect health and provide health benefits. (White wine was defeated as well.)

The beneficial effects of red wine occur through several pathways:

- Its antioxidant effect, that neutralizes free radicals and protects the HDL (the good cholesterol), preventing vascular and tissue damage. Its boosting of HDL levels (the higher the HDL, the lower the risks for heart attack).
- Its vasodilating effect (dilatation of small arteries).
- Its anti-clogging effect prevents the formation of blood clots that block the coronary arteries.
- Its relaxing effect decreases stress and psychological tension.
- The extraordinary amount of nutrients it contains, including flavonoids, antioxidants, and resveratrol, are anti-inflammatory, anti-clogging, and anti-cancerous.
- The daily consumption of one or two glasses of red wine does not appear to have any harmful effect other than adding calories to the diet.

Numerous epidemiological studies, including the Copenhagen Health Study, the Nurses' Heart Study, the Framingham Study, and the American Cancer Society Study, associate moderate red wine consumption with health and longevity. Much can be said about the excellent combination of red wine and olive oil. However, for the sake of time and space, we will focus on the entire Mediterranean Diet.

Natural antioxidants

One of the highlights of the Mediterranean Diet is its high content of natural antioxidants. The health benefits of antioxidants are well-known. They neutralize toxic free radicals, which are molecules that cause inflammation and damage in our tissues. Free radicals oxidize and neutralize the HDL (the good cholesterol) and cause damage in joints and injured areas, worsening arthritis, and pain. Antioxidants counteract these effects by blocking free radicals. Therefore, they enhance the healing and repair of injuries, decrease pain, and improve both arthritis and coronary inflammation.

Where are you going to get these natural antioxidants? Your shopping of course. You'll go through local markets and grocery stores and buy what you need.

The sources of these nutrients in the Mediterranean Diet are:
- Fresh herbs (basil, bay leaves, chives, cilantro, dill, fennel, garlic, marjoram, oregano, parsley, rosemary, sage, thyme, tarragon, and others). You can get them at the supermarket or in pots at garden stores
- Fresh raw fruits.
- Plant food, fresh legumes, and vegetables consumed raw, uncooked
- Red wine

-But doctor, what about my broccoli and my string beans?
-Are they cooked or steamed?
-Yes, but...
-No. Forget them!!

In addition to their protective effect on HDL and tissues, antioxidants also protect omega-3 fatty acids from being destroyed by free radicals. The intake of antioxidants in their fresh, natural state is mandatory and essential for good health. Awareness of this issue is very important. Antioxidants can be ingested through the foods we mentioned above, but frequently this consumption is not sufficient and the use of vitamins and supplements is, therefore, recommended. This will be explained further when we get to the basic concepts of the Jupiter Institute Omega Diet. Supplements and vitamins are needed and are discussed here and in the Supplements chapter. The reason they are needed is the lack of nutrients in the common foods available to us; hence, we have to get them from elsewhere.

In regards to taking antioxidants in pills or capsules, my advice to you is:

a) Don't take too many supplement pills, just two or three a day should be the basic dosage and should be plenty (unless you have a specific condition that requires taking more).

b) Take antioxidants in a combination with your MULTIVITAMIN - that is, take the best multivitamin you can that would contain some variety of essential antioxidants.

The Jupiter Institute Omega Diet in Brief

Foods That Are Best to Eat

Listed below are the food groups we recommend you eat. You will find plenty of omega-3 fatty acids and antioxidants.

1) **Protein** - White protein is best, found in fish, egg whites, lean chicken (white meat) (organic only), tofu, beef, pork, canned fish, veal, lamb, goat, wild meat is OK. Certain cold cuts, like ham, although not ideal, are acceptable.

   However, it is important to remember that the best way to eat all those protein choices is by alkalinizing and Mediterraneanizing them, that means to combine smaller portions with alkaline food, fresh herbs, raw vegetables, olive oil, and even raw fruits.

Again, I come with examples:

Baked lamb, green and black olives, with a large salad made with arugula, parsley, kale, sea salt, and olive oil.

T-bone steak with olive oil on top, olives, sweet potatoes, and a salad with carrots, cabbage, kalamata olives, lettuce, beets, and fresh herbs.

Baked pork, raw broccoli with toasted garlic and olive oil on top, rice, and a fruit salad with mango, pears, banana, strawberries, and pineapple.

Not appealing? Then make your own combination using the concepts I gave you.

Do you want some mac & cheese or cheeseburgers? Then figure out how to Mediterraneanize and alkalinize them.

How do you alkalinize and Mediterraneanize pork ribs with BBQ sauce and coleslaw? Go figure.

How do you do it with fried chicken, biscuit and fried onion rings? You don't! Don't eat it.

Remember that although you need protein every day you do not need a lot. Excess protein is not good, and neither is a protein-free diet. Brown rice combined with beans is a very good source of protein. We strongly recommend that you eat your protein with some vegetables and olive oil.

A word about turkey: I don't trust it. I think it is a toxic animal because of the way it is farmed. Stay away.

So, what do you do with mac & cheese, turkey burgers, and corn dogs? You just avoid them.

2) **Fish** - Eat fish regularly! The best kinds are oily fish: anchovies, bluefish, cod, halibut, herring, mackerel, salmon, sardines, tuna, and trout.

Raw fish is better than cooked, and cooked is better than canned. Canned fish in water mixed with additional olive oil is better than fish canned in oil.

Fish caught in the deep ocean waters contain much more omega-3 fatty acids than farmed fish because deep ocean fish feed on algae, which is rich in omega-3. However, they are not always easy to get. Market conditions, distribution, and price often make it more convenient and practical to obtain farm-raised fish. Although farm-raised fish are not a panacea, they are often subject to overcrowding, disease, and other deleterious conditions. Make sure you inquire about the source of your fish whenever possible.

The white, flaky, non-oily fish (such as grouper, snapper, mahi-mahi, and cobia from Florida), are good sources of protein but contain no omega-3. King mackerel, kingfish, and swordfish do contain omega-3, but I do not recommend them: they may be contaminated with mercury, don't eat them. Don't eat canned tuna more than once a week, it contains mercury and other toxins.

Variations in omega-3 fatty acids also occur in tuna. Tuna, when eaten raw and fresh, offers significant amounts of it, but canned tuna, which has been cooked at least twice in the process of packing, has much less.

3) **Olive oil and olives (green and black)** - Only extra virgin oil is recommended. We do not recommend light olive oil. One or two tablespoons of regular extra virgin oil twice a day is the current recommendation – uncooked oil that goes straight from the bottle to the food. Cooked oils are best to avoid as they do not have nearly the same health benefits as uncooked oils, and could be harmful. If you cook oil, make sure that it is fresh oil and that you are only cooking in it for a few minutes at most. Olives, either green or black, are strongly recommended, as a garnish for food, and as a snack.

For variety, you can flavor your oil, combining it with lemon juice, salt, thyme, and oregano, or with chopped fresh herbs. Alternatively, you can mix it with a little French mustard, ketchup, and horseradish, barbecue sauce, or fat-free mayonnaise, or mix it with a combination of dry herbs.

4) **Natural grains, beans, and pulses** - Recommended grains are rice, brown rice, couscous, quinoa, and even bulgur, as well as "pseudograins" such as quinoa and millet, that are not grains but seeds from plants. Recommended pulses (legumes) and beans are lentils and dried beans (canned beans are OK as long as they are plain), green beans, and string beans.

Green peas and chickpeas are allowed. Although hummus is a typical Mediterranean dish, it is traditionally consumed in small quantities. You should eat it only on rare occasions and in small amounts. The reason is the preparation: in Mediterranean countries, hummus is prepared with a large amount of fresh olive oil while the tendency in the United States is to use processed oils and other preservatives. Hence, because of its high omega-6 content, it is not recommended. This recommendation does not apply as strictly to homemade hummus prepared with fresh olive oil; still, care should be taken not to over-consume it.

Corn is full of omega-6s and should be avoided.

Consume grains in their natural forms. Avoid processed products of the grains we mention here, such as rice cakes, rice crackers, refried beans, bean dips, processed lentil soups, processed pea soups, and so on.

5) **Nuts** - Walnuts are the nuts that we recommend the most, although macadamia nuts, pumpkin seeds, almonds, and hazelnuts are also approved.

Brazil nuts, cashews, and pecans are not recommended. Peanuts are not nuts, and they are forbidden. Sesame seeds and sunflower seeds are seeds, not nuts, but they are accepted and their oils are accepted as well, although some authors don't agree. By-products of peanuts – peanut oil, peanut butter - and pecan products – are not allowed.

6) **Flaxseeds** - Flaxseeds, ground flaxseeds, flaxseed oil, and flaxseed gel caps are strongly recommended and should be liberally consumed. Feel free to use them as often as you want and in the quantities you desire. They are an excellent source of omega-3.

7) **Red wine** - Red wine is the only alcohol allowed in the Jupiter Institute Omega Diet. It is approved in quantities of 2-4 ounces at a time and with a meal only. One time a week, at home, at dinnertime is a good way to begin.

As with any alcoholic drink, one should be aware of the side effects and act responsibly. Consuming alcohol is not required for health. However, if you wish to drink wine, consume it always at dinnertime and in the stipulated quantities of 2-4 ounces. No driving is allowed after consumption. (Being aware of the adverse effects of using alcohol while on medication is the responsibility of the patient. You must consult your doctor.)

For those who don't like wine, scotch and good quality vodka, in moderation, are second choices.

8) **Herbs** - Herbs contain minerals and antioxidants that are not found in any other food and are crucial to our metabolism. Fresh herbs also provide valuable vitamins.

Here is a list of common herbs:

- Basil
- Bay leaves
- Chives
- Cilantro
- Coriander
- Dill
- Garlic
- Ginger
- Marjoram
- Mint
- Oregano
- Parsley
- Rosemary
- Thyme

Fresh raw herbs have a much higher concentration of antioxidants; that is why we recommend them. You can find them in plastic containers or bags in the vegetable section of the supermarket. You can also buy them in pots at garden stores and plant them in your backyard. Try getting into the habit of using fresh herbs regularly in your salad. Adding fresh herbs and olive oil to your salad is a very healthy habit. When fresh herbs cannot be obtained, dried herbs are acceptable.

9) **Raw fruit -** Raw fruit is strongly recommended. A variety of seasonal fruit is best. Your local market is one source but look for fruit that has been recently picked. Fruit that has been picked too many days in advance has lost much of its antioxidant and vitamin value. One of the best examples is the bananas found in local American markets, that have been picked green many days and even weeks ahead. By the time they are consumed by the public, by now yellow and soft, their vitamin and antioxidant content are very low. Other examples are mangoes and oranges. They, too, have been harvested too many days before reaching the market. Even though they have been refrigerated, their vitamin and antioxidant content are low. Each market in each state is different. The reader needs to take into account the possible local production and the origin of each of the

fruits they find. Again, local fruits in season and picked when ripe are best.

DON'T FORGET the concept of Nutrigenomics as you choose your food. When consuming fruits, veggies, proteins, etc., you need to take into account your genes, that is your origin, your roots, where your mom, your dad, and your grandparents came from. If you are Polish like me, Russian or German, then pineapple, coconut, kiwi, rum, tropical fish, and many other foods are not for you. If you are Sicilian, Moroccan, Iranian, Japanese, etc., take into account what your ancestors ate. Don't let your palate or local bad dietary habits mislead you.

10) **Vegetables** - Fresh and raw is best. Vegetables can be steamed, but just lightly. The more a vegetable is cooked, the lower its vitamin and antioxidant content. A variety of vegetables and vegetables of different colors are strongly recommended. Frozen vegetables are okay, but their vitamin and antioxidant content are also very low. All fresh vegetables are a source of good (complex) carbohydrates, natural vitamins, and antioxidants. Some have high omega-3 content that makes them desirable for those who follow our program. These omega-3 vegetables are:

• Alfalfa sprouts	• Cauliflower	• Mustard greens
• Arugula	• Collard greens	• Romaine
• Bean sprouts	• Kale	• Spinach
• Broccoli	• Lettuce	• Watercress

11) **Recommended vitamins and supplements** - These are capsules and tablets including omega-3 fatty acids (fish oil, salmon oil, flaxseed oil), gamma-linoleic acid (GLA), antioxidants, and vitamins.

I describe these supplements better in the Supplements chapter. Suffice it to say that I don't take or recommend any vitamin or supplement that is not produced by recognized laboratories. I don't believe in any wonderful website or health food store and especially I don't recommend any vitamins from pharmacies or supermarkets. We live in times of a lack of consumer awareness and protection. Imports of all kinds of supplements manufactured without oversight in unknown countries with high environmental toxicity that affects everything we take. I will be telling you in the Supplements chapter which brands I recommend.

12) **Avoidance** - Whatever is not listed above should be avoided – especially omega-6 food including fried food, sugary baked goods, and processed food as discussed later in this chapter.

Additional recommendations for the Jupiter Institute Omega Diet

1) **Snacks.** Learn to snack on things you can have – walnuts, olives, fruits, or a bit of bread dipped in olive oil. Canned mushrooms, canned beans, canned hearts of palm, and canned asparagus are also acceptable.

   Snacks to avoid. if you do not see an item on my list, ask your doctor or chiropractor, or contact us by phone, mail, or fax. Sugar, honey, and alcohol other than wine are not allowed.

2) **Beware of marketing.** Foods you see in television commercials are bad for you. If you see someone on television in a white coat pushing a particular food, he or she is being paid to mislead you. Much of the food advertising in magazines is misleading and manipulative. Be careful!

3) **Go easy on** soy sauce and diet sodas – these are OK, but only rarely. Pasta is allowed one to three times a month, and no more. Two slices of bread a day is allowed. A little fruit spread (with no added sugar) for your toast and a little milk for your coffee are also allowed. One or two cups of coffee in the morning are OK, but not more than that.

4) **Do eat fat!** But it must be good fat, like that found in nuts, olive oil, and avocado. Never eat fat-free meals and never touch deep-fried food! A bit of butter every day is good. Adding a bit of sesame oil to the olive oil is good too.

5) **Restaurants are dangerous.** With some exceptions, restaurants are dangerous for your diet. Do not waste your time, your money, or your health on such foods. Cruises are also not healthy because of the uncontrolled amounts of food that people tend to consume. Do not go to places where your dietary plan will be in danger.

6) **Read labels.** If the fat content of a food product you are buying is more than zero percent, then you can be sure it contains processed fat that is bad for your body.

7) **Not recommended:** Salami, pepperoni, mozzarella cheese, hamburger, milkshakes, pizza, fried chicken, potato salad, coleslaw, supermarket salads, hot dogs, pâté, cheeses, luncheon meats, sour cream, milk, frozen dinners, chain-restaurant "Mexican" food, chili, bagels, cream cheese, donuts, muffins, pastries, cakes, ice

cream, candy bars, peanuts, peanut butter, bakery products, butter, margarine, salad dressing, commercial sauces, liquor, beer, chips and dips, and any food from fast-food restaurants.

But that does not mean that you can't "cheat," right?

Besides, you can Mediterraneanize and alkalinize those products. Do you want some salami, pepperoni, and cheese? Well, serve them with olives over a bed of arugula and tomato and pour olive oil on top.

Want some donuts and peanut butter cups? No. Not good.

8) **Manufactured and processed food.** If the food was made in a factory or a restaurant, it was not made with your health in mind.

9) **Cereal products.** Whole wheat bread (not recommended because of the gluten: use gluten-free breads if need be), oatmeal, breakfast cereal, and granola are inventions to make you believe you are eating healthy. I do not recommend them. They are not included in the Mediterranean Diet.

10) **Certain oils.** Corn oil, sunflower oil, safflower oil, cottonseed oil, peanut oil are not good for you. They are even worse when cooked or fried.

The Jupiter Institute Omega Diet combines three key elements:

1) The Mediterranean Diet.

2) Avoidance of foods with omega-6s and activators of omega-6.

3) Supplements of omega-3s and carefully chosen antioxidants.

This diet is designed to elevate you into the omega-3/antioxidant state that we emphasize for reduced pain and inflammation. The foods we eat, the supplements we take, and our lifestyle habits (exercise, sleep, etc.) can balance the metabolism (what we call the omega-3/antioxidant state) or cause imbalance (what we call the pro-inflammatory omega-6/free-radical state). Both of these metabolic conditions work through activating – favorably or unfavorably – the eicosanoid system that we described earlier. In the omega-3/antioxidant state all metabolic functions work in harmony, so inflammation, cellular damage, and pain are decreased.

The Importance of What You Don't Eat

When it comes to healthy eating, what people don't eat is just as important as what they do eat. Meat, in general, carries a lot of saturated fat and other substances that pose a threat to health. Some of these substances are known to generate cardiovascular diseases and cancer.

Mediterranean people consume very little meat, if any, and avoid seed oils such as corn, sunflower, cottonseed, and soybean oil. They also consume very little butter and milk and avoid the dense fatty acids of margarine, processed food, frozen meals, and snacks. Foods such as cheese, pizza, cheeseburgers, a glass of milk, meat and potatoes, bagels with cream cheese, hot dogs, barbecued ribs, breakfast cereal, orange juice, mayonnaise, cookies, ice cream, and many other foods typical of the American diet, are not consumed by Mediterranean people. In general, they do not expose themselves to large steaks, pork products, large pasta dishes, shakes, luncheon meats, donuts, beer, chips, dips, and salad dressings. They do not embrace the typical American breakfast, brunch buffets, waffles, pancakes, and the great variety of breads and cereals commonly consumed in the United States. Therefore, they don't load themselves with saturated fat, fried food, processed foods that are high in refined carbohydrates, and trans-fatty acids, that are loaded with toxic, pro-inflammatory omega-6s. As compensation for a more simple and natural way of eating, Mediterranean people are rewarded with better health, fewer strokes and heart attacks, and less arthritis and cancer. They also live longer. However, Mediterraneans who depart from their traditional diet and adopt foods from other cultures – specifically Northern Europe and the U.S. – do not do well. The significant increase in omega-6 fatty acids causes Mediterranean people to develop the same diseases (atherosclerosis, inflammation, and vascular diseases) as the cultures who eat this way. When Mediterranean people – regardless of where they live – don't follow a Mediterranean Diet, their health suffers. So, if Mediterranean's eat like Americans, they die like Americans.

Processed Foods

I described them already, but it is worth reviewing them again because of their strong impact on health. Processed foods are made in a factory from once-natural and whole foods. It is food that has been created artificially by a corporation or a company whose primary purpose is to make a profit, not to make us healthier. Some examples are orange juice, canned syrups, frozen dinners, bread, yogurts, and cereals. In all of these products, different natural foods are taken, processed, mixed, combined with unnatural fats and/or unnatural carbohydrates, chemicals, flavor enhancers, color additives, and other chemicals like preservatives, and then packaged and sent to the market. They taste delicious and they provide enjoyment, but because of their omega-6s, their acidity, the free-radicals they generate, their absence of omega-3, their lack of antioxidants, and their poor nutrient value, they stimulate a chronic inflammatory response that leads to disease. Is this clear enough? If you are fighting inflammation, degeneration, weight issues, surgical recovery, injuries, severe arthritis, painful disorders, or any disease, YOU DON'T EVEN WANT TO TOUCH THEM, SMELL THEM OR HAVE THEM NEAR YOU.

Yes, besides increasing your weight and pushing you closer to diabetes, ultimately these products will make you ill.

Processed foods are divided into three main groups:

1) Fatty foods - Foods containing processed fat and vegetable oils. Processed fats are known as trans fatty acids: man-made fats that do not become rancid and are excellent for preservation. They are found in all kinds of packaged and canned foods. The problem is that both the trans fatty acids and vegetable oils are high in omega-6s, which means they are pro-inflammatory and toxic. Examples of these fatty processed foods are cheeses, spreads, dips, sauces, snacks, soups, frozen meals, cookies, hot dogs, muffins, etc.

2) Carbohydrate-containing foods. - Processed carbohydrates are carbohydrate-containing foods that have gone through a manufacturing process; their structures are broken-down, manipulated, cooked, and simplified "pre-digested" for ease of eating. Once eaten, they are absorbed quickly by the body, stimulating the omega-6 system and the production of insulin. In their original, unprocessed state, these foods could be good sources of omega-3s. But processing puts them on the omega-6 pathway where they become "foods" that cause obesity, inflammation, and diseases such as diabetes. Examples of this include tomato juice (from tomatoes), apple juice and apple jelly (from apples), orange juice, orange jelly and orange marmalade (from oranges), flour products, pasta and breads (from flour), breakfast cereals (from grains), grape juice and grape jelly (from grapes), potato chips, corn muffins, corn chips and corn tortillas (from corn). Also included in this group are beer, rice cakes, donuts, and sherbets.

Remember: Processed carbohydrates are omega-6 activators.

3) Combination foods - Food containing processed carbohydrates and processed fats represent our food industry at its worst. Food manufacturers' extremely successful effort to generate highly durable foods with a longer shelf life has created a toxic mess for the human body. This is evidenced by escalating rates of diabetes and other Occidental diseases like cancer. These combinations are packaged breads, cakes, frozen dinners, yogurt, candy bars, chocolate milk,

bakery products, ice cream, cookies, canned meals, canned soups, canned pasta, etc. Vegetable oils, trans fatty acids (synthetic fat), and processed carbohydrates are the lifeblood of the food industry but, sadly, at the root of our increasingly diseased society.

Remember that cocktail?

If you eat all kinds of processed carbs and processed fatty foods, without alkalizing your meals, without Mediterraneanizing them, you live in an omega-6, pro-inflammatory, anti-healing, state.

Well, how do you Mediterraneanize pizza? Place it on a plate, pour olive oil on it, then eat it with anchovies and olives and enjoy a simultaneous salad with arugula, tomato, onions, and some of the alkaline foods from the list.

How can you Mediterraneanize a donut and a cappuccino with whipped cream? You don't! Don't have them.

How do you Mediterraneanize a hotel breakfast with cereal, milk, oatmeal, bagel, donut, juices, wafer, pancakes, bread, butter, jelly, peanut butter, etc.? You don't! Don't touch those things. Have instead some bananas, apples, hard-boiled eggs or eggs any style, black coffee, ask for olive oil.

How do you Mediterraneanize fried chicken, coleslaw, corn, and mashed potato with gravy? You can't. Go somewhere else and get baked or grilled chicken over a bed of salad.

It is with substitutions and additions that you Mediterraneanize and alkalinize your meals.

Fats: the Bad and the Good

Another important food category to avoid occurs in both processed and unprocessed foods: saturated fat. This is the fat that comes from animals, especially from red meat. It is found mainly in beef, pork, veal, burgers, meat products, cold cuts, deli meat, sausage, salami, bacon, pâté, and also in the fat of chicken and turkey and all products cooked with lard or animal fats. Saturated fat tastes good, especially when fried or grilled. We, humans, have a pleasure center for fat and foods fried with fat. Nathan Pritikin described this very well in his books, and I recommend that you read them if you want to learn more about this issue. Apparently, as part of the evolution of primitive man, our ancestors developed a "fat instinct center" somewhere in the brain. This center, which is strongly associated with our instinct for preservation, caused primitive and non-primitive humans to gorge on fat whenever possible. Gorging on fat was a survival technique, providing people with large amounts of calories that would help them survive until the next time food became available. Since food was not readily available in those times, people whose brains had a well-developed "pleasure center" for the taste of fat survived through natural selection; those without this center would perish in the face of drought, famine, disease, frigid weather, and similar adversities. All of us, therefore, are descendants of those who survived. We all have this fat instinct in us, some more, some less. You experience the awakening of your fat instinct, for example, when you become hungry while driving past a hamburger place. You can also feel it when you get an uncontrollable desire to eat meat. Although in olden times, the generous consumption of meat and meat products, pork, organ meats, etc., was nutritionally important, nowadays it is no longer so. You should forget about how important this type of food was in the 18th century when the American colonies were fighting England, or in Europe 500 years ago, or now for struggling communities in Africa, and understand that the meat products that we mention here give you two bad things: saturated fat that clogs your blood vessels and coronary arteries, and excessive amounts of omega-6 fatty acids, that give you bad eicosanoids and excessive inflammation. Unfortunately, it gets worse. The pleasure center related to this fat instinct frequently wants to be satisfied, and can easily control a person. Fortunately, this does not happen to every human being, as the center is not the same for everybody. It is strong in some people while weak in others. But those with even a mild urge for fat do get the call for meat and other fatty foods. You can see them filling the steakhouses, hamburger places, and restaurants. You see them buying meat products. You hear them when they describe with pride how their freezer is full of meat. It is the same in every country – only the type of meat product varies. So, now that you understand this, you can see the conflict: the instinct of your body will call you to consume foods containing saturated fat, even though this kind of food hurts you. Consumption of foods containing saturated fat is without any doubt a source of health problems and should be restricted in everyone's diet, and particularly for those suffering from arthritis, inflammatory diseases, pains, and injuries.

The Three Bad Fats

Reviewing the above, the three bad fats with omega-6s are:

1) Saturated fat, that is the fat from animal products we've just described.

2) Fried foods or foods cooked with oil or fat.

3) Trans fatty acids or processed fat contained in processed foods.

The Good Fat

The good fats provide helpful omega-3s. This is the fat in fish, especially oily fish such as salmon, trout, tuna, cod, sardines, anchovies, bluefish, and mackerel. It also comes in olive oil, olives, flax seeds, flaxseed oil, avocados, walnuts, and walnut oil. Also, easy to take and recommended: concentrated purified fish oil (get the highest quality you can get).

Avoid Omega-6

Foods containing omega-6 fatty acids and those that activate the toxic omega-6 metabolic pathway should be avoided.

Sources of omega-6s:

- Meat and meat products (especially red meat: pork, beef, lamb, and veal) - Dairy products
- Poultry
- Sesame oil
- Corn
- Peanuts, peanut oil and peanut butter
- Vegetable oil (soybean, safflower, sunflower, corn, and cottonseed)
- The three bad fats: saturated fats from animal products, fat from fried food, and trans-fatty acids from processed food. Sesame oil, although it contains omega-6, is allowed in small quantities due to some of its metabolic benefits. Also, meat, although it contains the adverse omega-6, is needed for general nutrition, but there is a way to balance its adverse properties: eating it with alkaline foods and plenty of olive oil.

Activators of toxic omega-6s:

- Deficit of antioxidants (excess of free radicals)
- Excessive alcohol consumption
- Excessive quantities of coffee and sugar
- Flour products (bread, pasta, cakes, pastry, donuts, bagels, and bakery products)
- Fruit juices
- High simple-carbohydrate diets
- Processed carbohydrates (simple carbohydrates)
- Stress
- Uncontrolled diabetes

Let me give you some examples. Pork lo mein with a beer and dessert or pasta and meatballs with a couple of beers are all omega-6 meals. Chicken fried with corn oil, rice cakes with peanut butter, a breakfast with orange juice, cereal, and fat-free milk are all examples of omega-6 meals. Working under stress while drinking plenty of coffee and snacking on donuts and cake, or enjoying football on Sunday with lots of beer, chips and dips are omega-6 activators. A large hamburger with fries, a large steak with mashed potatoes, a typical Mexican meal, a large pastrami sandwich, a couple of cocktails with some peanuts, fettuccine alfredo, or bagels with cream cheese are all omega-6 activators. They are also acidic and they are lacking omega-3 and antioxidants. They all push you deeper into the pro-inflammatory omega-6/free radical state that, when chronic, shows up as ongoing disease, including pain and inflammation.

Cholesterol and CRP

Lowering levels of cholesterol and LDL, (the bad cholesterol) is very simple.

To lower cholesterol and LDLs (low-density lipoprotein), avoid omega-6 foods, and follow the Mediterranean Diet. Nevertheless, you may have a congenital tendency to have high cholesterol. If this dietary program does not work to reduce your cholesterol in six weeks, you may need a dietary adjustment, and if that does not work, you may need medications. See your doctor in this case.

HDL, or high-density lipoprotein, is the good cholesterol and works as a detergent, cleaning the pipes (arteries and coronaries). The higher the HDLs the better, since it prevents coronary disease, heart attacks, and strokes.

These are the recommendations to increase HDL:
- Regular exercise
- Nuts (mainly walnuts but also macadamias and pumpkin seeds; on occasion some almonds and hazelnuts)
- Olives, black or green
- Olive oil – at least one or two large tablespoons twice a day
- Mediterranean Diet
- Fish (mainly oily fish like anchovies, bluefish, cod, halibut, mackerel, salmon, sardines, trout, and tuna)
- Fish-oil gel caps, salmon-oil gel caps, or cod liver oil
- Ground flaxseeds and flaxseed oil, liquid or gel caps

- Omega-3 foods, such as algae and green leafy vegetables (alfalfa sprouts, arugula, broccoli, cauliflower, collard greens, kale, lettuce, mustard greens, romaine, spinach, and watercress)

To Lower Levels of CRP

C-reactive protein (CRP) is a marker for inflammation in the body, detected by a blood test. When elevated, it is an indicator of active inflammation and an ongoing disease or threat of disease. Just as lava can erupt from a volcano anywhere on earth, this inflammation may erupt anywhere in the body and may explode as colitis, heart attack, arthritis, or an injury that does not heal. It may also erupt as pain, severe atherosclerosis, lack of immunity, and many other metabolic disorders.

These are the recommendations to lower CRP levels. Same recommendations as before:

- Decrease omega-6 intake.
- Increase omega-3 intake.
- Get antioxidants, from either fresh food (fruits, vegetables, herbs) or high-quality supplements.
- If taking omega-3 supplements (fish oil, salmon oil) vitamins and antioxidant pills, take the highest quality possible and only the brands from laboratories recognized by the Academy of Anti-Aging and only the recommended brands. Avoid unreliable brands from supermarkets, pharmacies, etc. (I am sure you can find a local physician or chiropractor who can help you get them).
- Avoid the three bad fats.
- Consider taking supplements of GLA (gamma-linoleic acid).
- Control diabetes, infections, and dental diseases.
- Follow the Mediterranean Diet.
- Take high-quality olive oil twice a day.

A Few Things to Remember

→ Beefeaters don't last long.

→ Fat-free diets are dangerous; everyone needs good fats.

→ If omega-3 pushes your car to the west and omega-6 pushes your car to the east, you may not get anywhere.

→ The poker game called "your life" may depend on your essential fatty acid cards: Too many sixes and just a few threes and you lose, but plenty of threes and only a few sixes and you win. Some people cheat and win, but most of those who cheat lose it all. Do you want to gamble with your life?

The Anti-nutrient Lifestyle

Joints, heart, muscles, coronary arteries, and all the organs of the body are made of living tissue, fibers, cells, and complex proteins. Daily use causes wear and tear, and demands a daily supply of nutrients to help with the repair. A smoker who abuses alcohol, for example, lives in a state of permanent physical stress. As such, his or her system will contain excessive amounts of free radicals. In the absence of adequate nutrition from fresh fruits and vegetables, omega-3 fatty acids, proper protein, vitamins, and minerals, the excessive free radicals will not be neutralized by antioxidants, and tissue damage will occur. Additionally, if such a person eats too much saturated fat, and high amounts of sugars and flour products, dairy products, meat, fried food, fast food, frozen dinners, processed foods, processed fats, vegetable oils and juices (that are all factory or man-made foods instead of natural food), his or her diet will be full of the harmful omega-6 fatty acids, that generate bad eicosanoids. Even if this person eats a lot of food, he or she will be nutritionally deficient because there are few good nutrients in these foods. This is essentially an anti-nutrient diet and is damaging to the heart, joints, coronary arteries, cartilage, ligaments, muscle, and all the organs of the body. A person following this anti-nutrient diet is full of free radicals and bad eicosanoids that cause tissue damage, promote inflammation, arthritis, and favor heart trouble in the form of coronary disease and atherosclerosis. The situation worsens when the person is affected by the chemicals and additives found in these foods, processed meats, and soft drinks. Corn, corn products, fast food (like hamburgers, pizza, and hot dogs), peanuts, peanut butter, vegetable oil, fatty snacks, fatty dips, and dressings are particularly high in omega-6s, generating even more bad eicosanoids (bad prostaglandins) and inflammation. If you thought that meat and potatoes, orange juice, cheeseburgers, a bagel with cream cheese, cereal with milk, the milk you see in the commercial "Got Milk?" salad dressings, and the chips and dips consumed during Sunday's televised sports programs were any good for you, think again! They are all omega-6 foods, promoting arthritis and pain. They are also enemies of the heart. Like beer, bakery products, cookies, and cream, they are all pro-inflammatory. If all of this was not enough, certain kinds of foods create more acidity in the body making the damage to the tissues even worse. These foods are alcohol, cheeses, cocoa, corn and corn products, coffee, flour products, pasta, meat, sugar and sugar products (e.g. candies, pastries, and snacks), vinegar, peanuts, and peanut butter. These foods create acidity that will attack the organs and tissues of our bodies, doubling their adverse effects on tissues. Hence, they should be eliminated from the diet. More poor food choices (because of their omega-6 content) are cakes, canned creamy soups, donuts, fried food, frozen meals, margarine, mayonnaise, canned food with fat, bakery products (muffins, bagels, bread, pastries, cookies), chips, dips, take-out food, packaged bread, waffles, and processed meat products (salami, hot dogs, pepperoni, bologna, etc.).

Pro-inflammatory Foods

Certain foods are pro-inflammatory because they create acidity in the tissues, have excessive omega-6s, lack omega-3s or antioxidants, and any or all of these reasons. While I've mentioned them before, these pro-inflammatory foods need to be mentioned again: Foods with high levels of omega-6, foods cooked in peanut, sesame and sunflower oils, such as restaurant food, ethnic food, fried food, and fast food are considered pro-inflammatory, saturated fat that comes from animal fat, dairy products, butter, and tropical oils, trans fatty acids, that are man-made (factory-made) fats, found in processed foods, salad dressings, margarine, bakery products (cookies, bread, muffins, bagels, donuts, crackers, etc.), salsa and dips, processed carbohydrates such as flour products, sugars, sweet drinks, and juices, candies, snacks, dips, all bakery products, pasta, cereal, breakfast cereal, alcohol (beer, liquor), fast foods, and fried foods.

An Anti-inflammatory Diet

The Jupiter Institute Omega Diet is a program rich in omega-3 fatty acids, that are natural anti-inflammatory nutrients. They come from fish and fish products, fish oil, flaxseed, certain nuts, supplements, and vegetables. This diet provides olive oil, well-known for its anti-inflammatory properties, and also fresh herbs, fruits, and vegetables known for their powerful antioxidant effect. Antioxidants are seriously important because they neutralize those unhealthy free radicals that cause so much harm to the injured tissue. Moreover, antioxidants protect the Omega-3, which are a bit delicate and need some local protection to prevent them from disintegration.

One of our program's goals is to disengage the person from the food that provides omega-6 fatty acids, that causes inflammation in joints, tendons, muscles, and the other tissues and organs of the body. Just increasing the intake of the good omega-3s, however, is not enough. The intake of omega-6s needs to be decreased and the meal needs to be Mediterraneanized and alkalinized. If you have just eaten corn with margarine and fried chicken, you cannot fix it by having some spinach and olive oil when you get home. A few capsules of salmon oil CANNOT erase the adverse effects of two cheeseburgers with French fries. If you want to enjoy the benefits of the program and avoid the damaging effect of anti-nutrients, you must increase the intake of foods containing omega-3s while decreasing or altogether avoiding the intake of omega-6 foods. I'll say it again: you can't expect to feast on pizza and cake or French fries and beer and then come home and clean up your act by taking two tablespoons of olive oil and a few gel caps of salmon oil.

"Mediterraneanizing" Your Diet

This chapter aims to give you a bit more information about how to follow the Jupiter Institute Omega Diet, so you can improve your overall health. Being in the omega-3/antioxidant state will also help you fight your pain, arthritis, or injury more successfully. In previous chapters, I reviewed which foods are good to eat and which are not. Now I will complement the concept that some foods usually considered "bad" or "not OK" can be converted, "Mediterraneanized," to make them healthier. Yes, you may be able to go back to steak and pasta by following some simple rules.

The countries that surround the Mediterranean Sea have a rich tradition of fine food, a tradition that has been spreading throughout the world. Mediterranean cuisine has achieved international popularity not only because of its fine flavors and aromas but because it is recognized as being the healthiest in the world, in tune with modern trends in nutrition and health. Fifteen countries and three continents border the Mediterranean Sea: to the north, the European countries of Spain, France, Italy, Greece, and Turkey. To the east is the Asian continent with Lebanon, Israel, and Syria. To the south is the African continent with Morocco, Egypt, Libya, Tunisia and Algeria, and the island nations of Cyprus and Malta. Each of them is unique in their language, culture, tradition, and also in cuisines, spices, and food presentation.

Despite these differences in culture and cuisine, many ingredients, spices, and recipes are common to the entire region. Indeed, when reviewing books on Middle Eastern, French, Spanish, Italian and Moroccan cuisine, it is fascinating to see how some dishes have traveled around the region. Slightly modified, seasoned with local ingredients, given different names, they become typical dishes of many different areas.

Among the staple ingredients of Mediterranean cuisine are couscous, rice, vegetables, spices, olives, fish, and olive oil used copiously. Of all the Mediterranean countries, Greece is the country whose diet has been shown to offer the best health benefits. Accordingly, we are going to take Greek cuisine as the model Mediterranean Diet. Although dishes from other Mediterranean countries will be considered as well, dishes that deviate too much from the typical Greek style, or offer foods that are too far removed from the omega-3 stream, are not recommended even though they are considered Mediterranean dishes. This is the concept that differentiates the Jupiter Institute Omega Diet from the Mediterranean Diet: certain dishes, although they are Mediterranean and generally considered part of the Mediterranean Diet and Mediterranean culture, are so loaded with omega-6s and carbohydrates that we discourage their consumption. Examples are the pasta with meatballs and tomato sauce of Italy, the pork dishes of Spain, the cochinillo of Segovia, the falafel with hummus of Israel, and the tahini and pita of Lebanon and Egypt. The same goes for kebabs, kibbeh, fancy risottos, etc., and many fried dishes and desserts, including fried calamari, baklava, fried cheese, etc. Several typical Greek dishes are left out for this same reason: they deviate from the omega-3 stream. Caution: you can find many "Mediterranean Diet" books out there with wonderful dishes and enticingly beautiful photographs of foods. However, the fact that a dish is in such a book, or that a dish is labeled "Mediterranean," does not make it good for you.

Does the traditional-sounding creamy spaghetti alla vodka served in a restaurant sound Mediterranean enough? Would it be good for you?

I say no.

What about veal parmigiana or fettuccine alfredo? I said no again.

Lobster ravioli, prosciutto, fried calamari, escargot, shrimp with linguine alla vodka, will they be OK?

Again, I say no.

To understand why I say "no," read on.

Don't be misled! When choosing a Mediterranean dish in the books commonly found in libraries, bookstores and even on our website (www.jupiterinstitute.com) you must keep in mind the classifications we provided in this book. We classify the foods that provide omega-3s and antioxidants, and the ones that flood the body with omega-6s.

As you plan or prepare your food, remember the important principles of the Mediterranean Diet: the low level of omega-6s, the high level of antioxidants, and the abundance of omega-3s and omega-9s. As you learn about different Mediterranean dishes, you will analyze each recipe and adjust it to what we teach you here. Some dishes, such as fried dishes or pork dishes, you will not be able to use. Others, however, can be adjusted by replacing fried snapper with grilled cod, exchanging pasta for rice, replacing turkey for salmon, etc. Hence, you will "Mediterraneanize" the dishes to subtract omega-6s and add omega-3s and omega-9s (olive oil). I think it is easier to write and say "Mediterraneanize," so I will use that word from now on. You can even buy a Mediterranean Diet cookbook and write adjustments for each recipe. Where it says fry, write bake, poach or grill; where it says pork, scratch it out; where it says chickpeas or green peas, decrease their amount and add beans; and where it says pasta, substitute with rice. Increase the olive oil in each recipe. In short, "Mediterraneanize" the Mediterranean dishes – or maybe we should say "Mediterraneanize the dishes," sounds better.

Fried pork over a bed of fettuccine, not good. Lean baked pork over a bed of brown rice and arugula, with olive oil on top, is better. Changing the pork for salmon or sardines and olives is much better. See? You just "Mediterraneanized" your dinner.

But remember, it is not just important to increase the omega-3 and omega-9 (that's olive oil) in your food, you also need to reduce the omega-6. That's a better "Mediterraneanization." And it's even better if you eat your meal with salads and fruits rich in antioxidants.

But wait, it's not just that. You also need to make the meal less acidic and more alkaline. Therefore, you also need to "Alkalize" your meal.

I know, it gets complicated; but now you are closer to what I call a BETTER MEDITERRANIZATION: you apply the Mediterranean diet principles, you decrease the omega-6s, you increase your omega-3 and omega-9s, you alkalize your meal, you place on your plate foods rich in antioxidants, and you are getting ready to eat. Of course, you also need some energy, so you add some grains like beans, rice, brown rice, chickpeas, green peas, lentils, quinoa, etc.

But you won't Mediterraneanize your meals by following recipes of those supermarket magazines, "famous" doctor's magazines, newspaper recipes, etc.

Another word about pork. As I wrote above, you can do the same with pork, if you get very lean pork, grilled or baked dry, you add olive oil, and you eat it with plenty of alkaline foods rich in antioxidants, but do you think they will do this for you in a restaurant? Nope. Unless you are very careful and you know that restaurants are not safe places, RESTAURANTS ARE DANGEROUS FOR THE SUFFERING PERSON.

As you go through this process, I want to remind you of the reason why antioxidants are important: they protect your omega-3 essential fatty acids. If this is not taken into account, you may find yourself with a dish that contains a good amount of omega-3s but no antioxidants. Then a good chunk of the omega-3s you've consumed may end up being destroyed by omega-6s and free radicals. Therefore, it is important to consume the omega-3s accompanied by its "bodyguards," the antioxidants.

You will find antioxidants in the following foods:
- fresh raw vegetables
- fresh herbs (basil, chives, cilantro, dill, garlic, ginger, parsley, rosemary, thyme)
- fresh raw fruits
- red wine

You will find the good omega-3s and omega-9s in:
- oily fish (salmon, sardines, tuna, herring, cod, mackerel, bluefish, trout, and anchovies)
- nuts (walnuts, macadamias, hazelnuts, and almonds)
- avocado
- olives, olive oil
- omega-3 vegetables (spinach, arugula, lettuce, kale, collard greens, alfalfa sprouts, broccoli, watercress, cauliflower, and bean sprouts)

How can you "Mediterraneanize" a steak if it's all omega-6? Make sure it's grilled, not fried, and eat it with olive oil and a raw spinach and broccoli salad, or any colorful salad, and some fruit at the end.

How can you "Mediterraneanize" pasta? Eat it with olive oil and some of the good fish mentioned above. Or, mix it with a sauce made from olive oil, walnuts, fresh basil and a bit of Parmesan cheese.

Want to try this fettuccine? Have the fettuccine cooked and dry. Throw in a hot frying pan and pour some olive oil, once it's hot throw two cups of arugula and chopped tomatoes, quickly add salt and oregano, work fast, remove from fire, serve immediately, (so the veggies will not be cooked, just warm). Once on the table, pour some more olive oil. Ready.

What about turkey? No. In this and many other countries, turkey is a dirty animal, full of chemicals, toxins, and omega-6s. Don't eat it.

How can you "Mediterraneanize" fish? Have it poached, baked, or grilled, then once on the plate, drizzle with olive oil and eat it with fresh, raw vegetables.

How can you "Mediterraneanize" fried pork or fried chicken with corn? You can't. Just forget them, "Mediterraneanization" has its limits! Hot dog, hamburger, or pizza? Sorry, no.

Do you think any restaurant will be nice enough to prepare for you a dish "Mediterraneanized" as I specify? No, it won't. Most restaurants are unreliable unless you know them well. However, the problem with the general population is that a) going out to eat is a worldwide entertainment, relaxation and disengagement from daily and weekly work and people do it everywhere in the world, and b) the craving for tasty food, exotic preparations, a different kind of food, foreign style of cooking and challenging dishes, seems to be universal. I see this in every country. This creates a problem since people guide their decisions on the need for entertainment and the satisfaction of their taste buds. Young, middle-aged and old, most people want variety in dishes, flavors, etc., so I know it is hard to disengage from those factors, it is hard to keep a cool head and just choose "Mediterraneanized" dishes. It is hard for me too, but I do what I can. My advice to you is to do what you can, design a plan, establish some limitations, have a dialogue with family and friends about healthy choices. State aloud which restaurants you are not going to and why. Study the menus on the Internet before you go (have you noticed that many restaurants now write a description of every dish so people like us can tell whether it is good or not?). Work on it.

And here we offer some interesting news. There are ways to prepare Mexican dishes and Chinese dishes in a Mediterranean way. Japanese, Brazilian, and even New Orleans favorites can be adapted to the Mediterranean-Greek style and suddenly become transformed into healthy dishes. You can read a cookbook, especially my favorite "Joy of Cooking," and "convert" – that is "Mediterraneanize" – some of the recipes to make them acceptable. Let me give you an example: pasta with fried tomato sauce and meatballs is clearly out of bounds. But if you sauté chopped fresh garlic and onions in olive oil, let it cool, then add fresh basil and some olives, mix them well, and pour the mix over plain pasta that covers a bed of chopped raw veggies, then add a bit of grilled chicken and a bit more olive oil, you'll have "Mediterraneanized" your pasta and yes, you can eat it.

As a general rule, we recommend staying away from fried oils of any kind. But it is okay on occasion. Lightly steam some chopped vegetables, then mix them with brown rice and lightly sauté them with olive oil, soy sauce, Mirin, and garlic powder for "fried rice à la Mediterranean." Don't laugh! It's healthier than the standard version. You need to learn to make your dishes omega-friendly, which means to decrease the omega-6s and increase antioxidants, omega-3s, and omega-9s. Fried catfish with a glass of beer is not the same as poached salmon with a drizzle of olive oil and a glass of red wine. As you explore all of these concepts, remember that food from restaurants, cafeterias, take-outs, and fast-food restaurants, as a rule, are not Mediterranean; they are unsafe in terms of dieting and are generally unhealthy.

INTERCHAPTER REMARK: An 'alkalinized' Mediterranean diet, following the guidelines of food sensitivity and NutriGenomics, is ideal for the person struggling with pain, joint disease, fractures, after surgery, after orthopedic surgery, inflammation, back or neck pain, neuro-muscular disorders, neuropathies, disc diseases, etc. It will assist any and every modality of treatment the person chooses.

Hormones, Thyroid, and Adrenals

Through my research I have found four factors that have an impact on the cause and healing of painful disorders, joint disease, inflammation, injuries, and even recovery after surgery. They are the hormones, the thyroid function, the adrenals, and the toxins. If they are all bad, your chances of getting all the disorders I mention in this book are much higher and the recovery and healing from them are lower. These four factors have a strong effect on the whole metabolism.

After I wrote my first book and while I was doing research on topics of the Academy of Anti-Aging Medicine I came across the following information. It is very important and I must tell you now, and I will repeat later on, that even if you do everything well and "by the book," the four factors I here mention can still hunt you down and cause pain, inflammation and affect the way you recover from injuries.

Medical problems are not always caused by a well-defined agent and frequently the real enemy is hiding behind a curtain of invisibility. Unless you suspect and look for it, you will not find it. Let me give you an example. If you are a 55-year-old man, and you have a fair amount of stress and you live in a smoggy area, you may be doing everything correctly to treat your back and knee pain. But you will need to evaluate and replace your testosterone, adjust your adrenal gland, and engage in detoxification to enhance your healing, improve your whole metabolism, and start to see significant benefits.

As usual, and as I said before, not everyone is affected by these factors, but if YOU are, then you better find out.

The Hormone Factor

Gee, hormones? Why hormones? We were talking about joints and pains...and inflammation. What do hormones have to do with this?

Hormone decline is a natural and very normal process that affects men and women at a certain age. It is called menopause in women and andropause in men. I don't particularly like to use those terms because it is like putting a stigma on the forehead of people. I prefer to just call it "hormone decline," a much nicer term. As you well know, it happens in men and women at around the age of 45 to 50, or so, and it can bring on a multitude of symptoms. Although we know that this phase is part of normal life, several factors can cause this hormone decline to occur sooner, and sometimes much sooner. Some authors call this "early menopause," but from what I see, it can happen to men as well, therefore we now also have "early andropause." This occurs in our modern society apparently with increasing frequency. The way things are men and women are exposed to several factors that have an adverse effect on hormone levels. These factors are:

Stress - which might affect sex glands directly, or hurt the gut and contribute to dysbiosis, or adversely affect the adrenal gland causing adrenal dysfunction.

Nutrient deficit - because the fruits, vegetables, and the common foods we eat don't contain the vitamins and minerals they should (because of soil depletion, processing, and the timing of harvest, etc.).

Dysbiosis - because it triggers leakage of toxins into the bloodstream, that end up hurting all the glands of the body.

Diet – because of all the bad things people eat.

Food sensitivity – for triggering metabolic imbalance

Chemicals in food and beverages – so common in our society.

Toxins – of all kinds, and coming in the food, in what we drink and in the air we breathe.

Methylation – a complex cellular process through which our genes stimulate the cells to synthesize hormones and it becomes abnormal due to viruses, radiation, toxins, chemicals, etc.

This is not the place to deviate into analyzing the process of sex hormone decline or how methylation, toxins, chemicals, and each one of the above factors cause it. If you want to know more, let me know and I will either send you one of my papers or direct you to the right publication or website. Suffice it to say that it happens and that is the way things are.

Moreover, these factors affect the body in such a way, that lately we see a hormonal decline at much younger ages in both men and women. Symptoms of this decline vary from person to person, and it would take me too many pages to address the symptoms of the decline of each one of the hormones, but you need to know that there is a complex relationship between sex hormones and pain.

There is available evidence and publications that describe how sex hormone decline has a role in the feeling of pain, although the mechanism that causes it is not always clear. One of the pathways in which hormone decline can relate to increasing pain is through their effect on brain chemicals (known as neurotransmitters). Sex hormones can alter the chemical balance in the brain and nerves, alter their excitability, influence the nerve receptors, and thus enhance the feeling of pain. Which means that they can make a discomfort become an annoying pain by augmenting pain perception. Then a light joint ache can become a very painful joint.

Peripheral structures, like joints and ligaments, can suffer alterations in their structure or function, which can increase the sensation of pain. Estradiol deficiency causes a decrease in collagen structure and joint health that causes an increase in joint pain. Hence, it is likely that hormone decline can exert its effect on pain at many sites. This can explain, at least in part, the differences in pain experience between young men and women and peri and postmenopausal and andropausal individuals. This is saying that if you are fifty-five years of age, you will feel more pain from the same kind of arthritis or injury than a thirty-year-old. However, although this is known through observation and comparative studies, their mechanisms are complex and not well-understood. They happen but we don't know exactly why.

Studies have found that estrogens have an anti-inflammatory effect in the body and that when estrogen levels decline, chronic inflammation symptoms are increased. And not just estrogens, but progesterone and testosterone too. Many patients experience a decrease in their joint pain when these hormones are balanced.

For premenopausal women, maintaining normal levels of estrogen and progesterone appears to have a protective effect against many types of debilitating arthritis including rheumatoid arthritis. But as their hormones fluctuate during their cycle and plummet before their menstrual cycle, many of those women, if they already have some degree of osteoarthritis, report an increase in joint pain just before and during their periods, indicating a clear relationship between hormones, joint health and pain perception.

As these women advance in age and reach their perimenopause time, many of them start suffering from one joint pain or another for the first time, or aggravation of their already present joint disorder. As estrogen levels begin to decline, joints get less and less estrogen and a higher frequency and intensity of pain is often the result.

Some researchers have found that hormonal decline in women triggers not just osteoarthritis but a higher incidence of rheumatoid arthritis and fibromyalgia, that frequently go undiagnosed as women are told: "Well, it's just arthritis."

Again, exactly how biochemical processes cause chronic inflammation in the joints is not yet fully understood, but we do know that women and older people suffer more inflammatory illnesses. Researchers now state that the declining levels of hormones correspond to a rise of inflammatory molecules like cytokines (called inflammatory cytokines) and other pro-inflammatory chemicals. Estrogen affects joints by keeping inflammation down; therefore, as estrogen levels begin to decline during perimenopause, joints get less and less estrogen, and less inflammation suppression and pain is often the result.

And not only are the joints affected, but researchers also believe that inflammation is a particular issue for women during and after the hormone decline period. Inflammation caused by hormonal imbalance could be a reason why women suffer 75% of all autoimmune diseases. If this was bad already, now that women get hormonal decline at younger ages, they are also susceptible to inflammatory disorders and autoimmunity problems at a much younger age.

In addition to the above three hormones, estrogens, progesterone, and testosterone, the hormone DHEA (DeHydroEpiAndrosterone) is implicated in inflammation and pain control, and it also declines when menopause comes.

Therefore, there is a hormone-pain connection, for men and women. Not good.

Combination and cocktail - Many books describe how low levels of hormones for men and women can lead to generalized weakness, loss of muscle mass, weight gain, fatigue, depression, headaches, insomnia, and low libido. But you should know as well that deficient or fluctuating hormones for men and women can lead to all types of body pain, arthritis, and potentially increased sensitivity to pain. If the person suffers or has suffered a significant amount of stress, and carries on an omega-6 lifestyle, has significant dysbiosis and food sensitivity, the hormonal decline might happen sooner in life and the symptoms of inflammation and joint pain will show up sooner and will be more frequent and more intense. If that person now gets an injury or goes to surgery for whatever reason, the recovery and healing will be affected as well. This combination of adverse factors is what I call throughout this book THE COCKTAIL EFFECT.

And you better beware of the cocktail effect, that is, again, when several metabolic adversities combine. It can affect your quality of life, make your life miserable, throw you into disability, overwhelm you with chronic pain, and if that is not enough, increase your risk for a heart attack, stroke, cancer, and early death.

Pay attention to the different bad cocktails I describe throughout this book. In men, we know well that low testosterone can bring on mood disorders, fatigue, loss of muscle mass, low sex drive, etc., but it can also trigger aches, pains, poor healing, and increased sensitivity to pain. Men who have low levels of testosterone can all experience increased body, joint and muscle pain, and reduction of the ability to manage acute and chronic pain.

DHEA. This is another of the sex hormones affected by decline. This hormone plays a significant role in the antioxidant defense of the human body and has an important anti-inflammatory property. It has been known for a long time that DHEA can lower the levels of inflammatory cytokines, that are pro-inflammatory molecules. Hence, lower DHEA is associated with inflammation and decreased immunity. Inflammation brings on a higher incidence of painful disorders and a barrier to prompt resolution of injuries. If that is not enough, DHEA is a cardiovascular protector and a neuroprotector as well. A lot can be said and written about this hormone, but this is not the place. I am just addressing it due to its importance in the topics of this book. There is ample information on the Internet.

Consider having your hormones evaluated. If you have any kind of inflammatory process going on, or you get joint pains, even if it is in just one joint, you should get your hormones checked. As men and women are affected by a variety of metabolic and environmental insults, they should all think very seriously about this.

It is well-known that as hormones decline, inflammation, and disease increase. Don't close your eyes or your brain to this fact. I am not talking just about arthritis or pain here. Hormone decline increases the risk for cancer, stroke, and heart attack, the three major killers. There is ample information on the Internet and in libraries and bookstores.

I recommend that women and men over 35-40 years of age (or earlier if symptoms of pain, inflammation, and significant arthritis are present) be tested to determine what hormone level is deficient or imbalanced. Optimizing hormone levels at all ages and keeping them in balance naturally through either bio-identical hormones or natural supplementation will no doubt improve the ongoing pain state of any individual. It will improve inflammation and recovery after injury as well.

The Framingham Study published in 1998 looked at knees over an 8-year period in women over the age of 63 and found an astonishing 60% decrease in incidents of osteoarthritis in those taking Hormone Replacement Therapy compared to those who did not. Researchers in Denmark discovered a correlation between hormone intake and joint health, publishing their results in 2008. They concluded that Hormone Replacement Therapy significantly improved joint health and, in their opinion, should be considered for use to keep bone and cartilage healthy as we age.

a) When so many doctors remain oblivious to the problem of hormonal decline, refer to alternative medicine with disdain, and pay no attention to what good and bad nutrition are, but just give you pills and send you to the orthopedist, would YOU wait to take action?

b) In times when insurance, food, and pharmaceutical companies are controlling the health and nutrition market, would you just do what they say?

c) Or would you rather adopt an omega-3 anti-inflammatory kind of lifestyle, test and adjust your hormones, take the right supplements, and use some of the alternative therapies I mention in this book?

Hormone Replacement

This does not mean throwing a bucket of hormones at people, but checking the levels and replacing what is missing. Many publications show what bioidentical hormone replacement therapy can do, and how effective it can be in fighting degenerative and inflammatory diseases. The ideal treatment would be a combination of natural estrogens, like estradiol and estriol, combined with progesterone and sometimes, according to the laboratory test, some DHEA or testosterone. However, treatment should be evaluated and then prescribed by a physician. Only a doctor can determine if a person is a candidate for bioidentical hormone replacement treatment therapy.

WHAT TO DO? Go and see a gynecologist, a urologist, or an endocrinologist and discuss NATURAL hormone replacement. They may help you and advise you. If they give you a cold shoulder and deny, refuse, and ignore the use of NATURAL hormones, you will know they are stuck in the last century of medicine, so get out of there. Go to the Internet and search "compounding pharmacy near me," then ask the pharmacist about which practitioners near you offer this kind of service. Go and check them out, ask for credentials and training, meet the doctor, was he/she trained at the Anti-Aging Academy? Can he show you the certificate? If everything is OK, your hormones will be evaluated and the doctor will tell you what to do.

GENERAL WARNING: if you suspect that you might have hormone decline, thyroid disorder, or adrenal gland imbalance, your first step should be to consult with a physician. Don't diagnose yourself and don't take products without properly consulting a medical doctor.

Hormone Support

Certain products are known to assist the body in detoxification. Taken regularly they can help the body to get rid of some of the toxins that affect glands and organs. Combined with a toxin-avoidance attitude and an omega-3 lifestyle they can bring on HORMONAL IMPROVEMENT. As many toxins are endocrine disruptors, hormone disruptors, and estrogen contaminants, taking the following products every day may be very beneficial. Many authors recommend they be taken regularly.

For this purpose, you should only take products from laboratories associated with the American Academy of Anti-Aging Medicine. I just don't trust any other laboratory, health food stores, over-the-counter products, or any of those beautiful and promising websites. Contact your local doctor, chiropractor, or anti-aging practitioner to get them. Some compounding pharmacies also carry these products.

Here is a list of the laboratories and the corresponding product:

Laboratory	Web site	Products name
Douglas	www.douglaslabs.com	Detoxification Pack
Metagenics	www.metagenics.com	AdvaClear, UltraClear
NuMedica	www.numedica.com	HM Protect, Dual-Tox DPO
Nu-Vitals	www.jupiterinstitute.com	Bio-Detox, Vital-DETOX, Phyto-DETOX
Ortho Molecular	www.orthomolecularProducts.com	PhytoCore, Estro DIM
Pure Encapsulation	www.pureencapsulations.com	DIM Detox, HM Complex
Thorne Research	www.thorne.com	Detox Nutrients Packet
Xymogen	www.xymogen.com	XenoProtX, MedCaps DPO

These are all excellent products, but don't get them unless you are supervised by a professional.

Our office uses the following products:

Bio-Detox, in capsules, as it is practical and effective, sometimes alone or combined with

Nu-Vital Detox Program and Phyto-Detox

We found these products to be effective and well-tolerated.

Some of our patients do the whole Nu-Vital Detox Program and then continue with daily detox.

Thyroid

Studies show that thyroid hormone deficiency (especially T3 levels) can lead to increased body inflammation, which accentuates pain in the body. This happens regardless of the cause of thyroid decline.

An underactive thyroid gland triggers some metabolic changes that end up creating excessive deposits of certain proteins in connective tissues. When this happens in joints, it can cause joint inflammation and arthritis. Somehow abnormal thyroid-stimulating hormones, produced by the pituitary gland at the base of the brain, may cause excessive protein deposits in joints causing joint thickening, crystal accumulation, and fluid collection. Symptoms include slight aches and pains, but on occasion, patients can get significant osteoarthritis. The most affected joints are the ones in the limbs: hands, feet, knees, and ankles. This hypothyroid arthropathy can be light or very symptomatic.

The hypothyroid state can also affect muscles, making them weak and achy, and triggering diverse musculoskeletal symptoms like cramps and myalgias (intense muscle pains).

Nerves can also be affected, causing neuropathies that bring on numbness, tingling, and even achy wrists (carpal tunnel syndrome). Hence, neuromuscular symptoms are common in hypothyroidism, as hypothyroidism and inflammatory arthritis, neuropathy, and myopathy tend to coexist, but data on this association is sparse.

When hypothyroidism is caused by Hashimoto's disease, there is an association with rheumatoid arthritis. It is well-known that if a person has one autoimmune disease their risk of developing another is much greater compared to those individuals without an autoimmune disease. Individuals with rheumatoid arthritis are more likely to develop hypothyroidism due to Hashimoto thyroiditis, and vice versa. Rheumatoid arthritis is a condition in which the body's immune system wrongfully attacks its joints.

Without regard to the cause of hypothyroidism, neuromuscular and musculoskeletal manifestations with joint pain and inflammation can be observed in many patients with the condition. Some of the problems include general muscular weakness and pain, including cramps and muscle stiffness, joint pain, achiness, and stiffness, known as "arthropathy." Tendinitis in the arms and/or legs that involves pain, tingling, weakness, achiness, or numbness in wrists, fingers, or forearms. Also, tarsal tunnel syndrome, which is similar to carpal tunnel syndrome, and causes pain, tingling, burning, and other discomforts in the arch of the foot, and can potentially extend into the toes. Frozen shoulder, also known as adhesive capsulitis, causes pain, limited movement, and stiffness in the shoulder.

Now, this is not the place to get into a long thyroid explanation, but there are a few little things you need to know. We are witnessing a slow increase of thyroid disorders throughout our country and some writers claim that these conditions are affecting over 25 percent of the population. About half of those affected by this sluggish thyroid are undiagnosed, and many of those who are diagnosed are not being treated optimally.

When the thyroid gland is not working well, we call it "thyroid dysfunction" or "thyroid disorder," which only tells you that it is not working well, without pointing out whether it is under or overworking. When the production of thyroid hormones is not enough to satisfy the metabolic needs of the body the condition is called hypothyroidism ("hypo" means decreased). Hypothyroidism means that the thyroid is underactive, meaning it is underworking.

Millions of Americans have unrecognized thyroid disease, mostly in the form of subclinical hypothyroidism, and women are ten times more affected. Sub-clinical means that the symptoms and the lab tests are not enough to clearly show that the person has a strong case of hypothyroidism, but rather the symptoms are few and mild and the test for thyroid hormones is not fully abnormal.

Diseases of the thyroid gland are commonly encountered, and they are often challenging to diagnose, but satisfying to treat by those who understand them because of the usual good results. However, many conventional doctors are still stuck in the diagnostic protocols of the last century and are not accepting new thyroid management concepts.

Hypothyroidism has Several Causes

a) Hashimoto's Disease (caused by autoimmune dysfunction is the most frequent cause in the U.S.)

b) Thyroiditis (which is inflammation of the thyroid gland caused either by a virus, by postpartum stage, or it involves the "silent" thyroiditis" that occurs from unknown causes, although an autoimmune process is most likely the cause)

c) Congenital hypothyroidism (present at birth)

d) Surgical or radiation-related hypothyroidism

e) Malfunctioning pituitary gland (which fails to produce enough TSH)

f) Nutrition-related (such as lack of iodine)

g) Medication-related

h) Adrenal gland failure (chronic metabolic and environmental stress causes abnormal cortisol that causes the thyroid to fail)

i) And the modern cause that I will call "metabolic-wasting" in which complex interconnected events occur and slowly waste the thyroid gland (toxins, dysbiosis, food sensitivities, stress, cortisol, imbalance in the hormonal triangle, etc.).

The two main hormones of the thyroid gland are thyroxine (also known as "T4") and triiodothyronine (also known as "T3") and together they have a powerful impact in every metabolic aspect of the human body. They control heart rate, blood pressure, sleep, bone formation, weight gain, weight loss, muscle activity, muscular strength, mental alertness, fat deposition, thinking, intellect, digestion, sweating, stamina, the immune system, and they also interact and control the other glands and hormones. They control every function of the body and allow the cells of the body to use the body's fuel and energy supplies.

The secretion of T4 and T3 is stimulated by TSH, the Thyroid Stimulating Hormone, which is secreted by that little gland that we have in the brain called the pituitary gland. When the TSH is secreted less, then the stimulation to the thyroid is less, and the secretion of T4 and T3 diminishes. Insufficient TSH causes insufficient T4 and T3. Hence diminished secretion of TSH makes the thyroid underactive.

Low thyroid function is not always well-defined. Occasionally the symptoms and laboratory tests of low thyroid function are very clear and intense and the diagnosis of hypothyroidism is easy. However, on many occasions, neither the numbers in the laboratory tests nor the symptoms are very definitive, and the diagnosis is not so clear. This condition is called low-thyroid, or subclinical hypothyroidism, or slow thyroid or other names, and is very common. I prefer to call it SUBCLINICAL HYPOTHYROIDISM. Imagine Freddy, a 48-year-old man, overweight, with some depression, general tiredness, constipation, muscle aches, and insomnia. You do blood work and you find normal TSH, borderline low T4, and low T3. Freddy has subclinical hypothyroidism.

Low Functioning Thyroid Can Cause:

1) In the metabolism: weight gain, difficulty losing weight, inflammation, low blood sugar, coldness, cold intolerance.

2) In general: fatigue, chronic fatigue syndrome, edema, generalized weakness, painful joints, hair loss, headaches, brittle nails, infertility, anemia, decreased sexual interest, menstrual irregularities, and acne.

3) In the vascular system: low pulse, high blood pressure, heart disease, high cholesterol, palpitations.

4) Mentally: depression, poor memory, irritability, insomnia, mood swings, attention deficit disorder (ADD), decreased concentration, mental fog, easy crying, anxiety

5) In the digestive system: constipation, gas, bloating, decreased absorption of nutrients.

6) In the musculoskeletal system: carpal tunnel, weak muscles, muscle pains, joint pains.

7) Senses: worsening eyesight or hearing

Thyroid Medications

I am not going to extend too much into this because the treatment is between you and your doctor. If you have some of the conditions I describe in this book and your thyroid test shows low T3, you need to do something about it.

The medications used are essentially synthetic and natural, more or less. T4 preparations are and can be very effective for a lot of people, as long as they convert well the T4 into T3. Those T4 preparations are made of Thyroxine (also known as levothyroxine) and are called Synthroid, Levoxyl, and Levothroid.

They are almost the same. Almost. But some people do better with one and not with the other. Different people react differently to thyroid medications and nothing is carved in stone about it. Many people do well with the generic form, others don't. Some people on Synthroid can't be switched to other brands because they don't feel well. Others prefer Levoxyl and they get symptoms if they are switched to generic or other brands.

To find out whether they are converting or not they need to get a blood test for TSH, T4, and T3. For example, if before the treatment they TSH was high, the T4 was low and the T3 was very low, and then after slowly increasing the dose (doses have to be increased slowly), they reach a level of normal TSH, normal T4 and good level of T3 it means they are converting well.

Those who don't convert well need a supply of oral T3. T3 can be taken by itself. It's called Cytomel, but has a short half-life and needs to be taken twice a day. Its generic form is called Liothyronine.

TREATMENT MUST BE SLOW, DON'T RUSH. Whether you are just starting the treatment or you are having your dose being adjusted, this must be done with slow increments. Every change in the dose should be kept at that same level for ten or fifteen days or maybe a bit more. If you are just starting Synthroid, for instance, you should start at 12.5 to 25mcg ("mcg" means micrograms) for two weeks, and then see your doctor and review symptoms and tolerability. Then perhaps increase it to 37.5mcg for two weeks and later to 50mcg. I would suggest staying at the 50mcg level for a month before further change unless hypothyroid symptoms indicate larger doses.

T3 can also be taken combined with T4 in a T4-T3 combination preparation called Armor Thyroid, Nature-Thyroid, NP Thyroid, Westhroid, and Thyrolar. The best known of them is Armor Thyroid, which is a porcine-derived thyroid hormone. Again, some individuals do very well with Armor Thyroid, some others with levothyroxine, and some need to take both together in the morning to feel well. Also, some individuals have different a different response to the ingredients of different brands, so some will do better with Armor while others prefer Nature-Thyroid or Westhroid.

Remember to take them alone, in the early morning, and don't eat or drink for 30-45 minutes.

Thyroid Supplements

Certain nutritional deficiencies interfere with thyroid function or with the conversion of T4 into T3. Therefore, I recommend all thyroid sufferers do the following:

1) Check your B12, and if it's low, supplement it.

2) Selenium, 50 to 200mcg a day and Zinc 25 to 50mg a day, better if together in one pill combined with iodine

3) A good brand of multivitamin with minerals containing an adequate amount of B-complex, as well as magnesium, copper, vitamin C, and calcium.

4) Iodine tablets, I prefer the natural kind made from seaweed, kelp, nori, kombu, wakame, etc., 50 to 150mcg a day, that is approximately the daily dose required. I don't like or recommend large doses of Iodine. Somehow large doses of Iodine can further irritate the thyroid. People with Hashimoto's should not take natural or marine Iodine

Thyroid Helpers

This is a very important concept. Some supplements are known to be THYROID HELPERS since they provide the thyroid with nutrients to facilitate its physiology. They combine iodine, selenium, zinc, and other essential nutrients. I use them in my office with many of my patients and find that they allow better thyroid control with fewer medications. Some patients are even able to control thyroid function with no pharmacological agents. Again, because of reliability and quality, I only recommend products from laboratories associated with the American Academy of Anti-Aging Medicine. I just don't trust any other laboratory, over-the-counter products, beautiful websites, or health food stores. Contact your local doctor, chiropractor, or anti-aging practitioner to get them. Some compounding pharmacies also carry these products. You could buy them from any of the following companies but take them ONLY under the supervision of your physician (or run the risk of severe complications). They are not for "do-it-yourselfers."

Remember: never play with the thyroid, always see a physician. Don't diagnose yourself. If you suspect a thyroid condition, seek medical care first.

Here is a list of the laboratories and the corresponding product:

Laboratory	Web site	Product name
DaVinci laboratory	www.davincilabs.com	Thyroid Basics
Douglas	www.douglaslabs.com	ThyroMend
NuMedica	www.numedica.com	Thyrodex, ThyroMedica plus
Nu-Vitals	www.jupiterinstitute.com	Thyroid-Aid, Bio-Thyroid
Ortho Molecular	www.orthomolecularProducts.com	Thyrotain
Protocol for Life	www.protocolforlife.com	Ortho Thyroid
Thorne Research	www.thorne.com	Thyrocsin
Xymogen	www.xymogen.com	T-150

IN OUR OFFICE we only use the following two products:

Bio-Thyroid

Thyroid-Aid

They are two excellent nutritional supplements designed to improve thyroid function. Both are designed by laboratories recognized by the Anti-Aging Academy. They enhance the effect of thyroid medication and even improve thyroid control.

We have had good success with them.

Adrenal Gland Disorder

Well, here we enter in a real gray zone, as many doctors don't recognize that the adrenal gland could be under-working without really reaching the level of failure called Addison's disease. For these doctors, patients are either OK or they have Addison's, with nothing in between. The position of many other doctors and professors of the Academy of Anti-Aging Medicine is quite different, and they recognize that the function of the adrenal gland can deteriorate in slow stages. My experience taught me that they are correct, and taking that into account, with small, careful, individualized treatments, I have been able to improve the quality of life for a lot of people. Of all the names I have read, I like to call the low functioning of the adrenal gland "hypoadrenia."

So, let me explain a bit about adrenal function first.

The adrenal glands are situated on top of the kidneys and secrete a variety of hormones. One of these hormones is cortisol, which has an incredibly strong impact on metabolism and disease. Abnormal cortisol levels can lead to a condition of severe exhaustion known as Adrenal Fatigue (previously known as neurasthenia), which I like to call hypoadrenia. Cortisol can also cause high blood pressure, weight gain, sleep disorders, high sugar levels, and low sex drive. Most of the time Cortisol rises bringing its "sister" hormones with it: epinephrine, norepinephrine (which stimulates blood pressure and heart rate), and insulin (which causes weight gain and diabetes).

Adrenal response - The adrenal glands are the center of stress response, and they have been essential for our survival for thousands of years. During wars, famine, long winters, hunting, escaping, prisoner camps, etc., the adrenal response to stress has been our ally in the struggle for survival. Nevertheless, as society is today, this response is working against us.

We face different kinds of stressors nowadays: spouses, children, jobs, driving, excess of caffeine, bad diet, exams, school demands, addictions, responsibilities, etc. These stress events stimulate the brain to release its chemical messengers which then go to the adrenal glands to stimulate the secretion of cortisol and its "sisters," (epinephrine and norepinephrine). This starts when we are in high school, and keeps going throughout college, when we get a car, start working, start a family, start facing bills, and so on. It doesn't stop. Some get it worse than others, a difficult home life, complicated relationships, being abused, facing hardship, etc. Some provoke this in themselves with a high carb diet, or by alcohol or drug abuse, but the response is always the same. However, when we are young and strong, we can cope with it. We fight, we climb, we push ourselves, we go forward. On those days cortisol is abundant and its "sisters" epi, nor-epi and insulin, are flowing everywhere like a river full of fish. But as time passes on, the abuse to this system combined with the effects of environmental toxins, chemicals, dysbiosis and the lack of essential nutrients, creates a lack of regulation, abnormal responses, a phase of excessive or insufficient response, and finally the system wastes away (with a very low response because of fatigue to the system, known as Adrenal Fatigue). According to the type, length, and intensity of the stressors, this final phase may take 5 months, 5 years, or 50 years.

Stressors - In addition to those above, the factors that also affect the adrenals are fear, marital stress, lack of sleep, war, hurricanes, chronic illness, psychological stress, pains, allergies, emotional stress, toxins, grief, lack of relaxation, excessive exercise, abuse of flour products, sweets, carbohydrates, caffeine abuse, stimulants, and poor eating habits. Sound familiar? How many of them have you been through?

Anyone can be affected, and of course doctors, nurses, policemen, and paramedics can have the most stressors. Some professions are harder on the adrenals than others. But then come the students, bank workers, mothers, teachers, business owners, drivers, and many other professions.

Metabolic effect - Initially, the cortisol, epinephrine (adrenaline), norepinephrine, and insulin (the four sisters of doom) are abundant, proportional, and work well-coordinated. But when the system loses its fine regulation, bad things start to occur: mitochondria, the energy machine inside the cell becomes dysfunctional and starts sparking free radicals (which cause inflammation), insulin goes up (which is a cause of inflammation), hormones are over-consumed, wasted and decline, muscle mass declines; immunity goes down; metabolism is hurt in many places, and inflammation develops.

As the process advances, insulin abuse leads to insulin wasting, which combined with the other factors causes diabetes. The same process causes low thyroid function, elevated Reverse T3, low DHEA, low hormone levels, poor sleep, low muscle energy, decreased brain chemicals, bowel malfunction (which can be a cause or a consequence of the process) which causes lack of vitamins and nutrients and the result is FATIGUE. The factors leading to an excess of free radicals and inflammation are multiple. All this varies from person to person, and some individuals can have fatigue and no obesity, some may just have obesity, some may have both. But make a note of this: malfunctioning adrenals will harm your hormones AND your thyroid, and one way or another the combined effect throws the body into inflammation. Inflammation opens the door to pain, joint disorders, poor healing, and difficulty recovering.

But wait, it gets even more confusing. In some persons, low thyroid (for whatever reason) and/or low hormones (estrogen, progesterone, testosterone, etc.) caused by aging, toxins, bad food, etc., are the ones that are stressing the adrenals. Then all together they cause the metabolic disasters that lead to obesity and/or fatigue, and inflammation.

WORSE YET, the adrenal gland enjoys a high blood flow and because of this, if the person is exposed to environmental toxins and/or is affected by significant amounts of toxins coming from dysbiosis, THOSE TOXINS ARE GOING TO SHOWER ON THE ADRENAL GLAND EVERY DAY. Then, soaked with toxins, this "dirty" adrenal gland can't work well. Disengaging yourself from toxin exposure, detoxing the gut, dealing with dysbiosis, and doing a detoxification program might be needed.

Symptoms of Hypoadrenia

Overweight, obesity, fatigue, chronic fatigue, poor sleep, joint pain, lethargy, low sex drive, low ability to handle stress, poor immunity, frequent respiratory infections, inflammation, increased time to recover from illness or injury, depression, PMS, less enjoyment, mental fog, poor memory, pains, frequent bronchitis or asthma, frequent cough, inability to lose weight.

Additional Symptoms and Medical Problems

Coldness, feeling tired, no erections, hormonal disorders, breast problems. If brain-chemicals are affected then the person may get: pain, muscle pain, anxiety, fibromyalgia, muscle weakness and pain, cravings, poor alcohol tolerance, exhaustion, back pain, addiction, apathy, allergies, insulin resistance, high blood pressure, high cholesterol, high triglycerides, increased belly-fat, decreased serotonin (causing depression, craving and lack of satiety), stiffness, nervous stomach, indigestion, frequent headaches, easy fatigability, nervous breakdowns, chronic fatigue.

But sometimes the root of adrenal imbalance is not the job or relationships but the foods that a person eats. Eating the wrong foods and staying in what I called the omega-6 state can create the problem.

As Barry Sears, Ph.D. wrote in his books about The Anti-Inflammatory Zone, underlying hormonal changes occur when inflammation persists in the body, and these changes then perpetuate the body's inflammatory response. Dr. Sears says that eating the wrong type of fats and too many carbohydrates cause overproduction of two hormones: pro-inflammatory eicosanoids and insulin. High levels of these hormones cause the body to produce more cortisol which furthers the inflammation. Insulin is a hormone produced by the pancreas in response to food in our stomach. Because of our modern-day diet of low-fat, highly processed, and refined foods, the pancreas keeps pumping out more and more insulin. This excess of insulin functions as a pro-inflammatory substance.

Whether insulin triggered cortisol or cortisol triggered insulin doesn't matter much because these two sisters go together. In the end, you get inflammation, disease, pain, fat, and all the consequences.

Managing Adrenal Dysfunction

Easy as A, B, C, and D.

A) Find out the causes of your stress and do something about it. Is it your job? Your food? Money? Family?

You need to make a change, stay away from the TV and cell phone, then think and meditate. Examine your life and see what you can do. What can you plan, so you can bring on improvements to your lifestyle? Perhaps you don't like the word "meditation" so just "think about yourself."

Since we are talking about thinking, I want to make you aware of other kinds of thinking or meditation that are available out there.

- Transcendental Meditation
- Mindfulness Meditation
- Relaxation Meditation.

I recommend you research them through the Internet, libraries, or bookstores. They seek to provide a level of spirituality and an elevation of mental awareness to create a beneficial reduction in stress and have a positive effect on brain and adrenal functions. Meditation can increase self-efficacy and even provide a sense of control. The books of Dr. Deepak Chopra can be very effective as well.

Once you have taken the steps then focus on choosing and planning a strategy to examine and review your life, and see what changes you can make. You can use meditation as disengagement and stress management, which might help you in the process of relaxation and stress relief. It is well-known to help patients with chronic illness, to reduce the symptoms and improve their quality of life. As you are engaging in the process of learning about yourself, it may be a good idea to go to the library or the bookstore and spend some time examining the books on meditation. Some of these books were written by teachers of meditation and are very helpful. You may even find them on audio-books. Meditation is easy to learn, and it is a safe and easy way to learn about yourself. Some of the books you find may help you in your quest. Take a good look at the books of Chopra. I don't accept everything he says and you don't have to either, but it is a very good way to get yourself involved in the subject. Besides, he is a philosopher who brings ideas from another country, and his ideas may help you see how other people in other parts of this world view life and the human spirit.

As you advance in your readings, you will find out that Transcendental Meditation (TM), has very well-documented clinical studies showing its benefits in human physiology. It provides a tremendously deep state of relaxation, with subsequent benefits in mind and body functions. It increases intelligence and creativity, and even decreases cortisol.

After meditating, hopefully, you got some idea of what is going on with you and which stressors are affecting you. You then need to start reviewing all the stress management techniques to decide which one or ones you are going to use and which ones you are at least going to try. There are essentially two kinds of stress management techniques: active and passive. The active one is the one you do, and the passive ones are the ones you let somebody do to you, easy. Examples of active stress management techniques are meditation, jogging, exercise, going to the beach (my favorite), going to the mall for a walk, and aromatherapy, and there are plenty more examples. Passive techniques are massage and acupuncture for instance.

Don't nurture in your mind the naïve thought that relaxation is something you do once a month or when you are on vacation. Like taking a cruise twice a year. You better wake up before some unwanted medical condition wakes you up. Stress management needs to be read, explored, learned, and then practiced regularly.

You can do it every day, every other day, or 2 or 3 times a week, but you need to do it regularly. You need to have a plan, a strategy for it.

B) Practice some form of stress management every day. According to what you learn in step A, engage in some form of stress management. Read about choices on the Internet, in bookstores, or at a library. Learn different techniques. I tell my patients that a slow walk in the supermarket, or parking your car for 10 minutes in a park and stepping outside is stress management. You need to do some stress management every day. Naps, walking, window shopping, sitting in a coffee shop, or reading, are some ideas. Explore options. If it is not YOU for yourself, then who will do it for you?

And if you don't start today, then when?

C) Make sure your thyroid is balanced or it will place strain on the adrenal. And consider disengaging from environmental and food toxins as much as you can. Heal your dysbiosis, detox your gut, engage in a general detoxification program.

D) Read and learn about ADAPTOGENS, which are herbal products that improve adrenal function. There is a big variety out there, but you should NOT just buy them and take them. You need to be evaluated by a professional who understands adrenal dysfunction, has experience in managing it, and who will be able to test you and treat you.

In my office, I teach people the importance of this ABC and I try different adaptogens with different individuals.

Be cautious: don't buy over-the-counter adaptogens and especially don't buy from dubious websites. Use the internet for research and to gain knowledge but never buy anything from websites that have no accountability for the products they sell. BUY ONLY from companies and laboratories affiliated with the American Academy of Anti-Aging.

WARNING: Taking adaptogens without doing A + B is a mistake.

Taking adaptogens on your own, without professional diagnosis and assistance supervision is another mistake.

And some mistakes can be costly!

Adaptogens

A very important concept. They improve, balance, and support adrenal function. Some come with dehydrated bovine or porcine adrenal gland, adding strength to the formula.

They are all ADRENAL HELPERS, aiding in adrenal hormone production and supporting the body's response to everyday stressors.

Again, I repeat, because of reliability and quality, I only recommend products from laboratories associated with the American Academy of Anti-Aging Medicine. I just don't trust any other laboratory, over-the-counter products, beautiful websites, or health food stores, etc., and you should not trust them either. Contact your local doctor, chiropractor, or anti-aging practitioner to get them. Some compounding pharmacies also carry these products. You could buy them from any of the following companies but take them ONLY under physician supervision (or run the risk of severe complications). They are not for "do-it-yourselfers."

Remember: never play with your adrenal function, always see a physician. Don't diagnose yourself.

Here is a list of the laboratories and the corresponding product:

Laboratory	Web site	Product
DaVinci laboratory	www.davincilabs	Adrenal Benefits
Douglas	www.douglaslabs.com	Ora-Adren 80
NuMedica	www.numedica.com	AdrenaMed
Nu-Vitals	www.jupiterinstitute.com	Adren-AM, Max-Adren
Ortho Molecular	www.orthomolecularproducts.com	Adren-All, Adapten-All
Protocol For Life	www.protocolforlife.com	Adrenal Cortisol Support
Thorne Research	www.thorne.com	Cortrex
Vital Nutrients	www.vitalnutrients.net	Adrenal Support
Xymogen	www.xymogen.com	Adrenal Manager, Adrenal Essence

Our office combines different products and we usually start slow and low and observe how our patients feel and react since all individuals are different.

However, NO ADAPTOGEN will work if you don't do some form of stress management.

Let me give some examples

Mary

-Hi Dr. Nuchovich

-Hi Mary. Good morning. What is going on?

-I am tired, I get emotional, achy, I get shoulder pains and headaches. I don't sleep well, my sex drive is down, I gain weight, my muscles ache, I feel I am swollen.

-What do you do? What type of work you do?

-Well...I am a nurse, and I have more patients than I can handle. They rotate me, so sometimes I have to do night shifts. My supervisor is selfish and told me he may fire me.

Paul

-Hi Paul, what's up?

-Oh, I am tired Dr. Nuchovich, tired and achy, I get brain fog, headaches, knee pain, anxiety, I get low back pain and tingling down the legs, stress, and also muscle aches, indigestion and...and...

-OK, Paul, what do you do?

-I am a supervisor in the local supermarket, my wife left me so I have to take care of my three kids, my aunt lives with us and she's not happy, and our 12-year-old dog just died.

Peter

-Hi Peter, tell me what is happening to you?

-Oh, hi Dr. Nuchovich, well, I don't know what to do, can you give me something? I have neck pain, my elbows are aching, I have arthritis in my elbows and my shoulders are stiff, I don't feel well, I run out of steam rather easily. I am moody, I don't sleep well, I have a cough. I am also gaining weight and my sex drive is down. My blood pressure is up, my hips hurt, and my arms too. I am stressed out. I retain water because so I feel swollen. Can you give some testosterone and something for depression?

-Well, Paul, what type of work you do?

-I am a paramedic.

DO YOU THINK that we could fix Peter, Paul, and Mary with some adaptogens, some hormones, some pain medications, sleeping pills, etc.?

Yes, I could provide those treatments temporarily, I could support and help the three of them, but the main point is to sit down, talk, and with a clear mind start making some plans as to how they are going to fix their lives. What small steps need to be taken, etc.?

The adrenal glands of the three of them are in a state of over-function, under-function, or dysfunction, and something needs to be done, but for how long should we take adaptogens if the trigger problems are not fixed?

AND I WARN YOU HERE: IF YOU LOSE YOUR ADRENALS, YOU LOSE YOUR HEALTH.

In our office we have had success with specific adrenal products, that we use alone or in combination according to each different individual's needs:
- Max-Adren
- Adren-AM
- Adrenal Rebuilder
- Adrenevive

None of our patients get three of them, but rather different combinations of one or two of them, according to their specific needs. One patient may get half Adrenal Rebuilder combined with half Adren-AM four days a week, while the next patient may get one Max-Adren, a whole Adrenal Rebuilder, and two special vitamins to take three days a week.

Some may take Adrenevive at night, others don't. Most patients require an initial trial to see how they feel.

EVERYTHING HAS TO BE PART OF A WHOLE. Just taking adaptogens without doing stress management is not a good approach. Why would you care for your adrenals and take adaptogens if you still commute one and half hours to a highly stressed job, you eat an omega-6 diet, you abuse alcohol and donuts, overwork your body at the gym, and you won't use alternative therapies?

Will you just fix your adrenals while your thyroid is low, your sex hormones are down, your pain is annoying, you don't sleep, and your body is full of toxins?

I know, it is too many things to do. Where do you start? You will find the answer when you locate a quiet corner and meditate.

INTERCHAPTER REMARK: The adverse effects of a low functioning thyroid, hormone decline, and a dysfunctional adrenal gland are a big disadvantage for anyone struggling with the ailments I describe in this book. These imbalances will affect inflammation resolution, repair, and may impair the process of healing. Their adverse effects on the whole body and soul are well-known.

Patients need to request (demand) to have the levels of those hormones checked and properly corrected.

Toxins

"The world has changed, and those changes are affecting the water, the earth, the air, and also the food we eat."

Chemicals and toxins are now everywhere, and much of that cleanliness that once was is lost.

Toxins of all kinds have been a persistent and common environmental contaminant over the last several decades, and continue to be a permanent threat to human health.

And no, you are not immune.

Although "chemicals" is a name we give to compounds that may or may not be dangerous, depending on their type and amount, "toxins" is a general name we use for definitively harmful chemical compounds. Both chemicals and toxins come from multiple sources and invade our bodies regularly. They include pesticides, plastic particles, petrochemicals, colorants, herbicides, fertilizers, some food additives, metal particles (known as heavy metal particles), chemical discharges from industrial plants, multiple air pollutants, water contaminants, colorants in drinks and snacks, etc. It is common knowledge that 80-90% of most chronic health conditions are triggered by toxins.

OK, I agree, but why did you put this in your book, Doctor Nuchovich? Who cares?

You should care. The impact of those toxins on our bodies enhances our risk for inflammation, arthritis and affects the way we recover from injuries and surgeries. It even affects pain perception. That is why I put it in the book. Toxins are known to cause neuropathy and pain as well.

Think of it this way: if you don't learn this now, when are you going to do it? When it's too late?

Nobody is safe, from Florida to Alaska and from New York to California the water supply and the water in rivers and lakes is contaminated with chemicals of all kinds, and supermarkets carry vegetables and fruits contaminated with herbicides, pesticides, toxic fertilizers and foods prepared with chemical additives, colorants and even petrochemicals.

Toxins are so widespread that you can find them even in breast milk and in the umbilical cord blood of newborns.

Toxins and Health

Our bodies are not a miracle. They are the product of a complex evolution that has transformed them into self-sustaining and self-repairing entities, independent and carrying out intricate bio-electrical, digestive, and immuno-humoral activities. Almost daily the body must face multiple assaults from the outside world, including viruses, bacteria, chemical toxins, stress, and other challenges. As long as the body's internal environment is working well and the toxic exposure is not overwhelming, the body's detoxification system is capable of eliminating those incoming attacks. This detoxification system is natural to us, and we acquired it during evolutionary times, just like the heart and the brain, part of our natural metabolism, helping us to fight against internal and external toxins, helping us fight diseases and infections. Our inherited detoxification system has always been there, helping us survive, even when there weren't antibiotics or doctors around. But things changed. For many centuries the agents attacking our body were natural, simpler, and not coming in such large numbers. But among the many good things brought to us by the advances in science, industry, and technology, was a tremendous explosion of new toxins and man-made chemicals: new, not-natural, and in large quantities.

We now have a more modern world, and use and enjoy the improvements in sanitation, housing, medicine, food production, manufacturing, communications, electronics, etc., that have made living more modern and comfortable. We look back at the way people used to live two hundred years ago and we can easily see just how much mankind has advanced. We are astounded by some of these technological advances, by huge buildings, beautiful cars, progress in medicine, smartphones, new means of transportation, and the incredible variety of foods and cosmetics, etc. However, with that progress new dangers have come to hurt our health and well-being. We now have exposure to a huge variety of herbicides, toxins, metal particles, and chemicals, most of them artificial (that is man-made, not natural) against which our detoxification system is unable to operate. Often, our bodies are not able to detoxify all the large amounts and variety of chemicals to which they are exposed, leading to a continuous process of accumulation of toxins in our tissues and organs.

The accumulation of toxins causes damage in the cells of almost every organ in the body leading to an imbalance in the hormones that control our whole metabolism. Toxins, chemicals, pollutants, contaminants, metal particles (like lead, mercury, cadmium, etc.) and food additives slowly accumulate and end up CLOGGING OUR DETOXIFICATION SYSTEM and causing hormonal-disruption and metabolic-disruption. These adverse effects cause glucose elevation, nutrient deficiencies and immune disorders that cause weight gain, inflammation, very high glucose (which leads to diabetes), poor immunity (which leads to infections, respiratory diseases, intestinal illnesses and a variety of cancers), nutrient deficiencies (which causes the brain chemicals, known as neurotransmitters, to malfunction, causing depression, cravings, personality disorders), fatigue, painful disorders, and health decline. Hormonal and metabolic disruption causes pain, muscular weakness, disability, sterility, psychological disorders, stiff tender joints, headaches, allergies, food sensitivities, high cholesterol, and affects our healing from injuries. The combination of all these factors causes liver disorders, neuromuscular problems, accelerated atherosclerosis, increases the aging process, and ultimately increases the risk for coronary disease, heart attacks, strokes, and early death.

People need to come to terms with the fact that toxin accumulation and the metabolic-hormonal imbalance they produce causes health decline, accelerated aging, and a severe decline in both quality and length of life. Symptoms and diseases are reflections and warnings of this decline.

In 2008, the National Institute of Environmental Health Sciences (NIEHS) stated that there is a clear link between environmental exposures and adult diseases. They also address the concept of ENDOCRINE DISRUPTORS, which is one of the most important concepts I want you to get from this book. Endocrine disruptors are chemicals that interfere with the body's hormone system, producing adverse reproductive, metabolic, neurological, and immunological effects, and yes, bringing your thyroid, sex hormones, and your adrenal levels down.

So now you see that toxins can bring on inflammation, arthritis, and poor injury repair through more than one mechanism.

A wide range of substances, both natural and man-made, are thought to cause this endocrine disruption, including pharmaceuticals, dioxin compounds, polychlorinated biphenyls, DDT, pesticides, and plasticizers are involved. Some of these toxins can be found in many everyday products, like plastic bottles, canned foods, detergents, food, toys, cosmetics, over-the-counter products, and air pollutants.

Do you think you are an exception? Do you think this is like being in a war and as long as you are far away the bullets will not hurt you? There is no "far away" here, toxins are all around us, in the soil, vegetables, foods, and drinks. We all have toxins inside. And all the fish in the world are already contaminated.

The Environmental Protection Agency (EPA) publishes a list of the drinking water contaminants, which include arsenic, asbestos, antimony, cadmium, barium, benzene, carbon tetrachloride, dalapon, dioxin, phthalates, dichloroethane, endrin, fluoride, thallium, trichloroethane, oximal, nitrates, chlorobenzene, radium, mercury, lead, PCBs and nickel. These products come from additives, discharges from refineries and waste plants, ceramics, electronics, discharges from industries, corrosion of pipes and plumbing systems, runoffs from fertilizer deposits, sewage, erosion, chemical plants, the decay of man-made chemicals, discharges from plastic and rubber factories, residues from all kinds of electronic devices thrown in canals and rivers, etc. All these contaminate the drinking water throughout our country. Irrigation water is even more contaminated, and it is used to irrigate vegetables and fruits and is also given to the animals we eat.

IS YOUR TOILET CLOGGED? - Toxins accumulate in our bodies. Exposure to harmful substances comes from many sources but wherever they come from, these toxins and chemicals tend to accumulate in our system.

Although we all have a natural detoxification system that we inherited from our ancestors, this normally sufficient and very efficient system slowly becomes clogged and stuck when confronted with unusual amounts of unknown toxins and heavy metals. This system uses the liver as the main organ for detoxification. However, if you are exposed to an excessive amount of toxins or the foods that you eat cause a significant amount of dysbiosis and bowel toxins, the liver may end up overwhelmed and unable to eliminate all the toxins. The waste will then accumulate in your body and spread to other organs, hurting them and altering their functions. Now imagine all this happening in very slow motion, so slow that it might not be noticed until it is far advanced. Unaware of this you continue enjoying your alcohol excess, your bad food, your favorite restaurants where you eat a variety of the wrong foods and bad fats, while your dysbiosis advances and leaks toxins into your liver. Then after several years, you start to develop health problems, including joints trouble, back pain, weight and blood pressure issues, etc. You may then scratch your head and say, "I don't understand what is happening, why?"

So reader, tell me why. What happened?

The answer: The body suffers from the effects of an extremely slow but progressive accumulation of all kinds of waste clogging the liver and the detoxifications systems.

Poor health and illness caused by waste (toxins, chemicals, etc.) are progressive; it does not occur overnight. They are the result of a very slow accumulation of these products. The occurrence of inflammation and cancer have a lot to do with it. And yes, joint diseases, inflammation anywhere in your body, pain disorders, many metabolic problems, poor injury healing, neuromuscular disorders, and neuropathies may be strongly related to your exposure to nutritional deficiencies (because of your dietary deficit), pollution, excess of carbohydrates, consumption of bad fats and bad food, food chemicals and even food sensitivities all causing toxin accumulation.

BUT DON'T BLAME IT ALL ON THE ENVIRONMENT, BECAUSE TOXINS COME FROM DIFFERENT SOURCES:

1) For one, our daily exposure to toxins in our environment allows them to enter through skin absorption, liquids, and food. We should call them the Environmental Toxins as I explained above. Over 1,000 different chemicals and additives are put in the foods we eat and are not required to be printed on the label. Over 70,000 chemicals are being used in commercial products in the USA. The Environmental Protection Agency has classified 65,000 of them as hazardous to human health.

2) Secondly, we also eat food with toxins: the flesh of animals who have been accumulating toxins, like fish, chicken, and cattle. These animals have lived weeks or months eating contaminated grains and plants and even getting antibiotics, chemical injections, and even hormones. They have also been drinking plenty of contaminated water. This is a process called bio-accumulation: the animals, while alive, have been storing toxins in their flesh. As we eat those animals, we get their load of toxins.

3) The third source of toxins is a very normal one. We should call them the Normal Toxins. Normal cellular metabolism produces waste molecules that need to be eliminated. All mammals have a cellular waste elimination system and use the liver as the main detoxification

organ. Normally, human beings spend their lifetime eating, digesting and metabolizing nutrients and later eliminating from the cells the waste products which are then taken to the liver to be eliminated. We call this natural elimination "detoxification." The problem is that when the system becomes dysfunctional because of external toxicities, these waste products cannot be eliminated and accumulate as toxins.

As if the other two pathways of getting toxins were not enough, the interference within our natural detoxification system, clogging the system, obstructing the detoxification pathways in the liver and not allowing us to eliminate the waste products of our metabolism cause severe metabolic irregularities and hormonal disruption.

4) The fourth way of getting toxins comes from inside, and we can call them the endotoxins or inside-toxins or own-toxins. As I explained earlier when our gastrointestinal system does not work properly, neither digestion, absorption, or elimination work properly, and all kinds of complications occur. The combination of artificial (man-made) foods, excesses of carbohydrates, processed carbohydrates, stress, bad fat, food chemicals, yeast, food sensitivity reactions, enzyme deficit, and everything else I described in the Inflammation chapter, causes poor digestion, abnormal fermentation, and dysbiosis, with consequent production of toxins inside the intestine. This dysbiosis allows yeast and bacteria to overgrow, which in turn produces more local toxins. All these toxins (we call them endotoxins) start to leak through the wall of the intestine into the bloodstream, a process called Leaky Gut, increasing the level of toxins that accumulate everywhere in the body.

5) In junk food eaters, individuals with unhealthy lifestyle habits, coffee abusers, those who use frequent antibiotics, those who take large amounts of poor-quality vitamins, alcohol abusers, drug abusers, consumers of foods known to irritate the digestive system bring toxins into their intestine. These are called "Lifestyle Toxins."

6) Emotional events and stress when they become chronic and intense can affect our capacity to detoxify. Fear, anger, grief, work-related stress, driving stress, financial and family stress, divorce, and recurrent states of anxiety produce this effect. Working as a truck driver, policeman, nurse, doctor, soldier, or paramedic are just a few examples of high-stress occupations. Any of these events or

occupations, after a prolonged time, can and will interfere with the liver detoxification process allowing toxins to accumulate.

We can have toxins stored in our bodies for years without experiencing any negative symptoms. However, the progression of chemical overload continues until a critical point is reached, AND THEN COMES THE EXPLOSION: the accumulation of toxins finally reaches a critical mass, and then disease starts. Did you think that it would take days or weeks for this to happen? No, although sometimes it does happen, those are the cases of acute poisoning or acute intoxication. It usually takes years, sometimes 10-15 years, for the metabolic mess caused by the toxins to reach its "explosion" point, its critical mass as some like to call it. And then it happens just like it happens in nature: a volcano erupts here, a tsunami there and an earthquake later on. In people, we start seeing a disease here, another one there, some weight gains here, some arthritis and back pain there, some inflammation and chronic fatigue here, then headaches, pain, and rashes later on, then hormonal imbalance, poor sleep, some depression, or maybe allergies, recurrent respiratory infections, and so on. Or they get an injury (because of a fall, whiplash, etc.) and take too long to heal and need too many medications. If someone gets surgery, it takes longer to recover and more medications are needed. The events look unrelated, disconnected, and give no clue of what's brewing under the surface. In other individuals, the storm comes in the form of a heart attack or cancer in a seemingly healthy individual.

Hallelujah, the Laws of Salvation

Before I start with this topic, you need to understand the following: not everybody is affected the same...and some are not affected at all. Nothing affects everyone every time, and that's the first law of salvation, the "random effect." Some people live in an area of severe smog, drink horrible water, and eat contaminated foods and are slim, look great, enjoy good health, and live to age 98. Some men and women are exposed to all kinds of chemicals in their foods, drinks, cosmetics and the environment and they look fantastic even in their later 70's. On the other hand, we have teenagers dying of cancer, young men dropping from heart attacks, young women affected by severe depression or cancer, etc. How's that possible? How can we explain this? Well, we don't have a very clear explanation, things just happen that way. We do have some understanding of these differences. It has to do with our genetic background and epigenomics. Epigenomics is the outer part of the genes that interact with the environment. Individuals who have a significant amount of toxins of all kinds in their body, and who are POOR DETOXIFIERS (that is they don't detoxify these toxins through their liver well), AND carry a significant adverse genetic background, may have those toxins interacting with the "epigenes," causing the symptoms and diseases that affect those individuals. This brings the second law of salvation, the "gene effect," in which your genes decide whether you get the condition or not. Like if you don't have such and such adverse genetic background then the environmental toxins may not give you what your three co-workers got. Or if you have a certain genetic background then your genes will produce an enzyme that will protect you against the condition that your four neighbors got.

And here, just in time, is a very important concept and your third law of salvation. A sign of hope. Your fate is not sealed. If you change your lifestyle, you move out of the danger zone, change the way you eat, sleep and drink, adjust your nutrition, correct your nutritional deficits, work on eliminating free radicals and chronic inflammation, etc., then by changing the effects on your "epigenes," your risk may change. I am writing "may" because if you worked in a coal mine 25 years, smoked two packs of cigarettes a day, ate all the worst foods during those years, and then you win the lotto and you go to live in the Florida Keys and start eating only super fresh foods, your odds will still be poor.

Hence, as you read the chapter on adverse toxic effects keep in mind that not all the symptoms and conditions that I describe will happen to everyone who is loaded with toxins. The genes may protect or be conflicting, and that epigenetics (interaction between genes and environment) play a significant role in all of this.

How Toxins Hurt You

In a nutshell, toxins hurt the neurotransmitters, the mitochondria, the digestive enzymes, the thyroid, the hormones, the brain, and the liver. All the important functions of cells and organs are affected. They just cause a mess. They can age people faster, they can cause chronic diseases and they can kill with cancer, stroke, and heart attacks.

a) Toxins hurt neurotransmitters. Neurotransmitters (NT) are brain chemicals that brain cells (neurons) use to communicate with one another. Some of these neurotransmitters (NT) are called excitatory, like dopamine (important for memory, satisfaction, joy and muscle control), epinephrine (important for energy, motivation, and mental focus), and norepinephrine (important for alertness, hormone coordination, emotional stability. and alertness). Some other NTs are called inhibitory, like GABA (important for controlling the excitatory NT, for calmness and relaxation), serotonin (needed for regulation of mood, hunger, and sleep) and glycine (for control of calmness and decreasing excitatory responses). There are many other NTs, over forty of them, with numerous other functions, but I am limiting the information to just a few.

Imbalance in NTs causes mental and physical disorders and can increase the perception of pain. Yes, it is known that imbalances in NTs are associated with higher pain perception and nerve irritability.

Some excitatory neurotransmitters are capable of adversely affecting the joints and increasing the risk of arthritis.

If dopamine, epinephrine, and norepinephrine are overstimulated and are in excess, the person can get anxiety, stress, attention deficit, hypertension, a higher tendency for inflammation, insomnia, poor digestion, autism, psychosis, agitation and may even become obsessive. If these three NTs are low then the person can get fatigue, restless legs, lack of motivation, poor mood, pains, difficulty losing weight, cravings, and depression.

Toxins (that include chemical compounds, toxic waste, pollutants, endotoxins, environmental toxins, etc.) interfere with neurotransmitters production, causing a deficit in some and an excess in others, thus breaking the harmony among them.

b) Toxins hurt digestion. Toxins and heavy metals destroy the digestive enzymes we use daily in our digestion of food. The result is the improper digestion of food, which impairs the absorption of nutrients, vitamins, and minerals. The lack of vitamins and minerals affects the energy cycle of the cells throughout the body, producing energy deficiency and caloric deprivation to muscles and organs. Muscles get weak, glands don't secrete all the hormones they should, and metabolic imbalance is widespread.

The food, which was only partially digested, continues its path to the colon where the process of fermentation and putrefaction becomes excessive, causing a large amount of gas that distends the abdomen to find an inconvenient and noisy escape at the most unexpected moments. The process of SBI (Silent Bowel Illness) begins, allowing the overgrowth of bacteria and fungus. With the local irritation, inflammation, and SBI the whole process of Dysbiosis is established. The Dysbiosis process opens holes in the intestinal wall, allowing toxins, microbes, and even food particles to leak through (Leaky Gut) into the bloodstream, to wreak havoc wherever they go.

Thus, the person becomes chronically ill with dysbiosis and these toxins leaking through the gut open the door to countless free radicals, inflammatory molecules, inflammation, joint and muscular disorders, vitamin deficiencies, nutritional deficiencies of amino acids, and impaired healing in the face of injuries.

c) Toxins hurt the thyroid and disturb thyroid function, either by decreasing gut absorption of iodine, or by triggering the cascade of toxins, immune reactions, and thyroid-antibodies that end up attacking the gland. The effect is a low functioning thyroid.

Toxins and chemicals also affect the cells, not allowing the membranes to receive the full effect of thyroid hormones, an effect called thyroid resistance. Toxins are therefore thyroid disruptors. Maybe the person will get a low level of the T4–type of thyroid hormone, maybe the person will get a low T3, or maybe both will be low, and maybe there will also be thyroid resistance, but the result is the same: clinical hypothyroidism.

I reviewed above the adverse effects of a low functioning thyroid, but remember that toxins are thyroid disruptors.

d) Toxins affect hormones. Whether directly or indirectly, toxins hurt the production and actions of what we know as sex-hormones: estrogens, testosterone, progesterone, and DHEA. We reviewed these hormones earlier, so you already know that hormone decline can trigger inflammation, higher sensitivity to pain, arthritis, and musculoskeletal disorders.

e) Adrenal glands. Toxins also hurt the production and function of cortisol by the adrenal gland. As this adrenal gland becomes abnormal, the secretion of cortisol may be insufficient for the needs of the metabolism. The imbalance causes fatigue, lethargy, poor immunity, inflammation, joint problems, frequent respiratory infections, increased recovery time from injuries and surgeries, mental fog, poor memory, asthma, cough, poor alcohol tolerance, exhaustion, apathy, diabetes, addiction, stiffness, depression, intellectual and physical decline as well as a decline in productivity.

f) Toxins hurt the natural detoxification system. All humans have a natural detoxification system that takes the waste products of digestion and cellular metabolism into the liver, which is the main organ of detoxification. Toxins have an adverse effect on enzymes and the detox system, clogging and deactivating them.

g) Toxins cause obesity. When we analyze all the factors that cause obesity, we get an idea of how toxins cause metabolic interference that inhibits weight loss. The idea that obesity is caused by "eating a lot and not exercising" is old. It's not wrong, but it's not complete, and it's misleading. Obesity is much more complicated than that. Here are some of the factors that interact to cause obesity: hormone and thyroid imbalance, improper nutritional balance of vitamins, amino acids, good fat and minerals, food sensitivities, inadequate liver support, dysbiosis, and leaky gut, lack of exercise and good sleep, poor appetite control, clogged detoxification, poor adrenal-stress situation, neurotransmitter imbalance, dysfunctional mitochondria, excess of oxidative stress, excess caloric intake, omega-6 lifestyle, etc. But for whatever cause, obesity is an inflammatory state that also puts a strain on joints, muscles, and nerves, therefore, arthritis and pain are almost inevitable consequences.

h) Toxins hurt mitochondria. Mitochondria are little organs inside the cells, and it is inside them that the cells burn the glucose and the fatty acids to produce energy. They are like little electrical energy generators. The mitochondria consume the molecules of the food we eat to produce the energy the cell needs to function. Inside it, many chemical reactions digest and disintegrate the molecules using enzymes and cofactors. The end result is pure controlled energy. This energy will allow the cell to do what it is meant to do, contract if it is a muscle cell, secrete if it is a gland cell, protect if it is a skin cell, fortify if it is a bone cell, etc. Almost all cells of our body depend on properly functioning mitochondria to work.

Toxins are mitochondria disruptors. They hurt the mitochondria and interfere with its job, causing faulty function, which causes an energy crisis inside the cell. As the mitochondria function is disrupted, the breaking down of the fuel-molecules (like glucose) is affected and electrons may escape from the otherwise controlled reaction. Those free electrons are charged and they are like a flying spark, hitting other molecules and structures, damaging the mitochondria, hurting the cell membrane, in a frenzy that is called "oxidative reaction." The electron spark may bounce against other molecules making them free, an electron of their own, and causing many electrons to bounce around the mitochondria leading to damage. It looks like a pinball game with many simultaneous balls all bouncing like crazy. If this oxidative reaction is intense, it can even damage the cell permanently, or kill it. This very stressful situation for the cell is what we know as "OXIDATIVE STRESS," and it creates free radicals and inflammation, which are two well-known agents of disease. This process is called mitochondrial dysfunction. Dysfunction means that it is not working well, or is working abnormally.

REMEMBER THIS WELL:

MITOCHONDRIAL DYSFUNCTION IS THE ROOT OF MOST CHRONIC DISEASES. It is actually the very root of them. Toxins cause mitochondrial dysfunction, which is one of the roots of inflammation, tissue degeneration, neuromuscular disorders, joint disorders, and painful conditions.

Oxidative Stress gives the cell a double-punch: the cell can't function and it gets damaged at the same time. This is the root of many diseases including most chronic diseases. Hence, this cellular damage may end up causing brain disease, obesity, thyroid disease, muscular disease (which may cause muscular aches, pain, and poor muscular healing), joint diseases, gland failure, liver disease, and digestive diseases. As life goes on, the person starts to develop digestive symptoms, brain difficulties, muscle weakness, pains, heart problems, the effects of hormonal failure, more inflammation, immune deficiency, detoxification failure, eye problems, diabetes, neurotransmitter disorders, atherosclerosis, slowly developing multiple medical disorders. Later on in life, dementia, Parkinson's, Alzheimer's, and cancer come as a consequence of these mitochondria adversities.

Of course, not everybody is affected, and those who are affected don't get all the above conditions, but there is no way to tell who will be affected and who will not, or who will get which of the above problems.

Will Bob get early heart trouble, late prostate cancer, dementia, or nothing at all?

Will Mary get breast cancer at 34, very low hormones at 39, chronic fatigue and depression at 45, severe arthritis and osteoporosis at 60, or nothing at all and die at 98 in some nursing home?

How about you? How old are you? Do you feel lucky?

AS YOU CAN SEE, toxins can cause pain, inflammation, joint disorders, poor healing from injuries and surgeries, and they can cause that either directly or indirectly. Indirectly by altering brain chemicals, mitochondria, absorption of nutrients, hurting the liver, adrenal gland, hormones, and thyroid, which ultimately have control over all those disorders.

DO YOU THINK OR DO YOU HAVE THE ILLUSION that your sore joint will just get better if you are contaminated with toxins, your neurotransmitter and hormones are all in imbalance, your thyroid and your adrenals are functioning poorly, and your detox system is clogged? Do you think that if you have all that, a simple cortisone shot will just do the job? And if you have significant dysbiosis and continue eating poorly, then what? Do you think that your sore joint will heal?

WHAT CAN WE DO?

The answer is not easy, it is complex.
We need to:

a) Avoid whenever we can any further exposure to toxins (drink non-toxic liquids, avoid drinking multi-chemical drinks, eat organic foods, avoid processed foods, avoid smog, avoid foods of questionable origin, avoid exposure to chemicals, etc.).

b) Inform ourselves about the problem by reading on the Internet, or in libraries and bookstores. Learn about what is polluted, where pollution is, and how to avoid exposure.

c) Read and learn about which foods and drinks to avoid and why.

d) Consult via the Internet the main federal centers (FDA, EPA, etc.).

e) Correct the metabolic abnormalities that need to be corrected, such as using thyroid medication if needed, using natural hormone replacement if needed, fix your adrenals, correct dysbiosis, and leaky gut if you have them, balance the neurotransmitters, improve your immune system, take vitamins, antioxidants, and omega-3s if they are needed, get tested for food sensitivities, and improve liver function.

f) Adopt a Mediterranean style of diet, organic when possible.

g) Get tested for metabolic imbalances, toxic effects, gut disorders, hormone imbalance, mitochondria dysfunction, vitamin deficiencies, and possibly heavy metals.

h) And overall DETOXIFY! Engage in a well-designed professionally recommended detoxification program that will remove toxins from your body.

Yes, part of the solution is you. You cannot just depend on this book, or any book you read to work on detoxification. You can't just "follow what the doctor says," when you know that most doctors have no knowledge about this and may deny that toxins are a problem at all.

However, should you do all this? Isn't ignorance a blessing? Perhaps the less you know the less it will hurt. Why should you complicate your life, when you could just ignore all this and continue living your life the way you have been?

Well, let me answer that question with another question: Do you have a spare body?

In addition to your work and family, do you have anything better to do than to read, learn, and take action about all this? Will you just wait for things to happen? And let me rephrase that: are you just going to sit and wait?

I won't, and I already started my metabolic evaluation and my detoxification.

Let's start with this question: Do you need detoxification?

Detoxification

By definition, detoxification is the removal of toxic substances from the body. It is a widely used treatment in alternative medicine.

Perhaps I should emphasize this point. Detoxification is not mainstream medicine and is not part of conventional medicine. It is not part of the medical school academic protocol and it is not accepted in the mainstream of medical treatment. It is part of a different field, the wide world of alternative medicine.

As much as conventional and orthodox medical practitioners hold tight to their ignorance and medical conservatism and claim that alternative medicine is "bad-unapproved-medicine," the reality and practicality show that alternative medicine is very successful in providing relief and healing to a very large number of people. We have seen how the unapproved acupuncture, chiropractic, and homeopathy have been growing in our country because they were able to provide health benefits without the costly and lengthy conventional medical approaches. Despite this, many alternative medicine therapies were and still are resisted by the medical community in general and by what we call the medical establishment.

Have no doubt, alternative therapies have proven themselves over time to be incredibly beneficial. And perhaps as a testimony to that, we now find departments of alternative medicine within the National Institute of Health, Harvard Medical School, and other mainstream academic institutions. This is telling you that mainstream medicine recognizes alternative medicine and even teaches it in many medical schools around the country.

Detoxification got the same cold welcome as acupuncture, homeopathy, and many other alternative therapies: it was denied by many, unapproved, and criticized by many more, but became a healthy solution for many others.

However, there is nothing to welcome, because detoxification is not new. It has been around for many centuries. It has only gotten better, and whether doctors accept it or not, it is here to stay.

Detoxification, as I wrote above, is based on the principle that illness can be caused by the accumulation of toxic substances (toxins) in the body. Eliminating existing toxins and avoiding new toxins are essential parts of the healing process.

There is nothing new here. Many ethnic groups on the five continents have been practicing detoxification for centuries. The only new thing here is conventional medical physicians ignoring and denying it.

Let me invite you to explore the history of detoxification and to use the Internet to review the current knowledge about toxins and detoxification. Check FDA, EPA, NIH, AAEM, Toxicology organizations, but start by reading the New York Times where you will see how the problem of toxins, chemicals, heavy metals, herbicides, etc., is getting worse.

Starting Detoxification

Gut Restoration Program

The ten basic rules of healing the gut are known as the "10 Rs" of management:

1) Relax your adrenal glands, (they have a strong adverse impact in the gut). Explore the vast world of stress management and relaxation techniques and choose the ones you like. Read about these subjects and explore the amazing fields of adaptogens. This first step is mandatory, since stressful situations, including toxins and metabolic stress, can adversely affect the bowel, causing SBI and Dysbiosis, allowing toxins to leak through the wall of the intestine and into the bloodstream.

2) Retreat from bad foods, the wrong way of eating, bad habits, avoiding the food groups I described, and will describe later on in this book.

3) Review your family background to eat according to the Nutrigenomics principle.

4) Recognize that a Mediterranean Diet is the best way of eating, with acidic food mixed with alkaline, and with plenty of omega-3s and antioxidants.

5) Remove bad bacteria, toxins, heavy metals, and unwanted waste from your gut, through a detoxification PROGRAM.

6) Relieve the liver of its toxic overload and improve its functions and bile flow.

7) Remember food sensitivities.

8) Repair the gut with the necessary functional foods and supplements.

9) Replace stomach acid and enzymes if needed.

10) Re-inoculate the gut with friendly bacteria by taking probiotics and prebiotics.

And if you are still not better, go to the 11th"R."

11) Research your stools, trying to find out why your symptoms persist. This "R" is to be done if you are not getting better and therefore there could be a problem in your gut. In this test, we collect your stools for a special stool test. Stool analysis is not a typical stool test and it has to be done in a very precise way and only with specific laboratories, like Genova, Doctor's Data, etc. If done well, it should reveal whether you have a stomach acid deficiency, enzyme deficiency, and whether you are absorbing the amino acids and fats. It will also show what kind of dysbiosis you have, whether you have yeast or bacterial overgrowth and especially it will tell you about candida and dysbiosis. It will bring information about the agents that are hurting your bowels and are opening the doors for the invasion by toxins.

About Detoxification Programs

In this phase you start to restore the bowel integrity while reducing the incoming burden of toxins, supporting the process of toxin elimination and enhancing the liver detoxification pathways. This detoxification has three systems in one:

1) Phase 1, which is the removal of toxins from the tissues and making them enter the blood circulation to transport them to the liver.

2) Phase 2, where the liver captures them and throws them into the bile to be eliminated through the intestine and excreted with the stool.

3) Phase 3, when toxins go from liver to the gut and from there to the outside.

You will be taking a variety of compounds with phase 1, phase 2, and phase 3 properties during detoxification.

Detoxification is not and cannot be a "do-it-yourself" program, and should not be a "just follow the book" program. Proper and safe detoxification should not be "a little package with instructions" that you buy in the health food store. It cannot be something you do without proper training or someone explaining the process to you and supervising every step.

Proper programs use anti-inflammatory herbs and specific intestinal nutrients to decrease inflammation, repair the intestinal cells, heal the gut, improve bowel function, promote healthy secretion, and repair the damage caused by chronic aggressors.

Detox Products

Because of reliability and quality, I only recommend products from laboratories associated with the American Academy of Anti-Aging Medicine and the American Association of Naturopathic Physicians. I just don't trust any other laboratory, over-the-counter products, beautiful websites, health food stores, or else, and you should not trust them either. Contact your local doctor, chiropractor, anti-aging practitioner, or local dietitians or nutritional consultants to get them and take them correctly. You could buy them from any of the following companies but take them ONLY under professional supervision (or run the risk of severe complications). They are not for the "do-it-yourselfer."

Here is a list of the laboratories and the corresponding product:

Laboratory	Web site	Product
Designs For Health	www.designsforhealth.com	Original 14 Day Detox Program, Amino-D-tox, Detoxification Support Packets
Douglas	www.douglaslabs.com	Metabolic Rejuvenation Program, LivDetox, Metabolic Cleanse, Detoxification Pack
Metagenics	www.metagenics.com	Clear Change 10 day and 28 day Programs, UltraClear, UltraClear Plus, Metallo Clear, AdvaClear
NuMedica	www.numedica.com	7-Day Detox Program, 14-Day Detox Program with DualTox DPO, HM Protect, Thera PRP, ProToxi Clear Program Nu-Vitals Vital-DETOX program, Phyto-DETOX, Bio-Detox
Ortho Molecular	www.orthomolecularproducts.com	CORE Restore Program with PhytoCore
Protocol For Life	www.protocolforlife.com	ProtoClear Program
Pure Encapsulations	www.pureencapsulations.com	Detox Program with HM Chelate and Detox Pure pack, Pure Clear
Thorne Research	www.thorne.com	Medi-Clear Program with Basic Detox nutrients
Xymogen	www.xymogen.com	Opti-Cleanse and Opti-Cleanse Plus Programs, with XenoProteX and MedCaps DPO, Liver Protect

These are all excellent programs and products from reliable and very good laboratories. I have tried them all.

In our office, however, we have found the following products to be very well-tolerated, have a tolerable taste, and great acceptability. Using them is very practical and we feel very comfortable with the results:

-Vital DETOX and

-Vital DETOX 7- or 14-day program with PhytoDETOX and the special DETOX Vitamins

We frequently use Bio-Detox as a complement.

All the above products are based on current detox literature and research, and all laboratories adjust their formulas according to advances in detoxification knowledge. Following strict guidelines, we teach patients 1-to-1 about each product, diet requirement, and the "10 R" Gut Restoration Protocol.

You can buy these products on the Internet, but use them only under a physician's supervision.

INTERCHAPTER REMARK: Toxins should not be ignored since their presence in our environment is only getting worse. Whether coming from our gut, from water, air, food, etc., this toxin problem is affecting us all. Learning about them and practicing some form of detox has become a necessity for us all.

Sleep

"A circle of soreness: pain, injuries, inflammation and arthritis cause lack of sleep; lack of sleep adversely affects them all"

I am sure I don't need to tell you how important sleep is, and how problematic sleep loss has become in this country. Loss of sleep is a common problem in our modern-day society, affecting millions of individuals.

Good sleep is essential for numerous body functions and physiological pathways, and actually, sleep affects almost every tissue and organ in the body. Moreover, sleep is important to many brain functions, including how nerve cells (neurons) communicate with each other.

There is a lot to learn about sleep and its mechanisms, its stages, the brain sleep centers, etc., but these are extensive in their description and are not the object of this chapter. There are books, websites, and many articles you can consult to expand on the subject, so I invite you to explore these sources.

The main object of this chapter is to help you understand a few details about poor sleep and some of its management and especially to emphasize the key point: that sleep is affected by pain, arthritis, injuries and inflammation, and the other way around. These four conditions can also affect sleep. Sometimes you don't know which started first, but, for sure, if you are affected by those conditions, and your sleep is poor, you need to find a way to sleep better and longer.

Common conditions that often cause sleep problems include heartburn, diabetes, depression, pain, cardiovascular disease, hormonal imbalances, arthritis, kidney disease, injuries, mental health problems, tendinitis, neck pain, painful tingling in arms or legs, sciatica, neurological disorders, respiratory problems, nasal congestion, being post-surgery, medications, stimulants, inflammatory conditions, caffeine, thyroid disease, and other disorders. Anxiety, lifestyle, stress, irregular work hours, alcohol, certain foods, infections, and feeling overwhelmed can be the cause as well. Age and genetic tendencies play a role as well, and many individuals can describe how their sleep hours started to shrink after age 50-55. However, sleep problems have been expanding in the general population and younger people are now affected as well. I think the cause of this "insomnia epidemic" is a combination of stress and the effect of toxins and chemicals.

However, there are also some other causes of sleep disturbance, and these are not that easy to understand:

- adjustment sleep disorder
- anxiety disorders
- breathing disorders
- circadian rhythm sleep disorders
- food allergy insomnia
- food sensitivities
- obstructive sleep apnea
- parasomnias
- post-traumatic stress disorder
- psychophysiological insomnia
- psychosis
- stimulants related

As you can see, sleep disorders are a very complicated field. Again, I am just giving you a brief panorama of sleep disorders, and you should expand your knowledge through books, publications, and websites.

If you do have a sleep disorder, consider seeing a sleep specialist or a neurologist.

Some publications point out that a) exposure to heavy metals, b) toxic chemicals, and c) mild but prolonged stress over a long period can affect the brain and interrupt its normal sleep function. This effect caused d) an imbalance in the brain chemicals involved in sleep and e) abnormal hormonal levels, which in turn disturb sleep function. To these factors, we should add the effect of caffeine, lifestyle, work, and social anxiety, then we might have the right cocktail. But, guess what: it is not always easy to determine the cause of sleeplessness.

If that was not enough, we recently found out that it is during sleep that the brain detoxifies itself and eliminates some of the toxins acquired during the day. One of the most interesting discoveries in the last few years is that the brain clears out toxins when we are asleep. Apparently, at nighttime, the spaces between brain cells increase, allowing the brain to flush out the toxic waste. This means that those who already have bad sleep will get worse sleep as time passes because of toxin accumulation. It also means they need to engage in detoxification.

At any rate, it seems that once you lose your good sleep, those good old times may not come back. That's bad news.

Sleep plays an important role in adrenal gland health, hormonal balance, and general physical health. Lack of sleep affects not only your joints and muscles but also cardiovascular health, blood pressure control, brain function, and the digestive system.

Worse even is how people affected by pain, arthritis, and injuries easily fall in the vicious circle of pain affecting sleep and sleep affecting pain.

That is the crude reality, as I already emphasized above, problems like pain, arthritis, inflammation, and injuries affect the sleep pattern and the lack of good sleep affects how people heal from those problems. Painful disorders affect the sleep, sleep affects those disorders, just like that. That's what I mean by a vicious cycle.

Let's review some of this.

Adrenal gland. The function of the adrenal gland can be affected by toxins, stress, dysbiosis, and food chemicals. Since adrenal function affects the brain, adrenal dysfunction is one of the causes of lack of sleep.

During deep sleep, the adrenal gland, which is so important for energy and hormone control and general metabolism, recharges itself, prepares for the next day, and loads itself with hormones for the forthcoming day's journey. If sleep is not adequate, the adrenal gland will not be properly fit for the morning, and there will not be good energy, and in consequence, the metabolism (needed for activities and healing) will be sluggish. You may notice sluggishness if you already wake up tired. Worse even is the fact that a tired and dysfunctional adrenal gland has a pro-inflammation and anti-healing effect. That's more bad news.

Also, the deep sleep hours, especially between midnight and six in the morning, are the time when growth hormone, (GH) (also known as "the repair hormone") is secreted. This hormone is designed to fix whatever needs to be fixed. It is a super hormone. You may see its effects if you observe the following. If you go to bed with a fresh mosquito bite, a little wound, or a cut, and you get a night of good deep sleep, you should see that when you wake up in the morning the lesion has somehow healed a little, like if the tooth fairy visited you at night. That fairy was your growth hormone (GH).

This hormone has an anti-inflammatory and a healing effect, and if you enjoy prolonged, natural, deep sleep, it will help your arthritis, injuries, and other painful disorders.

Therefore, if your sleep is not good, you may not enjoy the healing effects of Growth Hormones or the benefit of waking up in the morning with a healthy, refreshed, fully-loaded adrenal gland. That's not good either.

Brain chemicals. A very important cause of poor sleep is the imbalance of brain chemicals, known as neurotransmitters (NT), which connect one brain cell with another. Some of those brain chemicals are known by the general public as GABA, serotonin, and melatonin. Some others are less commonly known, like glutamate, galanin, acetylcholine, glycine, histamine, norepinephrine, adenosine, etc., that when imbalanced can affect relaxation and sleep.

Falling asleep does not happen like flipping a switch in a small brain center somewhere. A whole combination of neurotransmitters is involved in switching off the brain, "disconnecting it," and then allowing it to sink into the sweet unconsciousness of sleep. While none of these neurotransmitters acts individually, they all appear to contribute in some way. Hence, there is not just one sleep center and just one neurotransmitter, but rather several control centers at the base of the brain that use a variety of chemicals and waves.

So, grasp this concept: neurotransmitter imbalances cause sleep disorders.

These neurotransmitters can go wrong for several reasons. They can be hurt by environmental toxins. They can be scarce because the intestine is not absorbing the basic nutrients needed to produce them (that is how dysbiosis hurts your brain chemicals). They can be unbalanced because of food sensitivity, stress, or viruses. They can be in disorder because of stimulants, medications, lifestyle, chemicals in food and drinks, and excess caffeine.

More about neurotransmitters. There is something else you need to know about the brain chemicals, and this is the time to learn it. The problem with neurotransmitters goes far beyond the sleep problems that the general population is facing. Mental disorders and neurological problems of all kinds are now affecting millions of Americans throughout our country. The problem is universal and it is rooted in the decline and imbalance of those BRAIN CHEMICALS known as neurotransmitters (NT).

It is a fact and a true concern: this wave of brain chemical disorders constitutes a new expanding epidemic that is currently affecting larger and younger populations. And yes, it is becoming more frequent.

Toxins, chemicals, stress, nutritional factors, biological substances, and genetic tendencies are combining to damage our neurotransmitter system, depleting our brain of these precious chemicals, and causing multiple diseases. The consequences are not just sleep disturbances but a multitude of disorders like bulimia, chronic fatigue, fibromyalgia, insomnia, cognitive decline, poor memory, anorexia, dementia, Parkinson's, depression, anxiety, panic, migraines, chronic pain, OCD, ADD, headaches, phobias, and many others. Multiple pharmacological therapies are only able to exercise some control, if any, on these conditions, but at the cost of overwhelming side effects and very limited efficacy. The truth is that current conventional medicine does not offer a good solution to these disorders, and this is because neurotransmitters are hard to reach and manage. The brain will not allow brain chemicals coming from outside to enter its cells. Various trials have been done to improve the amount and function of neurotransmitters (NT) and they have all failed.

This information is very important and you should share it with the people you know. I AM SURE people are suffering from the above conditions among your relatives and friends.

Keep in mind that patients suffering from any of the above conditions are NOT suffering from medication deficiency, but rather they are suffering from a nutritional deficiency involving serotonin and dopamine precursors. Those precursors are called amino acids. I am going to rephrase it. Patients suffering from the above conditions are not suffering from Prozac deficiency, Xanax deficiency, or any pharma deficiency; they are suffering from precursor-amino acids deficiency for the production of their brain chemicals. If a program could find a way to rebuild amino acids, those conditions would get better. Well, there is such a program, and it was designed by Dr. Marty Hinz.

We know very well that our brain controls every single function of our body, including walking, talking, typing, digestion, liver and kidney function, heart and lungs, hormones, body temperature, blood pressure, mood, glands, muscles, immune system, etc. through the use of neurotransmitters. However, their decline and imbalance have been hard to correct.

Until now.

The only way I have found to improve the neurotransmitters imbalance was through the program of a genius doctor named Dr. Marty Hinz, who provides products with high concentrations of purified neurotransmitters building blocks (amino acids), allowing the brain cells to grab them and build inside of themselves the necessary brain chemicals. No sleep will be as good or regenerative as the one brought to you by your own neurotransmitters (NT). Do your own research about neurotransmitters.

In our office, we have been doing the Brain Chemicals Improvement Program following the guidelines of Dr. Hinz, and we have found very interesting results and quite positive improvements. We follow a strict protocol, adjusting the special natural amino acids according to the particular problem of the patient. We don't use pharmacological agents. I invite you to contact those websites and search for a similar program near you. If you are unable, contact my office, tell me where you are and I will try to find a center close to where you are.

Hormones. Certain hormones, like progesterone and DHEA, are well-known to affect the sleep pattern, but actual disorders of thyroid hormone, testosterone, cortisol, and growth hormone can all cause sleep disorders as well.

Hormone decline is not just an age problem as it is seen in younger populations as well. In both men and women going through menopause and andropause, and also with those in their 40's and even 30's, the hormone progesterone is the first to decline, which frequently produces a decreased quality of sleep. Thyroid hormone decline has become a universal problem, most likely associated with toxin exposure, chemicals, and toxins in food and drink, food sensitivity, dysbiosis, etc., and poor sleep is very common in those affected. Whether those hormones and the others I mention above, decline because of stress, age, chemical exposure, environmental toxins, radiation, dysbiosis, poor nutrition or dietary causes, the resulting bad sleep is the same. What I find alarming is that these hormone declines seem to be becoming more frequent, more symptomatic, and spreading into a younger population.

And keep in mind that, in turn, sleep deprivation can affect hormone levels in a sleepless vicious cycle. Low estrogen in perimenopausal women and low testosterone in periandropausal men can cause sleep problems as well.

Toxins. Certain environmental toxins can be neurotoxins, although most of the time the accumulation of these compounds is extremely low and the person has no idea it is happening. These toxins can be present in food, water, air, and even in your garden. They can be present in the products you buy to clean your house, so you better inform yourself. Certain medications and over-the-counter products can have a neurotoxicity effect. Alcohol in liquor, wine, beer, and cocktails can be neurotoxic for most people. (What did you think "being drunk" means if not a brain disorder caused by alcohol?)

Electronics. Sometimes the fault is in your habits. Having your cell phone, clock, radio, or TV in the room could be the cause of your sleep disorder. Get them out of the room.

THE POINT YOU NEED TO REMEMBER IS THAT WHATEVER IS CAUSING THE SLEEP DISORDER, the lack of sleep will interfere with the healing of your arthritis, pain, inflammation, and injuries.

Hence, you need to find a way to improve your sleep.

Start with getting your room ready. Make your bed. Close the curtains. Make your bedroom a sanctuary, dark and free of noises and stressors.

Establish a routine for going to bed, and try to always go to bed at the same time.

Don't do anything stimulating before going to bed, except sex.

Remove all electronics, including the TV (Yes! Get the TV out). Keep the room clean.

Is your spouse snoring? Make him/her take care of that. If it's from sleep apnea, see your pulmonologist.

Avoid sugars and sweets within six hours of going to bed. Avoid drugs and stimulants, such as coffee and an excess of alcohol. A glass of red wine with or after dinner is okay.

Consider herbal teas for relaxation or to induce sleep, like chamomile or valerian tea. Many health food stores and even supermarkets are now selling different kinds of herbal sleep helpers. Sometimes they combine two, three, or four herbs to provide a better result, like adding passionflower to the above two. Try some of them and see if they can help you.

If no success, then consider all the following.

Over-the-counter sleep aids can be very helpful, but don't take them for a prolonged time.

Check the websites of the American Academy of Sleep Medicine (www. aasm.org) and the American Sleep Apnea Association (www.sleephealth. org) for information. Also, check (www.insomnia.net), the World Sleep

Society (www.worldsleepsociety.org), and the National Sleep Foundation (www.sleepfoundation.org).

Strongly consider consulting with a sleep specialist.

Certain pharmacological products can be of help, depending on the individual and his/her problem. Products like Valium, Ativan, Ambien, Lunesta, Xanax, Sonata, and Restoril, and their generic forms, can help many individuals achieve a good rest at night. I only recommend them for a very short course or to be taken perhaps only once, maybe twice, a week, no more. The reason for this is their short term and long term side effects when taken more often than that. On the one hand, they give you a very needed break, allowing you to achieve deep regenerative sleep. On the other hand, they have side effects. Don't take any sleeping pills without checking the side effects on the web. Be extremely careful, and ask yourself why is it that I very rarely prescribe those pills.

Strongly consider trying acupuncture. Studies show that patients receiving acupuncture get a rise in their nighttime melatonin production and a much improved total sleep time. The patients who received acupuncture also fell asleep faster, were less aroused at night, and were less stressed.

Acupuncturists have been successfully treating sleep disorders for centuries. According to Chinese medicine, there are several types of sleep disorders: general inability to fall asleep, poor sleep onset or difficulty falling asleep, waking in the middle of the night, late insomnia, sleep with disruptive dreaming. Each of these particular types of disruptive sleep is caused by a different imbalance in the circulating energy, or chi, and deserves a different acupuncture approach. Don't hesitate to try it.

Herbal sleep helpers. There are numerous herbal and plant products that produce sedation and sleep improvement. Jasmine, Lavender, Valerian, Passionflower, Chamomile, Bamboo palm, Peace Lily, Ashwagandha, California poppy, Hops, Skullcaps, and Kava are some of the most common. They can be taken alone, mixed or combined with L-Theanine (a mild sedative), or Phosphatidylserine (a brain-adrenal blocker) or melatonin (a synthetic hormone-like product that helps regulate sleep).

But be careful, you should not just buy these products without getting advice from a physician or alternative medicine professional. Don't underestimate the possible side effects of these products. And especially, DO NOT buy three, four or more of these products and take them combined as you please. Some of those products might be the right ones for you or they might not be. Who are you going to trust? Whose advice are you going to follow? A pill-pusher health food store employee with a very convincing speech? A beautiful website "that looks really professional" but irresponsibly sells garbage? One of those Internet doctors that "looks really great and seems to know a lot"?

Who?

All of these products need to be the right ones for you, must be in the right combination and in the right amount and proportion to provide beneficial effects without undesirable side effects. They need to be manufactured by responsible laboratories. And you don't find them in health food stores or the pharmacy near you. You will find them on the websites listed below, or in some compounding pharmacies, and some of the offices of health care professionals.

Don't buy these products on your own or you may face a lack of efficacy and possible unwanted side effects. You could ask the owner of the health food store for advice if you know that person and you have been there before. But be careful who you ask, as most health food store employees don't know much and will just try to push sales.

And again, don't buy them from websites, TV commercials, or some "new expert" who claims what he shouldn't.

Just like the other products I recommended before, I recommend the laboratories associated with the Academy of Anti-Aging Medicine and the Naturopathic Society, who have scientific personnel evaluating these products, analyzing their origin and purity, combining them in the right proportions and providing a product that might offer reliable benefits with minimized side effects. Moreover, as you visit their websites you may find some brief information about each one of these products. I encourage you to do so. Some are more for relaxation; some are more for sleep. Get yourself informed before you buy anything.

Here is a list of those laboratories, their website and some of the products I reviewed.

Laboratory	Web site	Product
Douglas Labs	www.douglaslabs.com	Seditol (Magnolia Officinalis, Ziziphus, chamomile, passionflower and Lemon Balm), Valsed (combination of magnesium, Valerian and Passionflower (passiflora), Melatonin 1mg Melatonin 3mg
Metagenics	www.metagenics.com	MyoCalm Plus (magnesium, Passionflower, Valerian, Lemon Balm), Benesom (magnesium, Skullcap, Passionflower, Lemon Balm, Valerian, Hops)
NuMedica	www.numedica.com	Sereni-T (traditional Chinese herbal formula).
Nutritional Frontiers	www.nutritionalfrontiers.com	Relaxation and Sleep drops (an interesting combination of Chamomile, Valerian, Lemon Balm,
Ortho Molecular	www.orthomolecularproducts.com	Adrenevive (an excellent product with hosphatidylserine (a brain-adrenal blocker), L-theanine (mild sedative), ashwagandha (adrenal relaxer), Skullcap, and the adaptogens Eleuthero and Rhodiola), Botanicalm PM (with Valerian, Jujube, L-Theanine, Passionflower, Hops), Cerenity PM (Taurine, 5-HTP, GABA and phosphatidylserine)
Prothera	www.protherainc.com	TheraSleep (Hops, Passionflower, Chamomile), Stress Support Complex (GABA, L-Theanine,

Ashwagandha, Valerian, Passionflower) Nu-Vitals Vital-Sleep (lemon balm, california poppy, theanine, melatonin, lavender), Comfortil (ashwagandha), Bio-Relax (unique blend of relaxing herbs)

Pure Encapsulations www.pureencapsulations.com..........Best Rest Formula (melatonin, GABA, l-theanine, valerian, lemon balm, hops, Passionflower, chamomile), Melatonin, Deep Solution (magnesium, l-theanine, melatonin)

Skullcap and Linden)

Xymogen...............www.xymogen.com...............SereneX (concentrated Chinese botanicals, including panax ginseng, jujube, schisandra, rehmannia, scrophularia, and others), Sedalin (magnolia and ziziphus)

These are all excellent products from reliable and very good laboratories. Still, you must consult with your doctor before taking these products.

WARNING: all those products can cause sedation and impair mental faculties. Don't drive, use electrical devices or any machinery after you take them. They are intended to be taken before bedtime. Take responsibly. Always consult with your doctor before taking them. They may interfere or cross react with your medications or alcohol.

Not being able to properly relax is a very common problem. Lack of sleep, too. Women and men of every age suffer from insomnia, unable to fall asleep or frequently waking up at night. These conditions have different roots, as I addressed above, which vary from individual to individual and therefore require different approaches that might not be the same from one person to the next. Let me rephrase that. What helps Bob sleep better might not help Martin.

Individuals need to try different modalities and sleep helpers until they find what helps them.

In my attempt to avoid pharmaceuticals, I have studied these problems extensively, and, as I remarked above, I have researched the laboratories recognized by the American Academy of Anti-Aging Medicine, and I am now able to offer some natural options (which, as a poor sleeper myself, I have tried them all)

a) **Bio-Magnesium**. A gentle form of magnesium, a mineral essential for metabolism. Supports normal mood and emotional well-being. In many individuals, it induces sleep and fights insomnia. It is also a muscle relaxant, reducing cramps and inducing calmness. Bio-Magnesium combines the malate and glycinate forms, which are the most recommended form of this mineral. Take one at night.

b) **Vital-Sleep**. Contains valerian and lemon balm, two of the most studied herbs to help support restful sleep. It also contains passiflora for the relief of restlessness and irritability, and California poppy extract combined with theanine, melatonin, hops, and lavender to enhance the sleep-inducing and sleep-maintaining effects of these two excellent products.

c) **Comfortil**. A purified form of ashwagandha, one of the best-known herbs to improve adrenal gland function and provide restorative benefits. It decreases stress, anxiety, fatigue, and even depression. It supports falling asleep and remaining asleep, and makes sleep more restful. It even offers rejuvenating effects and improves mental function and sexuality. It can be taken in the afternoon or evening for relaxation or at bedtime.

d) **Bio-Relax**. Contains a blend of plant extracts that help provide relief from stress and nervous tension. It also contains ashwagandha, valerian, passionflower, lemon balm, chamomile, l-theanine, and lavender. It counteracts tension, irritability, and anxiety while supporting normal physiological relaxation and promoting a balanced mood. It calms the mind, the muscles, and even the digestive system. It can be taken in the afternoon or the evening when coming home from work to help you unwind. It can also be taken two to three hours before bedtime to induce sleep.

INTERCHAPTER REMARK: Sleep problems are increasing and more and more people are affected. Those affected need to review the possible causes and provide themselves with a "natural products arsenal" to improve their sleep, so they will not resort to pharmaceuticals.

Finale

The main reason I wrote this new book is to help my patients in the process of understanding this complex combination that we call integration. Unfortunately, my practice has become way too busy and at the end of the day, I find myself wondering if I have explained to my patients with inflammation, injuries, pain, arthritis, surgical recovery, bursitis, neck disc disorders, etc., all the very important details regarding the root of the process and the options for management. I am grateful to my practice since it has led me to meet wonderful people, but time is a factor I cannot overcome. This has been a great motivator for me to write this book. I deeply hope it will help many of my patients and their family and friends.

Millions of people suffering from pain, arthritis, and injuries have embraced alternative therapies with excellent results. Although not successful in every case, alternative medicine offers us a chance to find relief from ailments without having to deal with the negative aspects of pharmaceutical drugs (and their side effects) and surgeries, so commonplace in conventional medicine. I want to emphasize, however, that there is no substitute for conventional medicine in the case of many health conditions. Alternative medicine should not replace proven medical treatments. As such we support and encourage alternative medicine, in cases of sepsis (infections), fractures, surgical conditions, heart attacks, pneumonia, heart disease, bleeding, strokes, and many other acute or chronic diseases. Conventional medicine cannot be replaced. Hundreds of diseases of the eyes, ears, nose, throat, chest, and abdomen can only be taken care of by what is still one of the most wonderful advancements of mankind: conventional medicine.

Nevertheless, there has been and continues to be a growing dissatisfaction with conventional medicine. Many call this healthcare system impersonal because doctors practice medicine influenced by attorneys, pharmaceutical companies, and even insurance and "other" regulations. Many also call it ineffective due to its lack of success in treating the chronic conditions plaguing us today, including lifestyle diseases such as cancer, arthritis, diabetes, obesity, and heart disease. The invasion of HMOs, the ever-increasing price of health insurance, and the growing disappointments on the part of both doctors and patients have only made matters worse. Citizens (including healthcare professionals) lament that the overall quality of medical care has been decreasing over the past several years and that the government and major medical companies have done nothing to fix it. Faced with these real problems – and in light of the positive findings related to alternative therapies – a growing number of patients find it hard to accept that most doctors do not recognize the benefit of alternative medicine. These disappointments have created a fertile ground for alternative medical therapies that have been growing steadily in the USA for years. People began looking into alternative therapies and discovered that in many cases the practitioner is usually a very pleasant person (unlike many doctors), and treatment is mostly comfortable and effective. Friends told their neighbors and relatives. As the news got passed on, the popularity of these therapies spread throughout the country, and even more studies are being conducted now to support their efficacy. The fact is that Americans are finding relief in alternative medicine that they often cannot find in conventional medicine. Whether used alone or in combination with mainstream medicine or other conventional therapies, alternative medicine offers tools and remedies that work. It provides relief from pain and other symptoms of conditions like arthritis while providing overall health benefits. Most people suffering from pain, arthritis, and injuries consult a physician first. This is still the best initial path, since a combination of prescription medications (NSAIDs, pain medications, etc.), physical therapy and sometimes a cortisone injection may provide significant relief from acute conditions while providing time to investigate the root causes of the disorder. In a few cases, this initial treatment may provide permanent relief. In the majority of cases, however, symptoms and conditions persist, particularly if the person is not consuming a Mediterranean Style Diet. That is a true "crossroads" – the right time to stop, think, and consider how alternative medicine can help. Both physician and patient may choose to continue on the conventional path, even after X-rays, lab tests, an MRI and an accurate diagnosis show that there are no major lesions or pathological disorders. On this path, after one, two, or three trials of medications, injections, or physical therapy, patients will be sent to specialists for more therapy, medications, nerve conduction studies, another MRI, perhaps, and additional lab tests.

While this could be the right path for some patients, it often brings more suffering. Subjecting a person to strong medication, unnecessary injections, excessively lengthy therapy, and a surfeit of tests can cause tremendous stress. All too frequently they lose hope of ever being cured. Many people who follow this path find themselves losing their independence and sometimes even their jobs and relationships. They bounce from one doctor to the next – without relief – and end up drowning themselves in a sea of narcotics. It is for these reasons that I created the Jupiter Institute Program. There is another choice at the crossroads. Both patient and doctor can acknowledge the value of alternative therapies, and that the condition will likely have a better chance for improvement by including them. At this point (generally the second or third visit), the doctor who is considering additional medications and conventional treatments should also contemplate integrating alternative therapies such as chiropractic care, acupuncture, and nutritional adjustment. Treatment protocols can be discussed between patient and doctor, and experts brought in as necessary.

WHY is it that many doctors refuse to acknowledge alternative therapies, that could bring so much relief, but have no hesitation in prescribing 90 oxycodone tablets?

WHY do many doctors disregard alternative therapies so much, but go and give the patient 100 tablets of Vicodin, or Xanax, Valium or sleeping pills?

I don't have those answers, but I know that there is enough scientific proof for the success of alternative therapies to support and encourage that option.

My message to patients and doctors alike is this: yes, there is another option – a new and extremely positive one – that is showing consistent promise and success. These therapists are not in competition with doctors or other therapists, and they can be extremely effective in helping doctors get their patients better, sooner. The problem that might arise is that there may not be a center like ours near you that will provide integrated treatment protocols. Practitioners of alternative medicine therapies may be scattered throughout your area or even in another town. The best advice, in this case, is to do what you can. Find high-quality alternative therapy practitioners in your local area and visit them. (Health food stores are generally a good resource.) Ask them how they would treat your condition and, if you feel comfortable, try their treatment. Chiropractors, acupuncturists, reflexologists, physical therapists and nutritionists can help establish an effective treatment program for pain conditions, as well as a myriad of other diseases and illnesses. Many of these consultants will be happy to share 10 minutes of their time to tell you what they do. Some may even provide treatment at no charge.

Ah, and don't forget to fight inflammation with a proper way of eating a good Mediterranean diet.

You can visit our center online at www.jupiterinstitute.com. We hope our initiatives in this area will give doctors in other areas the inspiration to create similar programs for their communities. Going beyond the orthodox boundaries of conventional medicine is wise and it pays because it prioritizes the common goal: to heal. We invite patients in other states to look for integrative medical centers such as ours. If they are not available, contact a local health professional with the reputation of being open-minded to coordinated care and management. We also invite patients and physicians to read some of the excellent books mentioned at the end of this book and found on the Internet.

Good luck.

Appendices

Resources for Your Health

The following is a list of organizations and sources of information that readers may contact.

American Academy of Anti-Aging Medicine, Boca Raton, FL, P: (561) 997-0112, info@a4m.com, www.a4m.com.

American Academy of Craniofacial Pain, Reston, VA, P: (703) 234-4087, central@aacfp.org, www.aacfp.org.

American Academy of Family Physicians, Leawood, KS, P: (800) 274-2237, www.aafp.org.

American Academy of Medical Acupuncture, Redondo Beach, CA, P: (310) 379-8261, info@medicalacupuncture.org, www.medicalacupuncture.org.

American Academy of Pain Management, Sonora, CA, P: (209) 533-9744, F: (209) 533-9750.

American Academy of Pain Medicine, Glenview, IL, P: (847) 375-2738, info@painmed.org, www.painmed.org.

American Alternative Medical Association, www.joinaaom.org.

American Assoc. of Acupuncture and Oriental Medicine, Washington, DC, P: (253) 851-6896, www.aaaomonline.org.

American Chiropractic Association, Arlington, VA, P: (703) 276-8800, www.americhiro.org.

The American Chronic Pain Association, Rocklin, CA, P: (800) 533-3231, ACPA@theacpa.org, www.theacpa.org.

American College of Rheumatology, Atlanta, GA, P: (404) 633-3777, F: (404) 633-1870, www.rheumatology.org.

American Fibromyalgia Syndrome Association, Tucson, AZ, P: (520) 733-1570, F: (520) 290-5550, kthorson@afsafund.org, www.afsafund.org.

American Headache Society, Mount Royal, NJ, P: (856) 423-0043, F: (856) 423-0082, americanheadachesociety.org.

American Massage Therapy Association Evanston, IL,
P: (877) 905-2700, info@amtamassage.org, www.amtamassage.org.

American Medical Association, www.ama-assn.org.

American Osteopathic Association, Chicago, IL,
P: (888) 626-9262, www.osteopathic.org.

The American Pain Society, Glenview, IL,
P: (847) 375-4715.

American Physical Therapy Association, Alexandria, VA,
P: (800) 999-2782, www.apta.org.

The American Society for Nutrition, Rockville, MD,
P: (240) 428-3650, F: (240) 404-6797, www.nutrition.org.

The Arthritis Foundation, Atlanta, GA,
P: (800) 283-7800, www.arthritis.org.

The Arthritis Society, Toronto, ON,
P: (416) 979-7228, F: (416) 979-8366, info@arthritis.ca,
www.arthritis.ca.

Fibromyalgia Network, Tucson, AZ,
www.fmnetnews.com.

Food and Drug Administration Rockville, MD,
P: (888) 463-6332, www.fda.gov.

The Foundation for Peripheral Neuropathy, Buffalo Grove, IL,
P: (877) 883-9942, F: (847) 883-9960, www.foundationforpn.org.

Insight Meditation Society, Barre, MA,
P: (978) 355-4378, www.dharma.org.

International Chiropractors Association, Falls Church, VA,
P: (800) 423-4690, info@chiropractic.org, www.chiropractic.org.

Mayo Clinic Health Information, Scottsdale, AZ,
P: (480) 301-8000, www.mayoclinic.com.

Mind-Body Medical Institute, Chestnut Hill, MA, P: (617) 991-0102,
F: (617) 991-0112, mbmi@mbmi.org, http://www.mbmi.org.

National Center for Complementary and Integrative Medicine,
P: 1-888-644-6226, www.nccam.nih.gov.

The National Center of Homeopathy, www.homeopathic.org.

National Certification Commission for Acupuncture and Oriental Medicine, Washington, DC, P: (888) 381-1140, www.nccaom.org.

The National Foundation for the Treatment of Pain, Monterey, CA, www.paincare.org.

National Headache Foundation, Chicago, IL,
P: (312) 274-2650, info@headaches.org, www.headaches.org.

The National Institutes of Health, Bethesda, MD,
P: (301) 496-4000, www.nih.gov.

Pain Connection, Tucson, AZ,
P: (800) 910-0664, www.painconnection.org.

The Qigong Institute, www.qigonginstitute.org.

Transcendental Meditation, www.tm.org.

U.S. National Library of Medicine, Bethesda, MD www.nlm.nih.gov.

World Health Organization, www.who.org.

More Information About Acupuncture

www.acupuncture.com, www.acsh.org, www.healthy.net.

American Association of Naturopathic Physicians, Washington, DC,
P: (202) 237-8150, www.naturopathic.org.

American Association of Oriental Medicine, Catasauqua, PA
P: (888) 500-7999, (610) 266-1433, www.aaom.org.

American Botanical Council, Austin, TX, www.herbalgram.org,
www.ahpa.org, www.amfoundation.org, www.medherb.com.

American Chiropractic Association, Arlington, VA
P: (703) 276-8800, (800) 986-4636, www.americhiro.org.

U.S. Pain Foundation, Middletown, CT, P: (800) 910-2462,
contact@uspainfoundation.org, www.uspainfoundation.org.

Schools of Naturopathy

Bastyr University, Kenmore, WA,
P: (425) 823-1300, www.bastyr.edu.

National University of Natural Medicine, Portland, OR,
P: (503) 552-1555, www.nunm.edu.

Southwest College of Naturopathic Medicine & Health Sciences,
Tempe, AZ, P: (602) 858-9100, www.scnm.edu.

References

Adebowale, A. O., & Cox, D. S. (2000). Analysis of glucosamine and chondroitin sulfate content in marketed products. *Journal of the American Nutraceuticals Association, 3*(1), p37-44.

Aker, P. D., & McDermaid, C. (1996, October). Searching chiropractic literature: a comparison of three computerized databases. *Journal of Manipulative and Physiological Therapeutics, 19*(8), 518-524.

Albert, C. M. (1998). Fish consumption and risk of sudden cardiac death. *Journal of the American Medical Association, 279,* 23-28.

Arnold, W., & Berman, B. (2001). Arthritis Foundation Guide to Alternative Therapies. *Arthritis Foundation Publications.*

Assendelft, W. J. (1992, October 15). The efficacy of chiropractic manipulation for back pain. *Journal of Manipulative and Physiological Therapeutics,* (8), 487-494.

Audette, J. F., & Ryan, A. H. (2004). The role of acupuncture in pain management. *Physical Medicine and Rehabilitation Clinics of North America, 15*(4), 749-72.

Backonja, M. M. (1998). Neuropathic Pain Syndromes. *Neurologic Clinics, 16*(4), 775-988.

Balch, J. F., & Balch, A. B. (1996). *Prescription for Nutritional Healing.* New York, NY: Avery Publishing Group.

Balch, J. F., & Stengler, M. (1999). *Prescription for Natural Cures.* Hoboken, NJ: John Wiley and Sons.

Barnard, N. D. (1999). *Foods That Fight Pain.* Danvers, MA: Three Rivers Press.

Barney, P. (1998). *Doctor's Guide to Natural Medicine.* Salt Lake City, UT: Woodland Publishing.

Berman, B. M., & Lao, L. (2004, December). Effectiveness of acupuncture as adjunctive therapy in osteoarthritis of the knee. *Annals of Internal Medicine, 141*(12), 901-10.

Böhn, L., Störsrud, S., & Törnblom, H. (2013, May). Self-reported food-related gastrointestinal symptoms associated with more severe symptoms, *American Journal of Gastroenterology, 108*(5), 634-41

Bove, G., & Nilsson, N. (1998, November). Spinal manipulation in the treatment of episodic tension-type headache. *Journal of the American Medical Association, 280*(18), 1576-79.

Brandt, K. D., & Doherty, M. (1998). *Osteoarthritis.* Oxford, UK: Oxford University Press.

Bresler, D. E. (1979). *Free Yourself From Pain.* New York, NY: Simon & Schuster.

Bushnell, M. C., Ceko, M., & Low, L. A. (2013, July). Cognitive and emotional control of pain. *Nature Reviews Neuroscience,14*(7), 502-11.

Carey, T. S., & Evans, A. T. (1996, February 1). Acute severe low back pain. *Spine, 21*(3), 339-44.

Cassidy, C. (1998). Chinese Medicine users in the United States. *Journal of Alternative and Complementary Medicine, 4*(1), 17-27.

Caudill, M.A. (2001). *Managing Pain Before It Manages You.* New York, NY: The Guilford Press.

Challem, J. (2003). *The Inflammation Syndrome.* Hoboken, NJ: Wiley Publishers.

Cloutier, M., & Adamson, E. (2003). *The Mediterranean Diet.* New York, NY: Avon Books.

Cochran, R. T. (2007). *Understanding Chronic Pain.* Hillsboro, KS: Hillsboro Press.

Coggon, D., & Reading, I. (2001). Knee Osteoarthritis and Obesity. *International Journal of Obesity and Related Metabolic Disorders, 25*(5), 622-629.

Credit, L. P., & Hartunian, S. G. (1999). *Relieving Sciatica.* New York, NY: Avery Publishing Group.

Cummings, A. (1999). *Glucosamine in Osteoarthritis.* The Lancet, 354, 1640-1641.

Curtis, B. & O'Keeffe, J. (2002, August). *Understanding the Mediterranean Diet.* Postgraduate Medicine Online, Vol. 112.

Dabbs, V., & Lauretti, W. J. (1995). A risk assessment of cervical manipulation vs. NSAIDs for the treatment of neck pain. *Journal of Manipulative and Physiological Therapeutics, 18*(8), 530-536.

Dalen, J. E. (1998). Conventional and unconventional medicine. *Archives of Internal Medicine,* 158, 2179-2181.

Darlington, L. G. (1991). Dietary therapy for arthritis. *Rheumatic Disease Clinics of North America, 17,* 273- 297.

Diehl, D. L., & Kaplan, G. (1997). Use of Acupuncture by American Physicians. *Journal of Alternative and Complementary Medicine, 3*(2), 119-126.

Dillard, J. (2001). *The Chronic Pain Solution*. New York, NY: Bantam Books.

Donati, S. (2001). *The Great Book of Mediterranean Cuisine*. Secaucus, NJ: Chartwell Books, Inc.

Drum, D. (1999). *The Chronic Pain Management Sourcebook*. New York, NY: McGraw-Hill.

Eaton, S. B., & Konner, M. (1983, January 31). Paleolithic nutrition: A consideration of its nature and current implications. *New England Journal of Medicine, 312,* 283-289.

Eisenberg, D. (2003, March). Integrating Complementary Therapies into Clinical Practice. *Harvard Medical School Department of Continuing Education*.

El-Salhy, M., Ostgaard H., & Gundersen D. (2012, May). The role of diet in the pathogenesis (Review), *International Journal of Molecular Medicine*.

Felson, D. T., & Anderson, J. J. (1988). Obesity and Knee Osteoarthritis: The Framingham Study. *Annals of Internal Medicine, 109*(1), 18-24.

Ferro-Luzzi, A., & Branca, F. (1995). Mediterranean Diet, Italian Style. *The American Journal of Clinical Nutrition, 61,* 1338S-1345S.

Fisher, H., & Thompson, C. (2001). *The Mediterranean Diet*. Lebanon, IN: Da Capo Lifelong Books.

Fleming, R. M. (2004). *Stop Inflammation Now*. New York, NY: Avery-Penguin Group.

Fontanarosa, P. B., & Lundberg, G. D. (1998). Alternative medicine meets science. *Journal of the American Medical Association, 280,* 1618-1619.

Ford, N. D. (1994). *Painstoppers: The Magic of All Natural Pain Relief*. Upper Saddle River, NJ: Prentice Hall.

Fugh-Berman, A. (1997). *Alternative Medicine: What Works*. Philadelphia, PA: William & Wilkins.

Fuhrman, B., & Lavy, A. (1995). Consumption of red wine with meals reduces the susceptibility of human plasma and LDL to lipid oxidation. *The American Journal of Clinical Nutrition. 61,* 549-554.

Garcia-Closas, R., & Serra-Majem, L. Fish Consumption, Omega-3 Fatty Acids and the Mediterranean Diet.

Garcia-Cela, E., & Kiaitsi, E. (2018, January 29). Interacting Environmental Stress Factors, Toxins *(Basel), (2)* 29,10.

European Journal of Clinical Nutrition. (1993). 47:S85-S90.

Germain, B. F. (1983). *Osteoarthritis and Musculoskeletal Pain Syndromes.* New York, NY: Appleton & Lange.

Gordon, G. (2000). *The Omega-3 Miracle.* London, UK: Freedom Press.

Gordon, N. F. (1992). *Arthritis: Your Complete Exercise Guide.* Champaign, IL: Human Kinetics.

Gore, M. (1997). *The Arthritis Book.* Sydney, AU: Allen and Unwin.

Green, S., & Buchbinder, R. (2005 April). Acupuncture for Shoulder Pain. *Cochrane Database of Systematic Reviews,* (2): CD005319.

Greenberg, D. (1993). *Clinical Neurology.* New York, NY: Appleton and Lange.

Griffin, M. (1995, December 4). Practical Management of Osteoarthritis. *Archives of Family Medicine, 4,*1049-1055.

Heine, H. (1988). Structure of Acupuncture Points. *Journal of Traditional Chinese Medicine, 8*(3), 207-212.

Hertoghe, T. (2002). *The Hormone Solution* New York, NY: Harmony Publishing.

Hiesiger, E. (2001). *Your Pain is Real.* New York, NY: Regan Books.

Hochschuler, S. & Reznik, B. (2002). *Treat Your Back Without Surgery.* Alameda, CA: Hunter House Publishers.

Hollon, M. F. (1999). Direct-to-Consumer Marketing of Prescriptions Drugs. *Journal of the American Medical Association, 281,* 382-384.

Holman, R. T. (1976). Significance of Essential Fatty Acids in Human Nutrition. *Lipids* 1,215.

Holt, S. (2002). *Combat Syndrome X, Y and Z.* New York, NY: Wellness Publishing.

Hooper, L., & Ness, A. R. (2001). Antioxidant Strategy. *The Lancet, 357,* 1705.

Hunder, G. G. (2002). *Mayo Clinic on Arthritis.* Broomall, PA: Mason Crest Publishers.

Ianucci, L., & Horowitz, M. (1999). *The Unofficial Guide to Overcoming Arthritis.* New York, NY: Macmillan.

Iso, H. (2001). Intake of Fish and Omega-3 Fatty Acids and Risk of
	Stroke in Women. *Journal of the American Medical Association,*
285, 304-312.

Jarvis, K. B., Phillips, R. B., et al. (1991). Cost per case comparison
of back injury claims of chiropractic versus medical management for
conditions with identical diagnosis codes. *Journal of Occupational
Health, 33*(8),347-852.

Jenkins, N. H. (1994). *The Mediterranean Diet Cookbook.* New York,
NY: Bantam Books.

Jenkins, N. H. (2003). *The Essential Mediterranean.* New York, NY:
Harper & Collins.

Jonas, W. B., & Levin, J. S. (1999). *Essentials of Complementary
and Alternative Medicine.* Philadelphia, PA: Lippincott William & Wilkins.

Kahn, H. S. (2001, July 3). Wine and Mortality. *Annals of Internal
Medicine, 135*(1), 66.

Kalauokalani, D., & Cherkin, D. C. (2005, September). A
Comparison of Physician and Nonphysician Acupuncture Treatment for
Chronic Low Back Pain. *The Clinical Journal of Pain, 21*(5), 406-11.

Kaptchuk, T. (2002). Acupuncture: Theory, Efficacy, and Practice.
Annals of Internal Medicine, 136, 374-383.

Katzenstein, L. (1998). Taking Charge of Arthritis. *Reader's Digest
Association.*

Kessler, R. C., & Davis, R. B. (2001). Long-term trends in the use of
complementary and alternative medical therapies in the United States.
Annals of Internal Medicine, 135, 262-68.

Keys, A. (1995). Mediterranean Diet and Public Health. *The
American Journal of Clinical Nutrition, 61,* 1321S-1323S.

Keys, A. B. (1975). *How to Eat Well and Stay Well the Mediterranean
Way.* New York, NY: Doubleday.

Killion, K. H., & Kastrup, E.K. (eds). (2003). *Drugs Facts and
Comparisons.* Baltimore, MD: Lippincott Williams & Wilkins.

Klatsky, A. L., & Friedman, G. D. (2003, September). Wine, liquor,
beer and mortality. *American Journal of Epidemiology, 58* (6), 585-595.

Koes, B. W. (1996). Spinal manipulation for low back pain. *Spine,
21*(24), 2860-2871.

Koopman, W. J. (1997). *Arthritis and Allied Conditions in Textbook
of Rheumatology.* Baltimore, MD: Lippincott Williams & Wilkins.

Kriegler, J. S., & Ashenberg, Z. S. (1987, December). Management of chronic low back pain: a comprehensive approach. *Seminars in Neurology, 7*(4), 303-312.

Kris-Etherton, P. M., & Harris, W. S. (2002). Fish Consumption, Fish Oil, omega-3 Fatty Acids, and Cardiovascular Disease. *Circulation, 106,* 2747.

Lane, N. E., & Wallace, D. J. (2002). *All About Osteoarthritis.* Oxford, UK: Oxford University Press.

Lautenschlager, J. (1997). Acupuncture in treatment of inflammatory rheumatic Disease, *Rheumatology, 56,* 8-20.

Leskowitz, E. (2003). *Complementary and Alternative Medicine in Rehabilitation.* London, UK: Churchill Livingstone.

Lesser, M. (1980). *Nutrition and Vitamin Therapy.* New York, NY: Grove Press, Inc.

Levy, A. M., & Fuerst, M. L. (1993). *Sports Injury Handbook.* Hoboken, NJ: John Wiley and Sons, Inc.

Li, Y. (2016). *The World's Simplest Tai chi.* Yongxin Li.

Liu, S. (2001, April) Mediterranean Diets. *American Journal of Clinical Nutrition.* (Vol. 73, No. 4, pp. 847).

Lorgeril, M. D., & Salem, P. (1999). Mediterranean Diet, traditional risk factors and the rate of cardiovascular complications. *Circulation,* 779-785.

Malfliet, A., Coppieters, I., & Van Wilgen P. (2017, May). Brain changes associated with cognitive and emotional factors in chronic pain, *European Journal of Pain, 21*(5):769-786

Mallon, W. (1990). *Orthopedics for the House Officer.* Baltimore, MD: Lippincott Williams & Wilkins.

Marcus, S. M. (2017). *Medical Toxicology: Antidotes and Anecdotes.* New York, NY: Springer Publishing.

McAlindon, T. E., & LaValley, M. P. (2000). Glucosamine and chondroitin for the treatment of osteoarthritis. *Journal of the American Medical Association, 28,* 1469-1475.

McAlindon, T. E., & Biggee, B. A. (2005, September). Nutritional Factors and Osteoarthritis. *Current Opinion in Rheumatology, 17*(5), 647-652.

Meeker, W. C., & Haldeman, S. (2002). Chiropractic: A Profession at the Crossroads of Mainstream and Alternative Medicine. *Annals of Internal Medicine, 136,* 216-227.

Mercier, L. (1991). *Practical Orthopedics*. Maryland Heights, MO: Mosby

Meydani, M., & Natiello, F. (1991). Effect of long-term fish oil supplementation on vitamin E status and lipid peroxidation in women. *The American Journal of Clinical Nutrition, 121*, 484-491.

Moller, I. (2005, August 15). Efficacy of Glucosamine Sulfate in Knee Osteoarthritis. *Arthritis and Rheumatism, 3*(4), 628-629.

Murray, M., & Pizzorno, J. (1998). *Encyclopedia of Natural Medicine*. Roseville, CA: Prima Publishing.

Myers, A. (2016). *The Thyroid Connection*. New York, NY: Little, Brown Spark.

Namey, T. C. (1990). Exercise and Arthritis. *Rheumatic Disease Clinics of North America, 16*(4), 791-1023.

Napier, K. (2001). *Power Nutrition for Your Chronic Illness*. New, York, NY: Macmillan.

Ness, A. R. (2002). Is olive oil a key ingredient in the Mediterranean Diet? *International Journal of Epidemiology, 31*, 81-482.

Nestle, M.(1995). Mediterranean Diets: Historical and Research Overview. *The American Journal of Clinical Nutrition, Vol 61*, 1313S-1320S.

Novey, D. W. (2001). *Clinician's Complete Reference to Complementary/Alternative Medicine*. Mosby.

Oliveira, F. R., & Visnardi, G. (2018, February). Massage therapy in cortisol circadian rhythm and pain intensity. *Complement Therapy Clinical Practice, 30*, 85-90.

Osborne, C. (1997). *Middle Eastern Cooking*, London, UK: Prion Books, Ltd.

Osfield, S. (2013). *Food Sensitivities Fast Fix Guide*.

Panush, R. S. (1991). Nutrition and Rheumatic Disease. *Rheumatic Disease Clinics of North America, 17*(2), 197-456.

Peirce, A. (1999). *A Practical Guide to Natural Medicine*. New York, NY: Stonesong Press LLC.

Pittler, E. E. (1999). Expert opinions on complementary and alternative therapies for low back pain. *Journal of Manipulative and Physiological Therapeutics, 22*(2), 87-90.

Pizzorno, J., & Murray, M. (1999). *Textbook of Natural Medicine*. London, UK: Churchill Livingstone.

Pommeranz, B. (1996). Scientific Research into Acupuncture for the Relief of Pain. *Journal of Alternative and Complementary Medicine, 2*(1), 53-60.

Powles, J. (2001). Commentary: Mediterranean Paradoxes. *International Journal of Epidemiology, 30*, 1076-1077.

Pressman, A. H. & Shelley, D. (2000). *Integrative Medicine.* London, UK: St. Martin Press.

Raj, P. (1995). *Pain Medicine: A Comprehensive Review.* St. Louis, MO: Mosby.

Rakel, D. *Integrative Medicine.* Philadelphia, PA: Saunders.

Rakel, R. E., & Bope, E. T. (2003). *Conn's Current Therapy.* Philadelphia, PA: Saunders.

Rao, J. K., & Mihaliak, K. (1999). Use of complementary therapies for arthritis among patients of rheumatologists. *Annals of Internal Medicine, 131*, 409-416.

Reginster, J. Y., & Deroisy, R. (2001). Long term effects of glucosamine sulphate on osteoarthritis progression. *The Lancet, 357*, 247-248.

Reiss, U. (2002). *Natural Hormone Balance.* New York, NY: Atria Books.

Rosenfeld, A. (2003). *The Truth About Chronic Pain.* New York, NY: Perseus Books.

Rudin, D., & Felix, C. (2000). *Omega-3 Oils.* New York, NY: Avery Publishing Group.

Russell, A. S., & Aghazadeh, A. H. (2002). Active ingredient consistency of commercially available glucosamine sulfate. *Journal of Rheumatology, 29* 2407-2409.

Sandmark, H., & Hogstedt, C. (1999). Osteoarthrosis of the knee in men and women in association with overweight. *Annals of the Rheumatic Diseases, 58*(3), 151-155.

Sarzi-Puttini, P., & Cimmino, M.A. (2005, August). Osteoarthritis: an Overview of the Disease and its Treatment Strategies. *Seminars in Arthritis and Rheumatism, 35*(1), 1-10.

Sears, B. (1995). *Enter The Zone: A Dietary Road Map.* New York, NY: Regan Books.

Shekelle, P. G. (1992). Spinal manipulation for low back pain. *Annals of Internal Medicine, 117*, 590-598.

Shils, M. (1994). *Modern Nutrition in Health and Disease.* Philadelphia, PA: Lea & Febiger.

Simopolous, A. P. (1998). *The Omega Plan.* New York, NY: Harper Collins.

Simopoulos, A. P., & Robinson, J. (1999). *The Omega Diet.* New York, NY: Harper Perennial.

Simopoulos, A. P. (1991). Omega-3 fatty acids in health and disease and in growth and development. *The American Journal of Clinical Nutrition, 54,* 438-463.

Simopoulos, A. P. & Herbert, V. (1986). *The Eat Well, Be Well Cookbook.* New York, NY: Simon and Schuster.

Stamatos, J. M. (2001). *Painbuster.* New York, NY: Henry Holt and Company.

Stenson, W. F. (1992). Dietary supplementation with fish oil in ulcerative colitis. *Annals of Internal Medicine, 116,* 609-614.

Stoddard, D. (1998). *Pain Free for Life.* Imperial Beach, CA: Torchlight Publishing.

Stoll, A. L. (2001). *The Omega-3 Connection.* New York, NY: Simon & Schuster.

The Medical Letter. The Medical Letter on Drugs and Therapeutics. The Medical Letter, Inc.

Theodosakis, J. (2002). The Arthritis Cure. St. Martin Griffin, *Toxins Journal.*

Trichopoulou, A., & Costacou, T. (2003, June 26). Adherence to a Mediterranean Diet. *The New England Journal of Medicine, 348,* 2599-2608.

Vernon, L. F. (1996, March). Spinal Manipulation as a Valid Treatment for Low Back Pain. *Delaware Medical Journal, 68*(3), 175-78.

Wayne, P. (2013). *Harvard Medical School Guide to Tai chi.* Berkeley, CA: Shambhala.

Wall, P. D., & Melzack, R. (1999). *Textbook of Pain.* London, UK: Churchill Livingstone.

Weiger, W., & Smith, M. (2002). Advising patients who seek Complementary and Alternative Medical Therapies. *Annals of Internal Medicine, 137,* 889-903.

Weil, A. (2000). *Eating Well for Optimum Health.* New York, NY: Alfred Knopf Publishers.

Weil, A. (1998). *Health and Healing: Understanding Conventional and Alternative Medicine.* Boston, MA: Houghton, Mifflin, Harcourt.

Weil, A. (2001). Integrated medicine. *British Medical Journal, 322,* 119-120.

Weinbrenner, T., & Fito, M. (2004, September). Olive Oils High Phenolic Compounds Modulate Oxidative/Antioxidative Status in Men. *The American Journal of Clinical Nutrition, 134,* 2314-2321.

Weiner, R. S. (1998). *Pain Management: a Practical Guide for Clinicians.* Boca Raton, FL: CRC Press.

Wiancek, D. A. (1999). *The Natural Healing Companion.* New York, NY: Rodale Publishers.

Willett, E. (1998). *Arthritis.* New York, NY: Enslow Publishers.

Willett, W. (2001). *Eat, Drink, and be Healthy.* New York, NY: Simon & Schuster.

Willett, W. C., & Sacks, F. (1995). Mediterranean Diet Pyramid: a Cultural Model for Healthy Eating. *The American Journal of Clinical Nutrition, 61,* 1402S-1406S.

Wilson, J. D., & Braunwald, E. (2000). *Harrison's Principles of Internal Medicine.* New York, NY: McGraw-Hill.

Witt, C., & Brinkhaus, B. (2005, July 19). Acupuncture in Patients with Osteoarthritis of the Knee. *The Lancet, 366*(9480), 136-43.

Woodward, S. (1995). *Classic Mediterranean Cookbook.* London, UK: Dorling Kindersley.

Yang, J. M. (1997). *The Root of Chinese Qigong.* Wolfeboro, NH: Ymaa Publication Center.

Yang, Y. L., & Wang, Y. H. (2018 January 4).The Effect of Tai chi on Cardiorespiratory Fitness, *Front Physiol, 8,* 1091.

Zou, L., Yeung, A., & Quan, X. (2018 January 25). A Systematic Review /for Alleviating Musculoskeletal Pain. *International Journal of Environmental Resource Public Health.*

About the Author

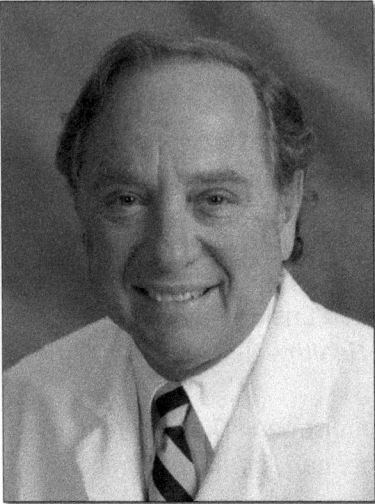

Dr. Daniel Nuchovich, MD was born in Uruguay and graduated as a Physician in Montevideo at the School of Medicine of the University of Uruguay, where being fascinated by human anatomy, he received the recommendation of the Dean of Students. This recommendation opened doors to a clinical research program at the Miami Heart Institute, Miami Beach, FL, which Nuchovich joined in 1982.

During that time Nuchovich got involved in other programs involving teaching and academics, and all the background he developed catapulted him towards higher degrees. Next, he was accepted and graduated in Internal Medicine at the Southern Illinois University School of Medicine, Springfield, Illinois, in 1989, after which he returned to Florida.

Daniel Nuchovich, MD

Very appreciative of the opportunities he received here in the USA, Nuchovich wanted to give back, so he joined the Palm Beach County Public Health Department, West Palm Beach, FL, serving and helping the poor and indigents for about 3-1/2 years. Thirsting for more action, he became a certified trauma doctor at the University of Miami and worked as an Emergency Room Physician in various southern Florida hospitals. "There, in those hospitals, amid sometimes horrible carnage, he also got to meet lots of people with arthritis, chronic pain, and injuries, and then realized how these chronic conditions are often not effectively treated by the conventional medical community."

Then Dr. Nuchovich took the intense and complicated course of "Integrating Complementary Therapies into Clinical Practice" at Harvard Medical School. "It took him over six months of intense studies to be ready." After this, he opened *Jupiter Institute of the Healing Arts*, where he brought together a chiropractor, an acupuncturist, a physical therapist, an orthopedic, a nutritionist, an exercise therapist, and a nurse practitioner proficient in alternative medicine to work together in harmony and coordination.

He wrote about his initial successes in his first book, *The Palm Beach Pain Relief System, 2013*, to later advance his studies and write a much more comprehensive manuscript that we now publish: *Advanced Alternative Medicine for Arthritis, Chronic Pain and Injuries*, We hope that it will reach the over-100 million people who struggle with those conditions.

www.ingramcontent.com/pod-product-compliance
Lightning Source LLC
Chambersburg PA
CBHW070233200326
41518CB00010B/1549